Client Education:
Theory and Practice

Mary A. Miller, PhD, RN
Dean Emeritus
School of Nursing, Aurora University, Aurora, Illinois
and
Associate Dean Emeritus
School of Professional Studies, Metropolitan State College of Denver
Denver, Colorado

Pamella Rae Stoeckel, PhD, RN, CNE
Assistant Professor of Nursing
Loretto Heights School of Nursing
Department of Online Nursing, Regis University
Denver, Colorado

JONES AND BARTLETT PUBLISHERS
Sudbury, Massachusetts
BOSTON   TORONTO   LONDON   SINGAPORE

World Headquarters
Jones and Bartlett Publishers
40 Tall Pine Drive
Sudbury, MA 01776
978-443-5000
info@jbpub.com
www.jbpub.com

Jones and Bartlett's books and products are available through most bookstores and online booksellers. To contact Jones and Bartlett Publishers directly, call 800-832-0034, fax 978-443-8000, or visit our website, www.jbpub.com.

Substantial discounts on bulk quantities of Jones and Bartlett's publications are available to corporations, professional associations, and other qualified organizations. For details and specific discount information, contact the special sales department at Jones and Bartlett via the above contact information or send an email to specialsales@jbpub.com.

Some images in this book feature models. These models do not necessarily endorse, represent, or participate in the activities represented in the images.

The authors, editor, and publisher have made every effort to provide accurate information. However, they are not responsible for errors, omissions, or for any outcomes related to the use of the contents of this book and take no responsibility for the use of the products and procedures described. Treatments and side effects described in this book may not be applicable to all people; likewise, some people may require a dose or experience a side effect that is not described herein. Drugs and medical devices are discussed that may have limited availability controlled by the Food and Drug Administration (FDA) for use only in a research study or clinical trial. Research, clinical practice, and government regulations often change the accepted standard in this field. When consideration is being given to use of any drug in the clinical setting, the health care provider or reader is responsible for determining FDA status of the drug, reading the package insert, and reviewing prescribing information for the most up-to-date recommendations on dose, precautions, and contraindications, and determining the appropriate usage for the product. This is especially important in the case of drugs that are new or seldom used.

Production Credits
Publisher: Kevin Sullivan
Acquisitions Editor: Amy Sibley
Associate Editor: Patricia Donnelly
Editorial Assistant: Rachel Shuster
Production Editor: Amanda Clerkin
Marketing Manager: Rebecca Wasley
V.P., Manufacturing and Inventory Control: Therese Connell
Composition: Datastream Content Solutions, LLC
Cover Design: Kristin E. Parker
Cover Image: © Peter Wey/Dreamstime.com
Printing and Binding: Malloy, Inc.
Cover Printing: Malloy, Inc.

Library of Congress Cataloging-in-Publication Data
Miller, Mary A. (Mary Alice)
    Client education : theory and practice / Mary A. Miller and Pamella Rae Stoeckel.
        p. ; cm.
    Rev. ed. of: Client education / Dorothy E. Babcock, Mary A. Miller.
c1994.
    Includes bibliographical references and index.
    ISBN-13: 978-0-7637-7412-7 (alk. paper)
    ISBN-10: 0-7637-7412-X (alk. paper)
    1. Patient education.   I. Stoeckel, Pamella Rae.   II. Babcock, Dorothy E. Client education.   III. Title.
    [DNLM: 1. Patient Education as Topic—Nurses' Instruction.   W 85 M649c 2011]
RT90.B3 2011
615.5071—dc22
                                                                        2009038845
6048

Printed in the United States of America
15 14 13   10 9 8 7 6

Dedication

Contents

Preface

This book is written for nursing students and professionals who teach clients. It is also written for practicing nurses and health educators interested in learning more about health education. Nurses have responsibilities for teaching not only clients, but also colleagues and other health team members.

The purpose of this book is to assist in further developing the knowledge, skills, and attitudes necessary for becoming effective client educators. We culled information most helpful to the reader. The text is thorough in covering the broad expanse of health education. It is organized so that professionals with limited time can readily find the information they need.

This text is extensively revised since an earlier iteration in 1994. New information is added to each chapter to reflect current knowledge, research, and approaches to health education. New examples that illustrate the material, and new practice exercises along with evidence-based research examples are added. A section on supplemental online resources is included in each chapter. One of the text's unique features is its emphasis on thinking within the framework of teaching and learning. The most significant change is the organizing framework. The Client Education Model is our view of health education. It forms the conceptual framework around which the text is written. The major components of the model are the Nurse as Educator, the Client as Learner, the Nurse/Client Relationship, and Client Education Outcomes.

We believe that teaching is an integral part of nursing care regardless of the employment setting. We identify the most common settings in which nurses are employed (healthcare institutions, public health, and health education programs), although we know there are multiple other settings in which nurses teach clients. Teaching is simply part of what nurses do as they engage in nursing care regardless of the setting. We believe that the client is anyone who needs health education. In our model we define clients as individuals, families, groups/communities, and health team members. This includes clients within the healthcare system or found elsewhere.

In any healthcare setting, it is the nurse/client relationship that is fundamental to the delivery of nursing care and health education. The relationship is critical if the educational goals are to be achieved. The nurse/client relationship integrates the nursing process, teaching and learning process, clinical judgment, and evidence-based nursing practice to achieve the client education outcomes. Although evidence-based research in health education is limited at this time, it will continue to expand and define nursing practice. We present a view of teaching that is balanced, comprehensive, clear, and sensitive to the needs of the reader as an adult learner.

Acknowledgments

When we began planning to revise and rewrite this text, there were three of us: Dorothy E. Babcock, Mary A. Miller, and Pamella R. Stoeckel. Shortly thereafter there were only two. Our dear friend and colleague, Dorothy E. Babcock, passed away quietly on October 17, 2007. She was active in nursing practice and nursing education and received many awards. She was widely recognized for her work and we miss her.

The history of this text is interesting. It represents the contributions of colleagues who have taught nurses how to teach clients since this subject was introduced about four decades ago. Dr. Mary A. Miller created the course (Clinical Teaching Methods) at Metropolitan State College of Denver and taught it for years to registered nurses enrolled in the baccalaureate degree nursing program. She continued to nurture its evolution through the years. Professor Dorothy E. Babcock greatly enriched the course while teaching it for another decade at the same college. Dr. Pamella R. Stoeckel has been a professional colleague for many years, during which time we have worked together on many professional projects. She is currently an Associate Professor in the Loretto Heights School of Nursing at Regis University in Denver, Colorado and has a strong interest in health education and teaching clients. She integrates health education into the online nursing courses that she teaches. She enriched the text by contributing to the conceptual framework, and the organization and content of the chapters. In addition, this book also has benefited from other faculty, nursing students, and practicing nurses who have added, questioned, challenged, suggested, and otherwise helped to fine tune the content.

Although we welcome this opportunity to express gratitude for all of our colleagues' contributions, we take responsibility for the book's content and our views of teaching and learning. Suggestions to improve its clarity, readability, and utility are earnestly invited.

PART I

A Framework for Health Education

CHAPTER 1

Overview of the Client Education Model

Knowing is not enough; we must apply.
Willing is not enough; we must do.—Goethe

OBJECTIVES

Upon completion of this chapter you will be able to:
- Explain the Client Education Model.
- Describe the nurse in the educator role in various settings shown in the Client Education Model.
- Discuss how clients are learners (individuals, families, groups/communities, and health team members) in the Client Education Model.
- Describe the relatedness of the Nursing Process, Clinical Judgment, and Evidence-based Nursing Practice as they apply to teaching and learning.
- Describe the components of Formative and Summative Evaluation.
- Explain why each component of Formative and Summative Evaluation is important.
- Discuss the importance of health education in a changing global environment.
- Discuss health education as a professional responsibility.

KEY TERMS

analyze	health team
assess	illness
client	implement
community	learner
evaluate	learning
family	model
function	plan
health	teaching

INTRODUCTION

This chapter introduces the Client Education Model as the conceptual framework around which this text is written. The model is supported by assumptions, concepts, and theories that are consistent with nursing as a practice discipline. We describe the model and its component parts and why it forms what we believe is the framework for health education in today's practice environment. We begin this discussion by examining the purposes and goals of health education and then move into a discussion of the Client Education Model itself. The four major components of the model are described and essential terms defined to fully understand the meaning and scope of health education. We introduce the Wellness/Illness Functional Continuum to help evaluate clients' perceptions of their health and illness state. This continuum presents individual health status in positive and negative degrees of physical and mental health that can be described incrementally on a continuum. Each of us defines our own wellness based on our individual circumstances and perceptions. We use the Wellness/Illness Functional Continuum as an assessment tool to help determine clients' personal perceptions of health and illness, and as a means of looking holistically at clients' health education needs. Finally, the chapter takes up a discussion of the context for and the national importance of health education. Our premise is that client education improves the health status of individuals, families, and groups/communities and directs them toward healthful changes in behavior. We begin by specifying the purposes and goals of health education.

PURPOSES AND GOALS OF HEALTH EDUCATION

The purposes of health education are to promote, retain, and restore health. They involve the prevention, treatment, and management of illness, and the preservation of mental and physical client well-being. Comprehensive client education includes maintenance and promotion of health, illness prevention, restoration of health and coping with impaired function. This view of health care can only be achieved by shifting the emphasis away from illness and cure, and integrating client education into a comprehensive approach to health maintenance, prevention, and promotion (Davidhizar & Cramer, 2002).

The goals of health education are to encourage positive, informed changes in life style. This involves encouraging behaviors that prevent acute and chronic disease, decrease disability, and enhance wellness. Nurses as educators empower clients to strive for optimal health and well-being. Individuals learn to make informed decisions about personal and family health practices and use health services in the community.

From a public health perspective, health education is intended not only to enhance individuals' abilities to make positive life style changes, but also to support social and political actions that promote health and quality of life in communities. Hall (2001) notes that effective community education is essential as individuals, communities, and the nation shift focus to wellness and illness prevention. The concept of community empowerment is designed to help individuals and organizations use their abilities and resources in collective efforts to address health priorities and their health needs. The ultimate goal of health education is for nurses as educators to help clients make changes in behavior that supports healthy living.

THE CLIENT EDUCATION MODEL

The Client Education Model provides the conceptual framework for understanding the essential, interrelated components of health education. The four major components of the model are: Nurse as Educator, Client as Learner, Nurse/Client Relationship, and Client Education Outcomes. The model assumptions are important to understand because they represent our fundamental beliefs about health education and its place in the context of today's health delivery system. The model has widespread application for teaching students how to teach clients and for practicing nurses implementing health education in their settings. In addition to the assumptions, each major component has supporting subcomponents that are essential to the delivery of competent and meaningful health education (Figure 1-1).

Model Assumptions

A model is a representation of something. Models are useful learning aids that conceptualize what is being represented through illustrations and figures rather than strictly textual information. They help learners grasp the larger picture and visualize relationships among component parts of something that would otherwise take many words to describe. For our purposes, models represent our view of client education in the context of professional nursing practice. Our assumptions for the Client Education Model follow. We believe that:

1. Health status can be improved for most clients through health education.
2. Nurses as Educators can help to promote, retain, and restore health.
3. Health status is affected by a variety of factors, such as life style, heredity, environment, and the availability of health care.
4. Clients' motivation and perceptions affect learning about health.

5. Clients can learn positive health behaviors.
6. Teaching appropriate prevention strategies are effective in dealing with health problems.
7. Clients are active participants in their health care, and are responsible for choices under their control that affect their health.
8. Nurses are responsible for health education in a variety of settings.
9. A therapeutic Nurse/Client Relationship is essential to achieve positive health education outcomes.

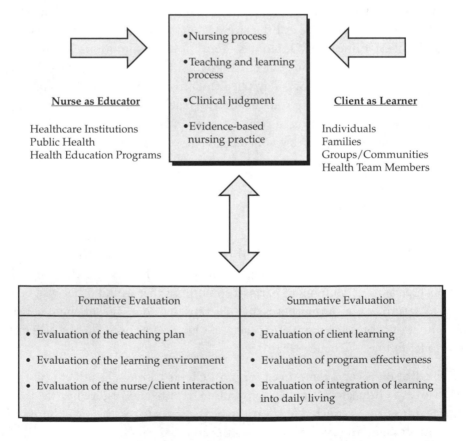

FIGURE 1-1   Client Education Model.

Components of the Client Education Model

The Client Education Model provides a framework for viewing the essential components of health education. The four components of the model, Nurse as Educator, the Nurse/Client Relationship, Client as Learner, and Client Education Outcomes provide the conceptual framework for this text. A discussion of the components follows.

Nurse as Educator

Nurses are professionals who plan, organize, teach, and direct health education to promote, retain, and restore health in a variety of settings. The model shows that nurses work in public health, healthcare institutions, and health education programs. These are not meant to limit nurses to those settings, only to identify the most common places in which nurses are employed. Nurses as Educators are fortunate to be employed in many areas beyond what we have identified; we list these only as examples.

Nurses work with other healthcare professionals, civic groups, and community officials to identify health needs, develop desirable health education goals, and evaluate the availability of health services. Nurses as Educators focus on promoting optimal health and preventing illness; but they also deal with social, cultural, behavioral, legal, and economic issues as they affect health.

Nurses' Role in Health Education

The teaching role of nurses has long been a recognized as a function of nursing practice. It has been within the scope of nursing practice since the days of Florence Nightingale. In 1918 the National League of Nursing Education (NLNE) defined nursing as the prevention of illness and the promotion of health especially in public health, child welfare, schools, home visiting, industries, hospitals, and social services. Health teaching was an expectation of nurses' responsibilities. Two decades later, in 1937, the NLNE stated that a nurse was essentially a teacher and an agent of health in whatever field nursing practice occurred. In 1998 the American Nurses Association (ANA) stated in the *Standards of Clinical Nursing Practice* that educating clients is a primary responsibility of nurses. The ANA continues its long-standing support for patient teaching as a primary component of nursing care. Today, all state nurse practice acts in the United States include client teaching within the scope of nursing practice. Further support for the role of Nurses as Educators is found in the Patient's Bill of Rights first adopted by the American Hospital Association (AHA) in 1973. The current bill was approved by the AHA Board of Trustees in 1992 and states that patients have the right to "relevant, current, and understandable information concerning diagnosis, treatment, and prognosis" (AHA, 1992, Right #2). The Joint Commission, the organization that accredits hospitals, recognized the importance of patient education and adopted nursing standards to address patient education as early as 1993 (Bastable, 2008; Joint Commission, 2009).

In addition to educating clients, nurses are considered to be the primary teachers of their colleagues and other health team members and are expected to have knowledge of health education (Donner, Levonian, & Slutsky, 2005). The Pew Health Professions Commission published a broad set of competencies in 1995 that projected the attributes that successful health professionals would need in the twenty-first century (Gragnola & Stone, 1997). The competencies include the admonition to "continue to learn and help others to learn."

Nurses are in an essential position to coordinate client health education because they are the healthcare providers who have the most continuous contact with clients. Because nurses are with clients at teachable moments, they are doing most of the health education. As a nurse, your educational background in anatomy, physiology, nutrition, psychology, sociology, anthropology, and other social and physical sciences makes you a very appropriate health educator. Your education has taught you how the body can and should function and about the interplay among mind, body, and spirit. In addition, you have access to behavioral and evidence-based health research that can help people learn healthy behaviors and reduce unhealthy ones. This same body of research can be applied to help people change and maintain those changes in their health behaviors.

First-hand knowledge about the consequences of various life styles will make you an authentic source of information. Nurses have earned the public's trust and by modeling healthy habits, they are more believable when they teach. Clients are entering the health system better informed about health issues. This means they will be demanding more knowledgeable caregivers, and they expect to be provided with current and scientifically sound information. Many clients have done considerable reading about their particular health problem and consequently ask informed, sophisticated questions. Your credibility will be established by your answers.

Client as Learner

We chose the word *client* to describe the learner in this text because the client is the consumer of health education and the focus of our teaching efforts. We define clients to be individuals, families, groups/communities, and health team members, which covers the scope of humanity. Clients are everywhere and include everyone in need of health information. The word *client* connotes someone who is free to come and go from your presence; someone who is free to refuse the services, counsel, and teaching that nurses offer. We view clients as responsible, thinking individuals who have the right to make choices about their health.

Contrast the view of the client with the view of the individual as a *patient*. When examined from this perspective, we think of someone who must depend on nurses for their care and sometimes even for their very survival. The term *patient* conjures up the image of someone who is dependent and in need of physical or psychological assistance related to health. The patient is in your presence, on your nursing unit, or in your service area, needing the health education that nurses can deliver.

Clients bring their individual and collective perceptions of what optimal health is to the Nurse/Client Relationship. Perceptions are influenced by their expectations, emotions, and needs. Perceptions about health are determined individually, culturally, environmentally, and socially. Clients' perceptions may not always be the same as nurses' perceptions. In the client education context, we perceive clients as active participants in health education to the extent of their ability and choice.

Nurse/Client Relationship

Between the Nurse as Educator and Client as Learner is the Nurse/Client Relationship. This is the point of contact between the participants and where the relationship between them is created. Of the many nursing interventions that nurses offer clients, we believe one of the most important is health education. A positive, respectful, and thoughtful Nurse/Client Relationship is essential if we are to achieve the goal of promoting, retaining, and restoring the health of clients.

The Nurse as Educator brings a formal, educational base to the Nurse/Client Relationship that is designed to promote, retain, and restore the health of clients. This includes preparation in the physical and social sciences, humanities, along with nursing arts and science. Nurses use this base of knowledge to understand human behavior, engage in clear communication, and commit to standards of ethical behavior that are the foundation of the Nurse/Client Relationship.

The Nurse/Client Relationship is therapeutic, promoting a psychological climate that facilitates positive change and growth. This aspect of the model is drawn from Hildegard Peplau's interpersonal nursing theory (1952) that stressed the importance of the therapeutic interpersonal process. Therapeutic communication between the Nurse as Educator and the Client as Learner is collaborative and focuses on the achievement of health education goals. It focuses on the client achieving optimal personal growth and the highest level of wellness possible given the client's situation. An

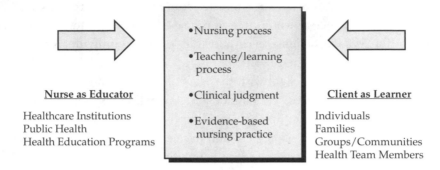

FIGURE 1-2   Nurse/Client Relationship.

explicit time frame, a goal-directed approach, and the expectation of confidentiality are important to the relationship. The nurse establishes, directs, and takes responsibility for the interaction. In this relationship clients' needs take priority over nurses' needs in the relationship.

Four goal-directed phases characterize the Nurse/Client Relationship: the *pre-interaction phase* occurs before meeting the client and involves gathering all available client information. This gives the nurse time to anticipate health concerns and plan for the initial interaction. The *orientation phase* occurs when the Nurse as Educator meets the Client as Learner and they get to know each other. The *working phase* occurs when the Nurse as Educator engages in health teaching and works with the client to solve problems and accomplish goals. Last is the *termination phase*, which is the process of ending the relationship (Potter & Perry, 2009).

Within the Nurse/Client Relationship, we believe two processes, the exercise of judgment and the application of research, are integral to each component of the Nurse/Client Relationship. These components are the Nursing Process, the Teaching and Learning Process, Clinical Judgment, and Evidence-based Nursing Practice. We describe each in order (Figure 1-2).

Nursing Process

The Nursing Process is the first component of the Nurse/Client Relationship. It is undoubtedly the most familiar to you as a student. It is the most common framework in nursing education and practice to conceptualize nursing practice and the nurse/client interactions.

The Nursing Process is a variation of the scientific reasoning process that allows you to organize your thoughts and systematize nursing practice. Its focus is to address client problems in professional practice in a variety of clinical settings. Steps in the Nursing Process include assessment, analysis, planning, implementation, and evaluation. Applied to health education, the steps of the Nursing Process relate directly to the learning needs of clients that are designed to improve clients' health knowledge and promote, retain, and restore health.

The steps of the Nursing Process are iterative as they may overlap or occur simultaneously. Reassessment, reordering of priorities, new goal setting, and revising the teaching plan continues as part of the process toward attainment of the health education goals. A discussion of the steps of the Nursing Process as they apply to health education follows.

Assessment

Assessment is gathering the essential information about the client to identify health education needs. As you assess the physiologic, psychological, sociocultural, developmental, and spiritual influences on each client, it helps to determine each individual's learning style and learning capacity. Assessment includes collecting subjective and objective client data, recording the data, and noting the data that affect learning. Subjective data include clients' perceptions of their condition and health status. How does the client view his or her situation? How does the client view his or her health? Is the client's situation conducive or obstructive to learning? Does the client show a readiness to learn? Do you have the requisite knowledge, skills, and attitudes to facilitate each client's learning in the situation at hand?

Analysis

The second step, analysis, is a careful examination and validation of the facts to identify the client's specific health education needs. When possible, you will collaborate with clients to diagnose their learning needs. A clear understanding of these needs become the basis for planning, implementing, and evaluating the teaching plan. This step includes analyzing both your perceptions and your clients' perceptions of the learning needs to validate them. Assessing and analyzing needs also includes determining the kind of learning clients want. For instance, in which domain are your clients deficient? Do they lack information? What do they want to know? Do they lack necessary skills? Is their developmental level a barrier to learning? Do they display attitudes that impair their optimum functioning?

When your client is a specific population, your assessment becomes complex. You may need to conduct a survey as part of the assessment. Another option is to form a focus group composed of individuals who are representative of the large group you are teaching. For smaller groups, interviewing selected members of the group may serve your purpose just as well. In all instances, it is important to avoid making assumptions about what clients need to learn. Ask them and be as thorough in your assessment and analysis as possible.

Another way to approach clients is from the perspective of potential growth. What information do they desire? What new skills do they wish to learn? What opportunities for growth are inherent in their developmental stages? What attitudes are they ready to exhibit? What attitudes do they already possess that could motivate further growth? What strengths of mind, body, and spirit do they manifest that can help them in the inevitable transitions of life?

A nursing diagnosis identifies the human response to the disease process. Standard classifications of nursing diagnosis used to identify dysfunctional patterns include North American Nursing Diagnosis Association (NANDA), Nursing Interventions Classification (NIC), and Nursing Outcomes Classification (NOC) (McFarland & McFarland, 1997). These diagnoses are applicable to health education.

Planning

Planning, the third step of the Nursing Process, is the development of the teaching plan. In this step you will outline the learning objectives based on the assessment and analysis of the findings. It involves identifying specific learning objectives and educational outcomes, establishing priorities, and selecting teaching strategies to achieve the outcomes. Planning is deciding what needs to be learned and what strategies and materials will most likely facilitate achievement of the learning objectives. Once these are selected, a written teaching plan is devised.

The planning step should involve clients and their families when appropriate. For example, if your client has Alzheimer's disease, then significant others, such as the caregivers, a spouse, or family members, must be included in the formation of plans. It is important to get feedback during the planning process about what is to be learned and how this is to be accomplished, to discover if you and the client are in accord.

Implementation

Implementing the plan involves acting to accomplish the learning objectives and educational outcomes. You and your clients will carry out the actions that are most likely to facilitate the desired learning. During this step, you will need to elicit periodic feedback and stay attuned to behavioral clues that indicate clients' feelings of success or failure. You will use a variety of teaching strategies and instructional materials to facilitate client learning. Ongoing reassessment and continued analysis are part of implementation and involve adapting to feedback as you enact the plan. Note the client's responses to your teaching and modify your approach as needed. Lastly, it is important to document the health education that you provide.

Evaluation

The evaluation phase is the final step of the Nursing Process. This is where you and your clients evaluate teaching effectiveness. Did the clients learn what was expected? Is their behavior more conducive to good health? Has the client's level of wellness improved? Are the problems with which clients needed help diminished, or are they coping with their problems more effectively? Two-way communication with clients helps you to summarize and interpret results.

Although evaluation is presented as the final step of the Nursing Process, evaluation takes place *throughout* the teaching and learning process. During the assessment phase, for instance, while identifying how clients perceive their problems, you will evaluate how well you communicated. Did you understand what the clients conveyed? To find out, repeat back your interpretation of what they said. Did clients indicate that they were understood correctly? Did clients indicate that your words and actions made sense to them? Such transactions are ongoing throughout each step of the nursing process. Evaluation involves determining the overall quality of health education.

Some suggest that the Nursing Process contributes to linear thinking. Chitty and Black (2007) state that, "The nursing process can be taught, learned, and used in a rigid, mechanistic and linear manner" (p. 194). However, we believe it can be used as a creative approach to health education by attending to feedback throughout the process. The Nursing Process used in health education is ongoing, with constant evaluation and reassessment to meet the ongoing learning needs of clients.

Teaching and Learning Process

The Teaching and Learning Process is the next component of the Nurse/Client Relationship. The process of teaching and learning means to engage with others to acquire new knowledge, behaviors, and skills. Nurses as Educators use "planned learning experiences based on sound theories that provide individuals, groups and communities the opportunity to acquire the information they need to make quality health decisions" (Wurzbach, 2004, p. 6). Learning is a process by which behavior changes as a result of experiences (Ormrod, 2008). In teaching, the Nurse as Educator chooses teaching strategies and selects instructional materials to assist the Client as Learner to make behavioral changes that promote, retain, and restore health.

Teaching and learning theories guide teaching practices. They are the foundation of the Teaching and Learning Process. Some learning theories are more applicable than others depending on the teacher, client, and the learning context. We examine the behavioral view of learning, cognitive view of learning, and the social cognitive view of learning in Chapter 3. These learning theories will be applied in Chapter 5 to the Child Learner, Chapter 6 to the Adult Learner, and Chapter 7 to the Older Learner. Learning theories are important and provide the foundation that guides you as you assume the role of educator. Together the Teaching and Learning Process and Nursing Process provide a holistic approach to address clients' health education needs.

Clinical Judgment

The third component in the Nurse/Client Relationship is the exercise of sound Clinical Judgment during teaching and learning. Clinical Judgment in nursing is the outcome of clinical reasoning, often referred to as clinical decision making. It is a characteristic way of thinking in the nursing discipline. You exercise Clinical Judgment as you assess clients, develop teaching plans, select teaching strategies and instructional materials, and evaluate the success of your efforts. Your judgments and decisions impact the outcome of health education.

Some nursing educators believe that critical thinking is "the brain's tool for developing the expert nursing judgment needed to improve patient outcomes" (Scheffer & Rubenfeld, 2006, p. 195). Others believe that forming clinical judgments in the delivery of nursing care is distinct from general critical thinking skills (Tanner, 2005). Regardless, it is essential for the nurse to exercise sound Clinical Judgment in the Teaching and Learning Process.

The Teaching and Learning and Nursing Processes provide the structural framework through which Clinical Judgment and clinical reasoning occur. Nurses engage in a variety of thinking patterns as no single pattern characterizes all situations. Tanner (2006) proposed a model with four aspects describing how nurses reason in the clinical area that is applicable to health education situations. The first aspect is *noticing*, whereby the nurse grasps the situation at hand. The second is *interpreting*, whereby the nurse develops an understanding of the situation. The third is *responding*, whereby the nurse decides on an appropriate course of action. The fourth is *reflecting*, whereby the nurse evaluates the effectiveness of the outcomes. These thinking and reasoning patterns occur within each step of the Teaching and Learning Process and Nursing Process to guide the nurse in the formation of Clinical Judgments related to health education.

Clinical Judgment in nursing develops as nurses gain experience and expertise in a practice area and expand their knowledge, moving from being a novice to being an expert. To become an expert in nursing, a beginning nurse passes through five levels of proficiency: novice, advanced beginner, competent, proficient, and expert (Benner, 1984). The *novice* has no experience in a situation, relies on rules, and is inflexible. The *advanced beginner* has more experience and has marginally acceptable performance. The *competent nurse* has 2 to 3 years of experience in similar situations and brings perspective, abstract, and analytic thinking to problem solving. The *proficient* nurse sees situations as wholes rather than specific aspects, and has learned from past experience what to expect in situations and what to do when things do not go as expected. The *expert* nurse has a deep understanding and intuitive grasp of situations and no longer needs rules or guidelines. This nurse sees the totality of situations, and quickly identifies the nature of the problem and how to solve it. These skill levels apply not only to the delivery of nursing care, but also to the delivery of health education.

Evidence-based Nursing Practice

The last component of the Nurse/Client Relationship is Evidence-based Nursing Practice as it relates to health education. Evidence-based Nursing Practice (EBNP) is the use of current best practices in making decisions about patient care by using a problem-solving approach. This approach incorporates a systematic search for evidence, clinical expertise, and patient preferences and values (Melnyk & Fineout-Overholt, 2004). It is the act of applying current research findings to clinical practice. Applying research to health education is an integral part of the Client Education Model. It means using the best available and pertinent research to make health education decisions.

The history of evidence-based research (EBR) goes back to Dr. Archie Cochrane, an English physician who, in 1972, confronted healthcare professionals about the lack of randomized control studies to support medical practice decisions. Because of his influence, the first electronic database of clinical trials was established in 1988. First called the Oxford Database of Prenatal Trials, it later became The Cochrane Collaboration (Bliss-Holtz, 2007). The Cochrane Collaboration is now an international database that disseminates research worldwide.

The concept of evidence-based practice was embraced by nursing and other health professions in the 1990s. The motivation behind this decision was the realization that many healthcare practices were based on intuition, experience, clinical skills, and guesswork rather than science. Evidence-based Nursing Practice (EBNP) uses a research-based, decision-making process to guide the delivery of holistic client-centered nursing care and health education. The specific steps involved in carrying out EBNP include: defining the problem and searching for evidence, critically appraising the evidence, applying the findings to practice, taking into account the client/learner's values and preferences, and then evaluating outcomes.

Although EBNP is accepted as a means of promoting best practices, differences of opinion exist among nurses regarding what types of studies constitute the strongest evidence and what weight to give them. The terms *levels-of-evidence* or *strength of evidence* refer to systems for classifying the evidence in a body of literature through a hierarchy of scientific rigor and quality. Several dozen of these hierarchies exist (Agency for Healthcare Research & Quality [AHRQ], 2002). The reviewers must select the most relevant levels-of-evidence to meet their needs. The following concise definitions of terms are used in describing the levels-of-evidence.

- Meta-analysis is a statistical analysis of a collection of quantitative studies.
- Systematic review is a research summary that searches the literature and critically appraises individual quantitative studies to identify valid, applicable evidence.
- Randomized controlled trial is a study in which subjects are randomly assigned to groups; one receives the intervention, the other is a control group.
- Quasi-experimental design is a modification of an experimental design in which there may not be manipulation of the independent variable, random assignment, or control group.
- Observational study is a study in which researchers have no control; instead, they observe what happens to groups of people.
- Case study (case report, single case report) is an uncontrolled observational study involving an intervention and outcome in a single situation.
- Descriptive study is a statistical study to identify patterns or trends in a situation, but not cause-and-effect.
- Cohort study is a study that involves the selection of a large population of people who have the same condition who receive a specific intervention and are followed over time and compared with a group not affected by the condition.
- Case-controlled study is a study that compares two groups of people—those with the condition and a similar group without the condition. It is also called a retrospective study.

- Expert opinion is a judgment by people who have experience with a particular subject.
- Qualitative study is a study focused on subjective experiences in naturalistic settings rather than under experimental conditions. There are different types of qualitative studies.

A diagram of the hierarchy of research evidence is included in Figure 1-3.

Figure 1-3 illustrates a research hierarchy in which the lowest tier includes the descriptive studies, case studies, case series, qualitative studies, and expert opinion. The highest tier includes meta-analyses and systematic reviews. Research at this tier has a greater chance of being generalizable to a group of clients.

Nurses as Educators should rely on substantiated, critically analyzed research to ensure that the most current and tested health education practices and teaching strategies are provided to clients. Nurses as Educators need a core foundation

FIGURE 1-3   Levels of Evidence in Research.

of health information that reflects quality care and best teaching practices supported by current research. Unfortunately, at this time, there is a dearth of research studies that focus on health education. Research is needed on the effectiveness of various teaching strategies and instructional materials for different population groups. The absence of such research affects health education practices. In addition to using the best available evidence, nurses are called on to exercise their best judgment in clinical and health education situations. Clinical Judgment and expertise are very important and should never be minimized in providing health education.

Interrelatedness of Components in the Nurse/Client Relationship

The components in the Nurse/Client Relationship (Nursing Process, Teaching and Learning Process, Clinical Judgment, and Evidence-based Nursing Practice) are interacting, interdependent. The components complement one another. During assessment and analysis the client's learning needs are assessed and analyzed to determine the extent of the client's need for health education. It is in this step that the nurse *grasps* the client's situation. It may involve looking for applicable literature specific to the client's situation or a group's health education needs.

Planning involves developing individualized care plans drawn from evidence-based research and setting priorities and learning objectives based on client health education needs. The nurse develops sufficient understanding of the situation and responds by involving the client in designing the teaching plan.

Implementation is carrying out the teaching plan. The nurse takes action and responds based on evidence-based research where it exists, but also reflects on client responses. Using judgment, the nurse is prepared to alter the teaching plan if necessary. The nurse uses judgment in selecting teaching strategies and instructional materials to meet the client's health education needs and preferences.

Evaluation reviews the successes and failures in meeting the learning objectives of the teaching plan. Teaching strategies may need to be modified to achieve the objectives. The nurse continually reviews the literature to update the teaching plan using current evidence-based research where available. Clients' achievement of the learning objectives is measured and reinforced to help ensure continued success.

The interrelatedness of these Nursing Process, Teaching and Learning Process, Clinical Judgment, and Evidence-based Nursing Practice components is illustrated in Table 1-1.

TABLE 1-1 Interrelatedness of the Nurse/Client Relationship Components

Nursing Process	Teaching/Learning Process	Clinical Judgment	EBNP Process
Assessment and analysis	Determine learning needs	Noticing	Define problem and search literature
Planning	Develop teaching plan	Interpreting	Appraise research findings
Implementation	Use teaching strategies	Responding	Apply to clinical situation
Evaluation	Determine behavior change	Reflecting	Assess the outcomes

Client Education Outcomes

Client Education Outcomes are achieved when health-promoting changes in knowledge, attitudes, and skills occur in clients. The last portion of the Client Education Model focuses on evaluation. To determine if health education efforts are successful, nurses must evaluate the results. Evaluation of Client Education Outcomes is measuring the degree to which the learning objectives are met. It is also the process of making judgments about the effectiveness of every aspect of health education as well as the teaching plan.

Evaluation consists of measuring how well the learning objectives were met. It looks at Client Education Outcomes on an immediate, short-term, and long-term basis. Consequently, the Client Education Model addresses both Formative Evaluation and Summative Evaluation. Both are essential aspects of evaluation that provide a holistic picture of what was achieved (Table 1-2).

Formative Evaluation is ongoing during teaching and learning activities. It is important to know if the learning activities are meeting the learning objectives as teaching is progressing. Formative Evaluation addresses three areas: evaluation of the teaching plan, evaluation of the learning environment, and evaluation of the nurse/client interaction.

In Formative Evaluation, the nurse gathers data in these areas on an ongoing basis and makes appropriate adjustments as necessary. Involvement of the client is

TABLE 1-2 Client Education Outcomes	
Formative Evaluation	**Summative Evaluation**
Evaluation of the teaching plan	Evaluation of client learning
Evaluation of the learning environment	Evaluation of program effectiveness
Evaluation of the nurse/client interaction	Evaluation of integration of learning into daily living

essential to the success of this process. Formative Evaluation is done early in the Teaching and Learning Process to avoid wasting time and resources. If weaknesses are identified, they can be changed right away. Formative Evaluation is very much process oriented. It asks questions such as, "Is the client responding to my approach and to the instructional materials?" "Is the client comfortable in this environment and is the environment conducive to learning?" "Does the client give evidence she or he understands the information?" "Am I communicating effectively with the client?" "In what ways is this learning activity contributing to learning and in what ways is it inhibiting learning?" Formative Evaluation seeks to know "how are we doing?" Chapter 12 goes into greater depth about Formative Evaluation.

Summative Evaluation occurs at the conclusion of the Teaching and Learning Process. It is directed toward measuring the degree to which the learning objectives and overall outcomes are met at the conclusion of the learning activity or program. It addresses three areas: evaluation of client learning, evaluation of program effectiveness, and evaluation of integration of learning into daily living.

Measurement of learning occurs not only at the conclusion of individual learning activities and programs, but also involves long-term follow-up of client learning. Results of systematically conducted long-term evaluations are important from an Evidence-based Nursing Practice perspective. Findings from evidence-based research can serve to guide future health education practices. Summative Evaluation is directed toward outcomes that determine whether clients have learned and if the activities and programs are feasible to continue in the future. Determining feasibility includes examining the effectiveness of learning materials, the costs, the time requirements, the degree of client satisfaction, and the long-term benefits of programs. Basically, Summative Evaluation wants to know, "How did we do?" Chapter 13 goes into greater depth about Summative Evaluation.

DEFINITIONS

The following definitions support the Client Education Model and broaden your understanding of health education. The most important terms to understand are: health education, health, illness, Wellness/Illness Functional Continuum, and the Health Belief Model.

Health Education

Health education enhances the quality of life for people worldwide. It is defined broadly by Green and Kreuter (1991) as any combination of learning experiences designed to encourage voluntary actions beneficial to health. Health education is achieved through the use of learning theories combined with teaching strategies to help individuals, families, groups/communities, and health team members to promote, retain, and restore health. It not only involves providing relevant health information, but also helps clients make appropriate health-related behavioral changes. The term health education also refers to the process of educating health team members to become more effective in their roles and responsibilities.

Health

Health, as officially defined by the World Health Organization in 1948 is "a state of complete physical, mental, and social well-being, not merely the absence of disease or infirmity" (WHO, 2004). Health is a dynamic state in which individuals adapt to changes in the internal and external environments to maintain a state of well-being in all life dimensions. This is the most popular and comprehensive definition of health worldwide and is applicable to individuals, families, groups, and communities. Clients bring their own definition and perceptions of health to the clinical situation. Their perceptions of what is and is not normal health influence their willingness to accept health education teaching.

Illness

Illness is a subjective perception of not being well. It is a mismatch between an individual's needs and the ability to meet those needs. It signals that the present balance to maintain health is not working. During illness changes may occur in the structure and function of a person's body and mind. Illness has a classifiable set of signs and symptoms resulting from disturbed body functioning. These are associated with characteristic preclinical findings, course, and etiology.

Wellness/Illness Functional Continuum

An individual's level of health is a constantly changing state that moves along a continuum from optimal functioning to a state of total disability. The basic premise of the Wellness/Illness Functional Continuum is that wellness and illness involve a variety of factors: social, physiologic, environmental, emotional, activities of daily living, and health access. The factors in the model can either enhance or distract from the client's health. Disease and illness are a failure of an individual's adaptive mechanisms to adequately counteract changes in functional and structural disturbances. Factors are displayed along a continuum showing incremental increases or decreases in health functioning. Each factor is plotted on the continuum moving from the center (score of 5 is neutral) either right (highest score of 10 indicates highest level of wellness) or left (lowest score of 0 indicates lowest level of wellness) showing changes in health state. High-level functioning or wellness involves increased ability to perform the activities of daily living. Low-level functioning is brought on by illness or disability, resulting in the decreased ability to perform activities of daily living.

This continuum is useful when working with clients to get a holistic picture of their functioning. Clients can place themselves on each factor's continuum to identify their strengths and weaknesses. Each person is unique, with different degrees of wellness and illness. Plotting the continuum for each factor helps the Nurse as Educator determine clients' health perceptions and needs. By using the Wellness/Illness Functional Continuum as an assessment tool when working with clients, you gain a more accurate picture of how the client perceives her or his state of health. The continuum can also be used to compare a client's previous level of health with the present level, but because of its subjective nature, it cannot be used to compare one client with another. The continuum illustrates the dynamic, ever changing, state of health (Figure 1-4).

Health Belief Model

The Health Belief Model (Rosenstock, 1974) was developed in the 1950s to explain why people did not use preventive health services such as immunizations. The model examines the relationship between a client's beliefs and behaviors and helps nurses understand these factors to plan teaching that effectively assists clients in promoting, retaining, and restoring health. An important assumption of using the model is that the nurse collaborates with the client to reach mutually agreed on goals by under-

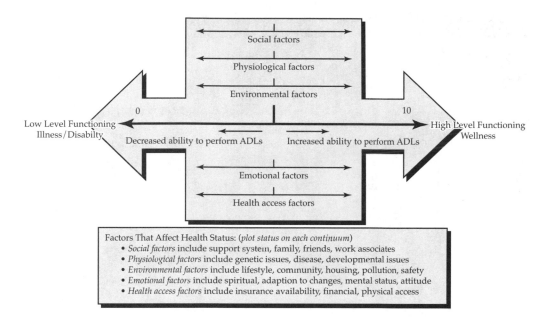

FIGURE 1-4   Wellness/Illness Functional Continuum.

standing the factors that influence health beliefs. The Health Belief Model identifies the following factors that influence health beliefs:

- Personal expectations regarding health and illness
- Perception of the seriousness of the illness
- Likelihood of following prescribed healthcare measures
- Perceived barriers related to such factors as cost, inconvenience, or pain

A criticism of the Health Belief Model is that it is based on the Western cultural health belief system and does not allow for other influences and for the fact that clients do not always act on their belief system. Our approach, shown in Table 1-3 uses the basic format of the model but includes questions that address the cultural aspects of client teaching. Our approach is a starting point for examining client decision making concerning health education and can be used to develop teaching plans. It is important for the nurse to understand client perceptions about health and the likelihood of adhering to health recommendations. This involves examining beliefs through a cultural lens. Communication is targeted at clarifying the nurses' and the clients' perceptions and beliefs. Based on this information, nurses use those strategies that are most effective to meet client health education needs (Table 1-3).

TABLE 1-3   Health Belief Model: Perceptions

Client Perceptions	Nursing Application
Need for care	• Clarifies client concerns and reasons for seeking treatment • Explores client experiences with health issues past and present • Asks about family and cultural factors affecting client perceptions
Seriousness and consequences of condition	• Clarifies client perceptions of harm the condition can cause • Clarifies client perceptions of consequences without treatment • Answers questions and clarifies prognosis; describes experiences with similar problems • Explores common and different beliefs and values
Value of health intervention	• Discusses treatment client is seeking • Describes treatment: medical treatment, behavior change (life style), medication (side-effects), costs, etc. and answers questions • Clarifies client perceptions of treatment

Effectiveness, cost, and barriers of treatment	• Prepares goals and timeline for client and nurse responsibilities
	  • Sets ground rules and boundaries for nurse/client relationship
	  • Outlines knowledge and skills for client and nurse
	  • Suggests and provides resources for knowledge and skill development
	• Clarifies client understanding of proposed plan

Adapted from Rankin, Stallings, & London, 2005.

CONTEXT FOR HEALTH EDUCATION

Nurses play a vital role in improving health on a local, national, and global scale. Nurses, in partnership with other healthcare professionals, facilitate delivery of health education in different venues to achieve positive Client Education Outcomes. In this section we address the importance of the wider scope of health education. Nurses should be aware that individual health affects the larger community and eventually affects global health.

National Importance of Health Education

The 1979 Surgeon General's Report, *Healthy People*, laid the foundation for a national prevention agenda. Every 10 years since that time, the US Department of Health and Human Services has provided science-based, 10-year national objectives for promoting health and preventing disease. Healthy People 2000 and 2010 established national health objectives that serve as the basis for the development of state and community health initiatives. Currently, Healthy People 2010 (2009) is leading the way to achieve increased quality and years of healthy life, and the elimination of health disparities (Box 1-1). The Healthy People 2020 objectives, to be released in the future, will reflect assessments of major risks to health and wellness, changing public health priorities, and emerging technologies related to US health preparedness. It will also provide guidance for achieving the new 10-year targets. This information will be available on a US government Web site. Core objectives will remain centered on prevention of illness and disease as the foundation of health. The Healthy People 2010 leading health indicators are shown in Box 1-1.

Living in an Interactive and Interdependent Global Community

Maintaining health is a global concern. Health issues have global consequences that not only affect the people of developing nations, but also the world community. Healthy, productive citizens are essential for global economic growth and security. Stable populations reduce pressures on global economies and the environment. Stable populations also reduce the number and risk of humanitarian crises. Programs to

---

BOX 1-1 Healthy People 2010 Leading Health Indicators

- Physical Activity
- Overweight and Obesity
- Tobacco Use
- Substance Abuse
- Responsible Sexual Behavior
- Mental Health
- Injury and Violence
- Environmental Quality
- Immunization
- Access to Health Care

(http://www.healthypeople.gov/LHI/lhiwhat.htm)

control the spread of infectious diseases reduce the threat of epidemics. With health-care services placing ever-greater pressures on state and federal health budgets, the economic burden of disease, as well as the burden to individuals and families, is a cause of great concern for governments and health systems. Health education not only affects the immediate recipients, but also future generations that will benefit from improved health habits and efforts to prevent illness. Eventually, improved health behavior will be ingrained when health education is widely available and an accepted part of health care. The prevention of illness and the promotion of health through the delivery of efficient and effective health education lie at the core of society's ability to affect health worldwide.

FUTURE CHALLENGES AND TRENDS FACING NURSES AS EDUCATORS

Future challenges in health care are difficult to predict, but current demographic and societal trends point to the increased need for Nurses as Educators. Demographic trends point to an increasing older population and a greater percentage of minority groups living in the United States that have unique health challenges. Societal trends show changes in social practices such as cohabitation, acceptance of gay relationships, and more single-parent families. Other trends point to greater access to reliable information using technology, more reliance on alternative medicine, and more questioning of medical advice. Nurses as Educators must be aware of demographic and societal trends. They must adjust to these trends and incorporate the challenges they present into their health education practices.

It is important for nurses to expand their knowledge of health education, their leadership abilities, and their involvement in health policy development. More collaborative networks with other healthcare providers are needed that foster accountability. This collaboration should occur not only on the local level, but also within the global community. Basing health education practices on research, demanding adherence to ethical standards, and promoting social justice are escalating challenges and trends. Doing it more, doing it better, and doing it with less are the future challenges (Breckon, Harvey, & Lancaster, 1998).

SUMMARY

This chapter introduced the topic of health education by introducing the Client Education Model. The Client Education Model serves as the conceptual framework around which this text is organized and written. The major components of Nurse as Educator, Client as Learner, Nurse/Client Relationship, and Client Education Outcomes were defined and explained. The role of the Nurse as Educator was clarified, described, and emphasized.

The nature of the Nurse/Client Relationship involves the Nursing Process, Teaching and Learning Process, Clinical Judgment, and Evidence-based Nursing Practice. The model concludes with an examination of Client Education Outcomes to include Formative and Summative Evaluation. Finally, the future challenges and trends facing Nurses as Educators were discussed. In this section we examined how health education can impact health, illness, and wellness in the local, national, and global health arenas. In the subsequent chapters of this book, we delve into greater depth about all of the components and aspects of providing health education.

EXERCISES

Exercise I—Philosophy of Health Education

Purpose: Develop a philosophy of health education.

Directions: Working with a small group of colleagues, write your philosophy of health education. This will take time, thought, and discussion. Your philosophy statement should be about two to three pages in length. Include your beliefs about the following:

1. The value of health education as an aspect of comprehensive healthcare
2. Teaching and what it means
3. Learning and its place in the human experience
4. The role of the Nurse as Educator
5. The role of the Client as Learner
6. The relationship that should exist between the educator and learner
7. The value of Client Education Outcomes

Exercise II—Ways to Promote Client Education

Purposes:

- Promote creative thinking.
- Raise consciousness regarding client education.

Directions: Form small groups and discuss the following situation. Take notes and prepare a report to be shared with the rest of your peers.

While carrying heavy patient care assignments and responsibilities, some nurses are managing to teach their clients in mutually satisfactory ways. What client teaching have you observed by your clinical instructors, supervisors, primary nurses, or other nursing personnel? What are you doing to promote client teaching? If you are not yet in the clinical area, seek out nurses in your school, hospital, or neighborhood and ask them what they are doing to promote health teaching. Draw on your experiences as a patient, client, relative, or observer. Upon reflection, summarize the nurses' role in client education.

SUPPLEMENTAL ONLINE RESOURCES

About the World Health Organization:
http://www.who.int/about/en/
Healthy People 2010:
http://www.healthypeople.gov/

REFERENCES

Agency for Healthcare Research and Quality (AHRQ). (2002). *Systems to rate the strength of scientific evidence. Summary, evidence report/technology assessment: Number 47.* AHRQ Publication No. 02-E015. Rockville, MD: Agency for Healthcare Research and Quality. Retrieved on May 30, 2008 from http://www.ahrq.gov/clinic/epcsums/strengthsum.htm.

American Hospital Association. (1992). A Patient's Bill of Rights. Retrieved July 25, 2009 from http://www.patienttalk.info/AHA-Patient_Bill_of_Rights.htm.

American Nurses Association. (1998). *Standards of clinical nursing practice* (2nd ed.). Washington, DC: The Association.

Bastable, S. B. (2008). Overview of education in health care. In Bastable, S.B. *Nurse as educator Principles of teaching and learning for nursing practice* (3rd ed.). Sudbury, MA: Jones and Bartlett.

Benner, P. (1984). *From novice to expert.* Menlo Park: Addison-Wesley.

Bliss-Holtz, J. (2007). Evidence-based practice: A primer for action. *Issues in Comprehensive Pediatric Nursing, 30*(4), 165–182.

Breckon, D., Harvey, J. & Lancaster, R. (1998). *Community health education: Settings, roles, and skills for the 21st century.* Sudbury, MA: Jones and Bartlett.

Chitty, K. K ., & Black, B. P. (2007). *Professional nursing: Concepts and challenges* (5th ed.). St. Louis: Elsevier.

Davidhizar, R., & Cramer, C. (2002). "The best thing about the hospitalization was that the nurses kept me well informed" Issues and strategies of client education. *Accident and Emergency Nursing, 10,* 149–154.

Donner, C. L., Levonian, C., & Slutsky, P. (2005). Move to the head of the class: Developing staff nurses as teachers. *Journal for Nurses in Staff Development, JNSD. 21*(6), 277–283.

Gragnola, K., & Stone, E. (1997). Pew Health Professions Commission December 1995 *Report Considering the Future of Health Care Workforce Regulation.* University of California, San Francisco.

Green, L. W., & Kreuter, M. (1991). *Health promotion planning: an educational and environmental approach*. Mountain View, CA: Mayfield.

Hall, A. (2001). Client education. In Potter, P., & Perry, A. (2009). *Fundamentals of nursing* (7th ed.). St. Louis: Mosby.

Healthy People 2010. (2009). US Department of Health, Education and Welfare, Public Health Service. Washington DC: US Government. Retrieved on May 23, 2009 from http://www.healthypeople.gov/LHI/lhiwhat.htm

Joint Commission of Accreditation of Healthcare Organizations (JCAHO). Retrieved on May 22, 2009 @ http://www.jcaho.org.

McFarland, G. K. & McFarland, E. A. (1997). *Nursing diagnoses and intervention, planning for patient care* (3rd ed.). St. Louis: Mosby.

Melnyk, B. M., & Fineout-Overholt, E. (2004). *Evidence-based practice in nursing and healthcare: A guide to best practice*. Philadelphia: Lippincott Williams & Wilkins.

National League of Nursing Education (1918). *Standard curriculum for schools of nursing*. Baltimore: The Waverly Press.

National League of Nursing Education. (1937). *A curriculum guide for schools of nursing*. New York: The League.

Ormrod, J. E. (2008). *Human learning* (5th ed.). Upper Saddle River, NJ: Pearson Education.

Peplau, H. E. (1952). *Interpersonal relations in nursing*. New York: GP Putnam's Sons.

Potter, P. & Perry, A. (2009). *Fundamentals of nursing* (7th ed.). St. Louis: Mosby.

Rankin, S. H., Stallings, K. D., & London, F. (2005). *Patient education in health and illness* (5th ed.). Philadelphia: Lippincott Williams & Wilkins.

Rosenstock, I. (1974). Historical origins of the health belief model. *Health Education* Monographs, 2(4).

Scheffer, B. K., & Rubenfeld, M. G. (2006). Critical thinking: A tool in search of a job. *Journal of Nursing Education, 45*(6), 195–196.

Tanner, C. (2005). What have we learned about critical thinking in nursing? *Journal of Nursing Education, 44*(2), 47–48.

Tanner, C. (2006). Thinking like a nurse: A research-based model of clinical judgment in nursing. *Journal of Nursing Education, 45*(6), 204–211.

World Health Organization (WHO). (2004). *About the World Health Organization*. Retrieved December 18, 2008 from http://www.who.int/suggestions/faq/en/index.html.

Wurzbach, M. E. (2004). *Community health education and promotion: A guide to program design and evaluation* (2nd ed.). Sudbury, MA: Jones and Bartlett.

PART II

The Learning Process

CHAPTER 2

Thinking and Learning

Thinking and learning are integrally related.
Thinking is learning.
Thinking is one of the most important aspects of human learning.
—Miller and Babcock, 1996, p. 33

OBJECTIVES

Upon completion of this chapter you will be able to:
- Analyze definitions of thinking and learning and formulate your own definition.
- Differentiate among cognitive, affective, and psychomotor domains of learning by giving an example of each.
- Give examples of how you have engaged in the following types of thinking in the context of health education: problem solving, nursing process, critical thinking, clinical judgment, creative thinking, intuition, reflection, fantasy, and reverie.
- Identify at least two ways to help clients as learners (individuals, families, groups/communities, and health team members) develop their critical thinking abilities.
- Describe the following styles of thinking and learning: Sternberg's thinking styles, Witkin and Goodenough's Cognitive-style Dimensions, Kolb's Experiential Learning Model: Learning Cycle and Styles, and Gardner's Multiple Intelligences.
- Describe how to apply the thinking and learning styles to client education.

KEY TERMS

affective domain	nursing process
clinical judgment	problem solving
cognitive domain	psychomotor domain
creative thinking	reflection
critical thinking	reverie
fantasy	thinking
intuition	thinking styles
learning styles	

INTRODUCTION

Learning is a purposeful activity with the goal of bringing about a necessary change. The teaching and learning process encourages clients to engage in activities necessary to acquire new knowledge, new skills, and incorporate new attitudes. Clients as learners do this by modifying and reorganizing knowledge already in place or by acquiring new knowledge. Clients as learners need specific, new information or assistance in learning how to use known information to best advantage.

This chapter introduces the broad domains of learning: cognitive, psychomotor, and affective. Next we examine thinking and the many ways thinking is categorized to include problem solving, nursing process, critical thinking, clinical judgment, creative thinking, intuition, and reflection. The chapter concludes by examining how thinking translates into various styles of learning and the implications this has for health education.

DOMAINS OF LEARNING

Clients learn as total beings, with all their senses. When they learn, they have thoughts about learning and experience feelings about what they are doing, thinking, and learning. The doing, thinking, and feeling aspects of learning are clearly related but they are not the same. When nurses help clients learn something, they select a domain(s) in which clients need to focus most of their energy. The three domains that have received the most attention in educational literature are the cognitive, affective, and psychomotor domains (Bloom, Engelhart, Furst, Hill, & Krathwohl, 1956).

The learning domains have been separated for research and study purposes but that separation is arbitrary. Human behavior includes components of each domain (Kretchmar, 2008). When providing health education to clients, the domains provide an organizational framework that is useful as educators contemplate what clients need to learn and what should be taught. Figure 2-1 illustrates the interactive, interdependent relationship among the three domains. The most effective learning occurs when all three domains are engaged in the learning process as illustrated by the center triangle (Goulet & Owen-Smith, 2005).

Cognitive Domain

Cognitive learning is concerned with intellectual activities such as thinking, remembering, reasoning, and using language (Merriam-Webster, 2007). It involves judging,

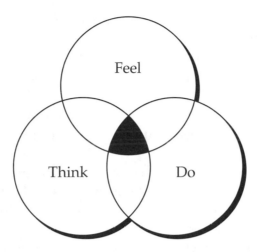

FIGURE 2-1   The interacting domains of learning: cognitive (think), affective (feel), and psychomotor (do) maximize learning.

considering, believing, reflecting, and recalling. It also means using the mind to exercise judgment, draw inferences, arrive at conclusions, and make decisions (Miller & Babcock, 1996). The cognitive domain was the first domain developed by Bloom et al. in 1956. It has received the most attention in educational circles and enjoys the widest application to learning, in part because of the emphasis of Western cultures on reason over emotions (Kretchmar, 2008). Cognitive learning objectives are concrete and reflect this emphasis on reason. They are relatively easy to conceptualize, write, and measure. Examples of cognitive objectives are found at the beginning of each chapter in this text.

Affective Domain

The affective domain deals with personal issues: attitudes, beliefs, behaviors, and emotions (Krathwohl, Bloom, & Masia, 1964). In the past educators believed that the affective domain was an area of learning that was too complex and fraught with conflicts. Research in this area, however, is changing that perception and educators are realizing the importance of integrating the affective domain into their teaching. Because the affective domain deals with personal issues such as attitudes, beliefs, behaviors, and emotions, it is increasingly integral to the provision of a comprehensive program of health education. Educational research indicates that there is a relationship between emotional intelligence and general intelligence in academic achievement. This research has implications for health education. Learning objectives in the affective domain focus on influencing attitudes, motivating learners, developing respect, and clarifying values.

Attitudes are acquired by associating with others and participating in satisfying experiences. Clients are influenced by nurses' attitudes. Role modeling, for example, occurs when nurses work with clients. Nurses are constantly observed by clients, who are influenced by their behavior. Characteristics of kindness, fairness, compassion, honesty, punctuality, dependability, and competence are evident to clients as they observe nurses working. These characteristics help clients determine their perception of the quality of care they receive. Some examples of the way that nurses display their values are by treating clients with respect such as providing privacy, adapting nursing interventions to their expressed concerns, and giving them undivided attention. It is important to include learning objectives in the affective domain as you provide health education for clients. Affective learning can also be facilitated by persuasion from other trusted authorities such as parents, teachers, scientists, spiritual leaders, and valued colleagues with special expertise. Participating in group discussions and role playing also helps promote affective learning.

Psychomotor Domain

Psychomotor learning encompasses many physical procedures that individuals use in their activities of daily living and the complex physical activities required for work and recreation. It also includes learning physical skills and procedures applicable to health care delivery. Psychomotor learning requires that individuals acquire information and store it in memory. During the initial practice of a procedure, skills are shaped and learned until they become automatic (Marzano & Kendall, 2007). This type of learning is the most concrete, and the easiest to teach, observe, and measure. Clients form a mental image of how a skill is performed and then translate that image into external behavior. An example of psychomotor learning is performing an insulin injection. This type of learning is usually done best in a step-by-step fashion, from the simple to the complex. Nurses show clients how to perform and then guide them through return demonstrations. Nurses correct errors and reinforce correct responses. Practice is encouraged until both clients and nurses are satisfied with the clients' skills.

THINKING

Thinking is categorized in different ways. In this section we look at definitions of thinking and types of thinking engaged in by nurses: problem solving, critical thinking, creative thinking, intuition, reflection, and other types of thinking. The nursing process and clinical judgment, also types of thinking, were discussed in Chapter 1 and not repeated here. Each type of thinking has a distinct focus as they overlap, are complex, and cannot be confined to distinct categories. They are described separately for purposes of this discussion to highlight the particular focus of each type of thinking.

Definitions of Thinking

To think is an activity of the mind that is essential to living. It involves a myriad of processes such as observing, recalling, remembering, reasoning, drawing inferences, reflecting, and deciding. It also encompasses beliefs, opinions, and judgments. Thinking has a subjective quality in that all past experiences influence how we see the world. It includes our personal knowledge, our interpersonal relationships, and our role as nurses (Miller & Babcock, 1996).

Ruggiero (2007) defined thinking as "any mental activity that helps formulate or solve a problem, make a decision, or fulfill a desire to understand. It is a searching for answers, a reaching for meaning" (p. 4). It also involves such mental activities as wondering, imagining, inquiring, interpreting, evaluating, and judging. Thinking can be concrete referring to physical materials or objects (What instructional materials do I need to teach this information?) or abstract referring to a quality of something (What value do instructional materials have in learning?). Thoughts can be about the past (What worked best yesterday in teaching Ms. Jones about diabetes?), the present (How shall I best present this material on smoking cessation?), or the future (How shall I use client feedback to improve my teaching?).

Thinking is complex, multifaceted, dynamic, and involves the creation of images (Halpern, 2003). For example, when you wonder if the intravenous solution is about to run out, you picture what the fluid level in the bottle looked like the last time you were in the room and you think about the amount of time that has passed. In this sense, thinking is imagery accompanied by silent, internal speech.

Thinking is described as directed or nondirected (Halpern, 2003). Directed thinking is a conscious mental focus on a problem or issue with a desired outcome. It is purposeful and goal directed. Directed thinking has an evaluation component that considers the effectiveness of thinking outcomes; that is, were the decisions effective. For example, asking yourself, "did I make a good decision in this situation?" In contrast, nondirected thinking occurs as a result of routine habits such as getting up in the morning, going to work, school, etc. Many aspects of life involve nondirected thinking.

TYPES OF THINKING

Problem Solving

The most common type of thinking is problem solving. Problem solving is a process of developing, testing, and evaluating a method for overcoming an obstacle by identifying a problem and finding the best alternative to solve it. Problem solving consists of these steps: identifying the problem, analyzing aspects of the problem, collecting pertinent information, hypothesizing about its cause(s), generating possible solutions, trying out one of the hypotheses, and evaluating the results.

In the process of problem solving, individuals use critical thinking skills to understand and solve a problem. Sometimes a situation requires considerable thought and contemplation (Should I attend school full or part time?) and at other times it is relatively simple (What shall I do this weekend?). Problem solving is conscious, focused thinking over which individuals exert control.

Problem solving requires being open to new ways of thinking, reflection, and clinical judgment. Nurses use problem solving most effectively in working with clients, assisting them to think through their health problems, and finding workable, realistic, and appropriate solutions.

Critical Thinking

Critical thinking is a specific type of thinking. The word *critical* often connotes a negative image, whereas the intended meaning of the word is analytical. To be a critical thinker is to be analytical, reflect constructively, and evaluate fairly. Ideas about critical thinking come from educators in the fields of philosophy and education (Brookfield, 1991; Ennis, 1985; McPeck, 1990; Paul, 1990; Ruggiero, 2007; Watson & Glaser, 1980). They define critical thinking as a rational process of thinking and knowledge acquisition with attitudes that support clear thinking. Lipman (2003) calls critical thinking, applied thinking.

Nursing lacks a widely accepted definition of critical thinking (Brunt, 2005; Riddell, 2007; Walsh & Seldomridge, 2006), but nurse educators see rational, logical thinking as central features (Walthew, 2004). Gordon (2000) compared how nurse educators perceived critical thinking skills and dispositions with non-nurse scholars in other disciplines. Although nurse educators and non-nurse educators agreed on many critical thinking skills and dispositions, they disagreed on others. Nurse educators were more focused on research, problem solving, decision making, and planning as important components of critical thinking in nursing. Scheffer and Rubenfeld (2000) conducted a study to define critical thinking in nursing with input from an international panel of nurse experts on critical thinking. They identified both cognitive and affective dimensions of critical thinking in nursing. Their consensus definition is:

> Critical thinking in nursing is an essential component of professional accountability and quality nursing care. Critical thinkers in nursing exhibit these habits of the mind: confidence, contextual perspective, creativity, flexibility, inquisitiveness, intellectual integrity, intuition, open-mindedness, perseverance, and reflection. Critical thinkers in nursing practice the cognitive skills of analyzing, applying standards, discriminating, information seeking, logical reasoning, predicting and transforming knowledge. (p. 357)

Because of the research supporting this definition, we believe it best represents the meaning of critical thinking in nursing.

Creative Thinking

To create is to bring into being; to cause to exist (Merriam-Webster, 2007). It is the ability to go beyond current knowledge and think in a new way. Creative thinking has both a creative and judgmental phase (Ruggiero, 2007). Individuals have creative thoughts and ideas and then proceed to judge them as they look for solutions to problems and answers to questions. This thinking moves back and forth between creating ideas and then judging them, the former being creative thinking and the latter being critical thinking. According to Halpern (2003), creative thinking has two aspects, novelty and quality, or appropriate and useful. Thus creative and critical thinking are intertwined.

Creative thinkers are curious, adventurous, resourceful, undaunted by the prospect of failure, and independent in the sense that they are willing to speak freely, not needing a lot of approval from others (Ruggiero, 2007). Creative thinkers tolerate ambiguity and uncertainty, adjust easily to new and changing situations, and freely abandon old assumptions when confronted with new evidence. Creative thinkers are willing to be different, to think "outside the box." In problem solving, creative thinkers propose multiple options to consider that are appropriate to the context rather than immediately focusing on one.

Santrock (2008) described the creative process as a five-step sequence, the first of which is *preparation*. In this step, a problem or issue arouses interest and curiosity. The next step is *incubation*, whereby individuals think about the problem and mull over ideas. The third step is *insight*, that moment when the pieces of the puzzle seem to fit together. The fourth step is *evaluation*, when individuals bring their judgment to bear on a tentative solution to determine if it is workable and realistic. The final step is *elaboration*, the most difficult step requiring the most time. These steps move back and forth and do not follow a linear, sequential path. For example, insight and incubation can occur throughout each step, and evaluation is ongoing.

Intuition

Intuition is quick and ready insight, knowing things without conscious reasoning (Merriam-Webster, 2007). It is information that is not acquired by rational, analytical processes; rather, it occurs outside of conscious thought. Its source is from within the person and is based on life experiences and accumulated knowledge. It is the "aha" experience that occurs with sudden insight. For example, nurses sense something important about a client, often described as a gut feeling or a flash of insight, but are unable to verbalize it or verbalize it with difficulty. However, based on that insight, nurses adjust their teaching and care to be more suitable for the client.

Intuition was once thought to be characteristic of only expert nurses (Benner, 1984). However, intuition is now known to be used by nurses at all levels of expertise, including the novice (Ruth-Sahd & Hendy, 2005). The primary difference between novice and expert nurses is their knowledge, expertise, and years of experience. Those with greater knowledge, expertise, and experience bring more to assessment, intervention, and evaluation when working with clients (Faugier, 2005). Thus, intuition has somatic, affective, and cognitive components, but further research is needed to understand how these components are integrated (Hodgkinson, Langan-Fox, & Sadler-Smith, 2008). Your intuitive knowledge is important to take into consideration when making health education decisions. However, you should validate your intuitions through evidence-based research, as many psychologists have found that spontaneous, intuitive approaches to solving problems are frequently wrong (Halpern, 2003).

Reflection

Reflection results from meditation (Merriam-Webster, 2007) and is an important aspect of thinking. The word *reflective* comes from the Latin word *reflectere*, meaning bending back, casting back, introspecting, and deliberating. Reflection helps to clarify thoughts and values and how they affect problem solving and decision making. It is important to reflect on health education activities and consider what is and is not effective. If nurses fail to reflect, it reduces the self-correction that comes with evaluating teaching effectiveness.

Reflective skepticism is an important aspect of critical thinking. Reflective skepticism requires thinking about the universal truth of statements rather than immediately accepting or rejecting them. Rather than accepting or rejecting statements at face value, reflective critical thinkers ask questions, analyze responses, reflect, and evaluate the merits of statements. This process is not cynical or dismissive of new ideas; rather, it is a process of analyzing and determining what to believe. Reflective skepticism requires reflecting on beliefs, assumptions, and intuitive responses to clarify thinking (Brookfield, 1991).

Reflection is described as an important parameter of clinical judgment (Tanner, 2006). Saylor (1990) describes reflective thinking as essential for self-evaluation and improving clinical performance. Reflection is viewed overall as a form of systematic inquiry that is used as a means to improve practice or as a way to make sense of learning, evaluation, and promotion of learning. Reflection may be a solitary process or involve collective reflection with colleagues, teachers, or interaction with theoretical literature.

Three different aspects of reflective practice are: reflection-before-action, reflection-in-action, and reflection-on-action. *Reflection-before-action* is anticipatory reflection involving the careful consideration of what to do and why to do it before engaging in action. The nurse develops a rationale for actions, organizes and prioritizes a vision for future action, and examines core beliefs and values. Reflection-before-action gives the nurse an opportunity to deliberate about possible alternatives, decide on a course of action, develop plans, and anticipate what the experience will be like for the nurse and client.

Reflection-in-action refers to reflective thinking as one is "doing the action." Reflection-in-action in health education refers to the nurse's thinking about the teaching and learning process while directly engaged in teaching. Reflection is usually stimulated by a problem that the nurse is facing. The process of analysis includes asking questions such as how the problem was perceived, what action was taken, and why this course of action was chosen. The nurse evaluates how the client is responding in the situation and then takes the opportunity to adjust the interventions based on that assessment. During reflection-in-action the problem is restructured and approached differently. This enables the nurse to reshape what they are doing while they are doing it.

TABLE 2-1 Reflective Practice Questions		
Reflection-Before-Action	**Reflection-in-Action**	**Reflection-on-Action**
Anticipatory Reflection	*Evaluation in Action and Revision*	*Analysis of Past Actions and Rationale*
What do I want?	What is effective and what needs to be different?	Why did I act as I did?
What outcome do I want?	What is the client response?	What was the client outcome?
What is my plan?	What other options are available?	What actions did I take?
What is my rationale?	What is the plan revision?	Why did I respond as I did?

Reflection-on-action occurs after the experience has taken place. The nurse looks back on experiences to analyze learning that occurred in light of the client outcomes. It means recalling the client's response and the evidence of client learning. It means assessing the client's satisfaction with the interaction. The act of reflecting-on-action enables the nurse to spend time exploring why they personally acted as they did and what was happening. In so doing, the nurse engages in self questioning and considers ideas about how activities and practices could be done differently. Reflection-on-action may involve colleagues who observe, engage in critical conversations, and help the nurse become aware of aspects of their practice they have not thought about. Table 2-1 summarizes reflective practice questions.

Other Ways of Thinking

Other ways of thinking include fantasy and reverie. Fantasy is the free play of creative imagination, the realm of the wild, visionary, or fancy (Merriam-Webster, 2007). It is a mental image, a capricious or whimsical idea or notion, a dramatic fiction characterized by highly fanciful or supernatural elements. Fantasy is useful in mentally working through difficult situations. For example, suppose you want more time to devote to teaching clients and anticipate that the supervisor will resist this idea. Fantasizing the supervisor's arguments helps you prepare to counter them.

Reverie, a synonym for daydream, is similar to fantasy and means dreamy thinking, imagining, or fanciful musing (Merriam-Webster, 2007). In general, reverie has a more meandering, less vivid quality to it than fantasy. An example of reverie occurs when a lecture is boring and learners' minds wander to something more engaging, like what they did last night or what they will do tonight. Fantasy, however, is more directed; for example, helping a client in labor to relax during contractions by focusing her mind on warm, soothing waves of water rushing over her body.

REFLECTING ON YOUR THINKING

Nurses are encouraged to become aware of their thinking processes. Thinking about thinking is called metacognition (Ruggiero, 2007). Nurses enhance their effectiveness when they reflect on the results of their thinking and decisions. For example, was a decision effective? Was there sufficient information on which to base good decisions? Were the inferences accurate? What were the underlying assumptions and how did these affect problem solving? What influence did beliefs and values have on how the problem was framed and approached? Were the generalizations justified? Once nurses internalize critical thinking skills, they are more effective in helping clients think more clearly.

How nurses think and go about their professional responsibilities are important insights. Although thinking per se is difficult to define, nurses will become skillful thinkers and increase their efficiency if they monitor their thought patterns. It is important to develop clear, analytic thinking habits. As nurses verbalize and critique their thoughts and practice clear thinking, they will develop confidence in their critical thinking skills (Miller & Babcock, 1996).

PROMOTING THINKING IN CLIENTS

Before nurses can promote critical thinking in clients, they need to be good listeners. Nurses in the educator role should listen to what clients say they want to learn. Frequently clients know what they need to learn and will verbalize it if they think the nurse is interested. Listen to how clients view their illness, what they think caused their health problem, and what home remedies they have taken to treat it. This will give the nurse multiple clues for situation-appropriate health education. If the clients are team members, listen to what they already know and want to learn and then make teaching plans accordingly.

Just as important as listening is respecting clients and colleagues. Showing respect is fundamental for promoting critical thinking skills. Seeing life from the perspective of the other person creates a safe environment for that person to experiment with new thoughts and behaviors. As nurses go about their responsibilities, they serve as role models for critical thinking.

When assisting others in their thinking processes, nurses should note the client's frame of mind and their readiness to entertain additional information and develop new insights. Remember that as an educator, nurses cannot completely change a client's thinking framework. Nurses can, however, promote small, incremental growth, and expand clients' perceptions of their circumstances, options, and facilitate problem solving.

When clients share insightful information or engage in critical thinking, nurses should reinforce their behavior. Praise clients for their thinking processes as well as the decisions they make when appropriate. Reinforce clients even when they question your procedure or teaching. Responses, such as, "I am glad you asked," and "Let me think, that is a complex question," and "That is a good point," are ways to reinforce thinking.

When conversing with clients, it may be helpful to mirror their attitudes, rationalizations, and habitual ways of thinking and behaving. As you reflect your observations back to them, monitor their responses. Ask yourself how your comments are being received. Are your comments annoying clients? If you encounter resistance, stop your intervention and assess what is happening.

Nurses should ask questions as they teach. As clients answer, it tells you if your comments are understood. It also provides opportunities to stimulate thinking. For example, ask, "If that is so, then how do you feel about. . . ?" or "Will you explain. . . ?" Another fruitful line of questioning that helps clients anticipate consequences is, "What will you do if. . . ?"

When teaching stress management, pain control, weight reduction, blood pressure control, and management of other stress-related diseases, make good use of the imaginative forms of thinking, fantasy, and reverie. Nurses who specialize in counseling and psychotherapy make use of these strategies. A nurse used fantasy to help a client who was under stress to relax. The client found the sounds of surf soothing, so the nurse used this image and said, "Picture the waves of the ocean rolling over you. Flow with the waves. Listen to the surf. Smell the salty air. Feel the warm mist on your skin."

Role playing is based on recall and fantasy. It is an excellent diagnostic tool for discovering the client's way of thinking and approaching interpersonal problems. Role playing is also helpful to the client who is learning to be more assertive. When used by the nurse psychotherapist, role playing may take on more intensity, such as that encountered in gestalt exercises, sociodrama, and psychodrama.

The Socratic method uses creative questioning to enhance critical thinking skills. In Socratic teaching the focus is on asking questions, not giving answers. Nurses model what it means to have an inquiring mind by continually exploring a subject by asking questions. Socrates described the true teacher as one who is the midwife to another person's discovery of truth. Socratic learning is joining in discussions with others, asking questions, thinking and reasoning clearly, and discovering answers (Paul, 1990). Questions elicit new ideas and make connections with previous knowledge and experiences. Questions expose the truth and bring unconscious beliefs to the surface of self-awareness.

STYLES OF THINKING AND LEARNING

Learning styles refer to how individuals prefer to processes information and learn. Styles develop from life experiences in the family, school, and work and result in preferred ways to learn. Consider how you learn best. Is it by reading a book, creating a mental image, watching a video, or hearing an explanation? Is it by working alone on a project or with a study group? Is it in a quiet environment or with music in the background?

In this section we examine several ways that thinking and learning styles are conceptualized. Styles are unique to each person and should be taken into consideration when providing health education. Keep in mind that one style is not better than another; styles are simply characteristics that individuals bring to the situation. Also keep in mind that individuals may change their style preference depending on the demands of the learning situation. They are not confined to only one style.

Sternberg's Thinking Styles

Robert J. Sternberg (1997) distinguished between thinking ability and thinking style. Style refers to how an individual uses the abilities she or he possesses. Sternberg draws an analogy between how individuals think, which he called mental self-government, and civil government. He uses the descriptive terms of the latter to describe his model of thinking styles. For example, *Legislative* individuals are creative and prefer to decide for themselves what they will do and how they will do it. They like problems that are not already structured and prefer to create the framework themselves. They prefer to solve problems, apply rules to problems, apply lessons based on other people's work, and enforce rules. They tend to be nonconforming individuals.

Executive individuals like problems that have some structure so they can address problems within that structural framework. They like guidelines and prefer to follow directions. These individuals are usually successful as students and employees because they do as they are told and like being evaluated on that basis.

Judicial individuals like to oversee, analyze, and evaluate existing rules, procedures, and ideas. They like to critique, give opinions, and judge people and their work. These individuals prefer positions in which they can evaluate the effectiveness of programs, tasks, and human endeavors.

Sternberg distinguishes between *Global* versus *Local* individuals. Global thinkers see the forest rather than the trees; that is, they prefer to deal with relatively large and abstract issues, whereas Local thinkers are more pragmatic, preferring to focus on details. Sternberg also distinguishes between the thinking of *Internal* individuals, who tend to be introverted, task-oriented, and prefer to work alone, and *External* individuals, who tend to be extroverted, outgoing, and people-oriented. Individuals have a profile of thinking styles and may use more than one.

Witkin and Goodenough's Cognitive-Style Dimensions

Field preference is another way to conceptualize how individuals learn and process information. Developed by Herman Witkin and Donald Goodenough, it is a bipolar continuum with traits of field dependence and independence at opposite ends. *Field* refers to how individuals perceive their surroundings. It is important to view field dependence and independence as relative dimensions, not fixed ones. Although individuals favor a particular cognitive style, no one is exclusively one way or the other. The cognitive style dimensions are value neutral; each has qualities that are adaptive in particular circumstances (Witkin & Goodenough, 1981). Knowledge of these dimensions is useful for nurses as educators in planning health education activities.

Field dependent and independent individuals have different perceptual and intellectual qualities (Cassidy, 2004; Claxton & Murrell, 1987; Garity, 1985; Noble, Miller, & Heckman, 2008; Witkin & Goodenough, 1981). Individuals who are relatively field dependent rely on an external frame of reference rather than imposing their own. They see the whole situation and its context rather than focusing on the smaller aspects. They are sensitive to their surroundings and open to external sources of information. They show more social behaviors, which contribute to effective interpersonal relationships. They pay attention to social cues in the environment by looking at others' faces and listening to verbal messages to sense what others are thinking and feeling.

In a learning situation, field dependent learners prefer the spectator role and are influenced by authority figures. They like structure, guidance, and clearly defined learning goals provided by the educator. They are motivated by extrinsic rewards rather than intrinsic ones. They enjoy interaction with other learners and prefer to cooperate and collaborate. They are sensitive to criticism; when they talk they refer more to others and less to themselves. They are holistic in their approach to problem solving but often unable to see the smaller components of larger problems, thereby making them less efficient.

Individuals who are relatively field independent are more autonomous and have a strong sense of self and differentiation from others. By having an internal frame of reference, they grasp the whole situation and its component parts. They are self-reliant, intrinsically motivated, and have their own learning goals. They are less sensitive to the social environment and less inclined to conform to group pressure.

In a learning situation, field-independent learners prefer to structure their own learning and study strategies. They are analytical, interested in abstract and theoretical concepts, and question opinions, ideas, and hypotheses. In learning situations they are able impose their own structure. They are less affected by criticism and make more "I" statements. They tend to be better at problem solving. Table 2-2 summarizes these characteristics.

Kolb's Experiential Learning Model: Learning Cycle and Styles

Many educators believe that education, work, and personal development are closely linked in a process of learning called *experiential learning*. They believe that learning is an ongoing, continuous process that occurs as individuals adapt to their social and physical environment. The emphasis of experiential learning is on the learning process itself, rather than on the behavioral outcomes; it is grounded in experiences as the individual adapts to the world (Kolb, 1984).

Based on this philosophy, David Kolb (1981, 1984) proposed an experiential learning model with a four-stage cycle with four adaptive learning modes: concrete experience, reflective observation, abstract conceptualization, and active experimentation (Figure 2-2).

The experiential learning model describes the learning cycle; that is, how experience translates into concepts that guide the choice of new experiences. Entry into the cycle begins with concrete experience (CE) followed by reflection and observation (RO). The third stage is abstract conceptualization (AC), which becomes the basis for ideas and theories that guide future behavior. In the fourth stage, active

TABLE 2-2   Field Preference Characteristics

Field-Dependent Individuals	Field-Independent Individuals
External frame of reference	Internal frame of reference
See the whole situation	See both whole and parts of a situation
Sensitive to surroundings	Less sensitive to surroundings
Open to external sources of information	Strong sense of autonomy
Social and people oriented	Impersonal orientation to others
Attend to social cues	Less sensitive to social environment
Prefer the spectator role	Prefers active learner role; self-reliant
Influenced by authority figures	Analytical, tests opinions and ideas
Prefer structure and guidance	Enjoys abstract and theoretical concepts
Prefer clear learning objectives	Sets own learning goals
Motivated by extrinsic rewards	Structures own learning
Prefer group work and discussions	Intrinsically motivated
Sensitive to criticism	Less sensitive to criticism

FIGURE 2-2   The Experiential Learning Model. Courtesy of Jossey-Bass/Wiley Publishers.

experimentation (AE), the individual tests the implications of new concepts and theories in different and more complex situations. By experimenting and applying new learning, individuals again engage in concrete experiences and so the cycle continues. As the knowledge base expands, the learning experiences become increasingly complex.

Based on heredity, past experiences, and the demands of the present environment, individuals develop a unique, preferred style of learning. Based on his learning cycle, Kolb (1981) identified four learning styles: *converger*, which combines AC and AE, *diverger*, which combines CE and RO; *assimilator*, which combines AC and RO; and *accommodator*, which combines CE and AE. Their strengths are shown in Table 2-3.

Teaching strategies can be employed that are suitable for the different learning modes (Burris, Kitchel, Molina, Vincent, & Warner, 2008). For example, clients favoring *concrete experience* benefit from small group discussion, specific examples, practical exercises, and role playing. Clients favoring *reflective observation* benefit from creative problem solving, personal journals, discussion groups, and thought questions. Clients favoring *abstract conceptualization* benefit from hearing lectures, analogies, and questioning. Clients favoring *active experimentation* benefit from case studies, projects, and psychomotor activities.

Gardner's Multiple Intelligences

The study of intelligence originated when the French government commissioned Alfred Binet to develop a measure of intelligence. In 1904 Binet produced the first measure that assessed a broad range of skills and performances. The findings were reduced to a single score, called the intelligence quotient or IQ (Slavin, 2009). IQ testing of school children was widely adopted in the United States. It is often used as a tool to place students in ability groups or tracks in the educational system.

Howard Gardner, Professor of Cognition and Education at Harvard Graduate School of Education, is critical of quantifying actual or potential intelligence by using a single number expressed as the IQ score. In the early 1980s Gardner began looking for other ways to measure intelligence and developed the theory of multiple intelligences (Gardner, 1983). Gardner has a pluralistic view of intelligence and believes that all humans possess these intelligences in varying degrees, with several of them working together. Where people differ is in the degree to which they possess the intelligences and the unique combinations in which they appear in each individual (Gardner, 2006).

Gardner defined intelligence as a biopsychological potential "to process certain kinds of information in certain kinds of ways" (Gardner, 2006, p. 64) and "the ability

TABLE 2-3   Kolb's Learning Styles

Learning Style	Strength
Converger: (AC and AE)	• Applies practical application of ideas • Focuses on specific problems • Is relatively unemotional • Prefers dealing with things rather than people • Has a tendency to narrow interests • Specializes in physical sciences
Diverger (CE and RO)	• Has good imaginative ability, generates ideas • Sees multiple perspectives • Is interested in people; emotional • Has broad cultural interests • Specializes in the arts and humanities
Assimilator (AC and RO)	• Creates theoretical models • Reasons inductively, logically sound theories • Is interested in abstract concepts • Has less interest in people • Focuses less on practical use of theories • Specializes in basic sciences and math
Accommodators (CE and AE)	• Likes to do things (plans, experiments, new experiences); willing to take risks • Adapts well to specific immediate circumstances • Solves problems intuitively, trial and error • Relies on others for information rather than self • Likes people; sometimes impatient • Specializes in technical or practical fields, e.g. business

Source: Kolb 1981, 1984.

to solve problems, or to fashion products, that are valued in one or more cultural or community settings" (Gardner, 1993, p. 7). The phrase *fashion products* includes things such as writing a symphony, creating a painting, staging a play, building up and managing an organization, and carrying out an experiment.

Gardner (2006) added an eighth intelligence, naturalist intelligence, to his original seven and is considering adding existentialist intelligence. The original seven intelligences are pertinent to health education and are described here. The first two are highly valued in United States society, as much academic testing and employment is based on verbal and mathematical skill (Moran, Kornhaber, & Gardner, 2006). The next three intelligences are associated with the arts, and the last two are personal intelligences. Each type of intelligence is important and has equal status with the others.

In most individuals, the intelligences work together to solve problems. Most vocations involve several intelligences working together to be successful. Most individuals possess several intelligences, although they may be able to process information better in one area than another. In terms of health education, a person may have difficulty learning in one area but be successful in another, so it is unfair to assume because clients are not understanding in one area, they cannot grasp the information in another way. Gardner's (2006) multiple intelligences follow.

Linguistic Intelligence

People with this intelligence are sensitive to sounds, rhythms, meanings of words, and have a facility with words. They are interested in language and sensitive to its different functions. They like to read, write, and tell stories. Linguistic intelligence is universal and constant across cultures. Poets, orators, and journalists possess this intelligence.

Logical-Mathematical Intelligence

People with this intelligence have the ability to discern logical or numerical patterns and are skilled at handling long chains of reasoning. These people have a passion for abstraction and ideas that are characteristic of scientific thinking. In gifted individuals, the process of problem solving is often rapid, and frequently a solution is found before it is articulated. Mathematicians and scientists possess this intelligence.

Spatial Intelligence

People with this intelligence rely on the sense of sight, whereas the visually impaired rely on tactile ability to achieve spatial understanding. These individuals have the ability to see things accurately in their environment. They are also able to create mental images, visualize objects, and re-create past visual experiences at will. They like to design and create things. Sculptors, architects, navigators, inventors, and land surveyors possess this intelligence.

Musical Intelligence

People with this intelligence can produce and appreciate rhythm, pitch, timbre, and the many forms of musical expression. Music is integral with life. This intelligence emerges earliest in life. Composers and musical artists possess this intelligence.

Bodily-Kinesthetic Intelligence

People with this intelligence have the ability to control their bodily movements to express an emotion (dancer), play a game (athlete), or create a new product (inventor). They like physical activities and have the ability to skillfully use body cues and motions for expression, handling objects, and goal-directed purposes. Athletes, actors, craftsmen, and surgeons possess this intelligence.

Interpersonal Intelligence

People with this intelligence have the ability to understand others through social interactions. They notice differences in moods, temperaments, motivations, and intentions. This allows them to understand and work with others. They have many friends and like to talk to others. Helping professionals (nurses, doctors, therapists) and gifted sales persons possess this intelligence.

Intrapersonal Intelligence

People with this intelligence focus inwardly on their feelings, talents, interests, etc. They are able to discriminate among their emotions, label them, and use them to understand and guide their behavior. It is the most private intelligence. They like to work alone and follow their interests. Persons with in-depth self-knowledge possess this intelligence.

Multiple intelligences theory is a challenging view of learning because of the many ways that intelligence is expressed in different individuals. People learn differently and cannot be so easily assigned or confined to categories. Table 2-4 offers some suggestions for how nurses as educators can work with clients who appear to fit this theory. To determine what kind of learner clients are, ask them how they best learn.

Implications for Health Education

How does knowing about thinking and learning styles help nurses as educators? It is not possible to give clients a battery of tests to determine thinking and learning styles, so talk with clients and get a sense of how they learn. For example, do they become informed by reading, watching videos, talking with a professional, taking classes, or observing others performing (Chang & Kelly, 2007)? Ask if they have hobbies and what they enjoy doing in their spare time to gather clues to clients' thinking and learning styles. As you work with clients, be especially observant to note what is and is not effective in helping them learn. In working with clients in a nurse-managed center, Kessler and Alverson (2003) found that 82% of clients surveyed preferred hands-on instruction, 63% preferred reading, and 59% preferred listening.

TABLE 2-4 Multiple Intelligence and Teaching Strategies		
Intelligence Type	**Learns By**	**Teaching Strategies**
Linguistic	Reading, writing, talking	Use handouts, pamphlets; encourage client to verbalize or write about experiences; encourage client to keep a journal if appropriate; discussion.
Logical-mathematical	Reasoning, computing, problem solving	Use case examples; ask questions; identify problems to solve ("how would you handle . . ."); encourage critical thinking in pondering solutions.
Spatial	Forming mental images	Draw pictures, especially helpful with children; mind mapping, visualizations are helpful.
Musical	Listening to music	Background music; comfortable learning environment; use rhythm or songs to aid memorization.
Bodily-kinesthetic	Touching, moving	Handle and manipulate equipment; develop skills.
Interpersonal	Sharing with others	Form groups to discuss common health problems or develop projects; group activities.
Intrapersonal	Working alone	Use programmed instructional software; computer assisted instruction; self-paced learning; individual learning projects.

Adapted from Holland, 2007; Miller and Babcock, 1996.

Nurses also are learners with their own preferred style of thinking and learning. It adds to their effectiveness if nurses are aware of how they think and learn. Nurses in the educator role have a tendency to teach in ways that are consistent with how they themselves learn. When the clients' thinking and learning styles fit with the learning setting, the task at hand, and the teacher, clients thrive. When clients' thinking and learning styles do not fit with these factors, clients may have difficulty grasping the health message (Dunn, 1983; Sternberg, 1997).

Rassool and Rawaf (2007) found that undergraduate nursing students preferred the reflector learning style. Noble, Miller, and Heckman (2008) found that nursing students were more field dependent than students in other health-related disciplines. When there is a mismatch between educator and learner, educators tend to attribute the problem to learners, assuming that they were not motivated or could not grasp the concepts. When that occurs, educators should consider that the problem may be with themselves and their failure to accurately assess clients. It is the responsibility of nurses as educators to evaluate the effectiveness of their teaching.

Nurses move beyond their concern with learning styles by creating a rich learning environment that provides many choices for clients (Moran et al., 2006). Having abundant reading materials (books and pamphlets), pictures, videos, interactive instructional materials, demonstrations, and resource persons available are helpful. Multiple choices allow clients to select among the learning options the one that best suits their learning style.

SUMMARY

This chapter introduced thinking and learning processes and how that knowledge increases the effectiveness of nurses as educators in working with clients. The three domains of learning—cognitive, affective, and psychomotor—provide a framework for developing learning objectives. Cognitive domain involves intellectual activities; affective domain deals with attitudes and values; and psychomotor domain involves learning motor skills. Thinking underlies these domains, and a summary of types of thinking was discussed. These types include problem solving, nursing process, critical thinking, clinical judgment, creative thinking, intuition, reflection, fantasy, and reverie. It is important to understand your own thinking and ways to promote thinking in clients.

This chapter also examined several styles of thinking and learning, including Sternberg's thinking styles, Witkin and Goodenough's cognitive-style dimensions, Kolb's experiential learning model, and Gardner's multiple intelligence view of learning. Each view of learning provides insight into how clients learn and how nurses as educators can best promote learning.

EXERCISES

Exercise I—Learning Domains

Purpose: Distinguish among cognitive, affective, and psychomotor learning domains.

Directions: Working alone, examine the learning objectives for the course you are taking. Place each objective into one of the learning domains. Then form small groups and compare your answers. Was each learning objective categorized correctly?

Exercise II—Affective Domain

Purpose: Examine the affective domain in teaching and learning.

Directions: Reflect on a client situation where the client's attitudes and beliefs were different from your own. Journal the following:

1. What was the difference between your attitudes and beliefs and those of the client?
2. Did the difference affect how you felt about the client?
3. How did you respond to the client when you became aware of the difference in attitudes and beliefs?
4. Do you think your client was aware that your attitudes and beliefs differed from theirs?
5. What effect did it have on the care you delivered?

Exercise III—Thinking

Purpose: Examine the various factors that influence your thinking.

Directions: Divide into small groups and discuss the following:

1. Identify factors that influence your present thinking. Consider your parents, siblings, close friends, schools attended, religion, music, and the media.
2. Under what circumstances do you do your best thinking? Consider factors such as noise level, time of day, activity you may be engaged in such as driving, gardening, sports, or watching TV. Why is this so?

Exercise IV—Types of Thinking

Purpose: Examine the types of thinking presented in this chapter.

Directions: Divide into small groups and discuss the following:

1. Share examples of how you have used these types of thinking: problem solving, nursing process, critical thinking, clinical judgment, creative thinking, intuition, reflection, fantasy, and reverie.

2. Share examples of observing these types of thinking in others (classmates and clients).

3. Identify ways you can stimulate thinking with your clients.

Exercise V—Critical Thinking

Purpose: Examine the impact of different frames of reference.

Directions: Divide into groups of four or five and discuss the following situation and answer the questions. After you have discussed the questions, rejoin the larger group and compare your group's answers with the answers of the other groups. How were your answers alike? Different? Discuss why the differences occurred.

A 23-year-old Hispanic woman had given birth to her second child and subsequently experienced kidney failure. On her fifth day of peritoneal dialysis, the client asked the nurse what the doctors left in her body that they were trying to wash out. She understood neither what the treatment was, nor why it was necessary. Had she not asked the question, her misperceptions would never have been known. Pretend you are the nurse in this situation and answer the following questions:

1. Restate the problem from the client's perspective, and from the nurse's perspective.
2. How is the nurse's frame of reference different from the client's?
3. What is the significance of this situation?
4. What is the nurse's goal in this situation? What is the nurse trying to achieve?
5. What assumptions has the client made? What assumptions has the nurse made?
6. What evidence does the client have? What evidence does the nurse have?
7. How has the client interpreted the evidence? How has the nurse interpreted the evidence?
8. What inference(s) did the nurse make?
9. What value judgments did the nurse make?
10. What are the implications of this situation for the client? What are the implications of this situation for the nurse?

Exercise VI—Creative Thinking

Purpose: Conceptualize your creative thinking.

Directions: Divide into small groups and have each participant draw a picture of how she or he thinks.

1. Is your thinking scattered and free associating? Is your thinking goal directed and focused? Do ideas pop into your thinking when you are thinking about something else?
2. Compare your drawings with your group members. How similar and how different are they?
3. How did this exercise help you understand your thinking? Did it give you insight into how others think?

Exercise VII—Creative Thinking

Purpose: Generate creative solutions that are both novel and appropriate to the situation.

Directions: Divide into small groups of three to four. Have each participant describe a recent clinical situation with a client that required problem solving. Before stating how each problem was solved, have each group members describe how they would have handled the problem. Finally, share how the participant solved it. Discuss the following:

1. How were the problem solutions alike? How were the problem solutions different?
2. Which problem solution were the most novel?
3. Were the solutions appropriate (useful)? Were some more appropriate (useful) that others?

Exercise VIII—Intuition

Purpose: Examine intuition in teaching and learning.

Directions: A client was due to be discharged and needed instruction on how to change a dressing. When the nurse talked with the client, the client was distracted and busy collecting her possessions for discharge. The nurse had a hunch that the client was concerned about something else rather than learning how to change a dressing. How would you handle this situation? What is the appropriate use of intuition in this situation? Is there a difference between how you and others in your class would handle this situation?

Exercise IX—Learning Style

Purpose: Reflect on your own learning style.

Directions: Write about the following in your journal:

1. When you want to learn something, how do you go about it? Consider visual (movies, pictures, videotapes, TV), auditory (lectures, discussions, tapes, records, radio), and kinesthetic (hands-on, demonstrations, games, trips experiments) modalities.
2. Under what circumstance do you learn best (study groups, individual learning, exam pressures, meeting with instructor)?
3. What environmental conditions help you learn (quiet, music, lighting, study area, snacks)? Hinder your learning?
4. What subjects/topics are easiest for you to learn? What are the most difficult?

SUPPLEMENTAL ONLINE RESOURCES

Learning domains:
http://honolulu.hawaii.edu/intranet/committees/FacDevCom/guidebk/teachtip/
    domains.htm
http://serc.carleton.edu/introgeo/assessment/domains.html
Overview of critical thinking:
http://www.coping.org/write/percept/critical.htm
Foundation for Critical Thinking:
http://www.criticalthinking.org
OpenCourseWare on critical thinking, logic, and creativity:
http://philosophy.hku.hk/think/critical/ct.php
Dunn and Dunn Learning Styles Assessment:
http://www.learningstyles.net
Experiential Learning (Kolb) at Learning Theories.com:
http://www.learning-theories.com/experiential-learning-kolb.html
Howard Gardner multiple intelligences and education:
http://www.infed.org/thinkers/gardner.htm
Multiple Intelligences:
http://www.thomasarmstrong.com/multiple_intelligences.htm
Journal of Technology Studies. Learning styles:
http://scholar.lib.vt.edu/ejournals/JOTS/Winter-Spring-2001/sutliff.html

REFERENCES

Benner, P. (1984). *From novice to expert*. Menlo Park, NY: Addison-Wesley.

Bloom, B. S., Engelhart, M. D., Furst, E. J., Hill, W. H., & Krathwohl, D. R. (Eds.). (1956). Taxonomy of educational objectives: *The classification of educational goals. Handbook I: Cognitive domain*. New York: David McKay.

Brookfield, S. D. (1991). *Developing critical thinkers*. San Francisco: Jossey-Bass.

Brunt, B. A. (2005). Critical thinking in nursing: An integrated review. *The Journal of Continuing Education in Nursing, 36*(2), 60–67.

Burris, S., Kitchel, T., Molina, Q., Vincent, S., & Warner, W. (2008). The language of learning styles. *Association for Career and Technical Education*, Research Report, February 1, 44–48.

Cassidy, S. (2004). Learning styles: An overview of theories, models, and measures. *Educational Psychology, 24*(4), 419–444.

Chang, M., & Kelly, A. E. (2007). Patient education: Addressing culturally diversity and health literacy issues. *Urological Nursing, 27*(5), 411–417.

Claxton, C. S., & Murrell, P. H. (1987). *Learning styles: Implications for improving educational practices* (ASHE-ERIC Higher Education Report No. 4). Washington, DC: Association for the Study of Higher Education.

Dunn, R. (1983). Can students identify their own learning styles? *Educational Leadership, 40*(5), 60–62.

Ennis, R. H. (1985). A logical basis for measuring critical thinking skills. *Educational Leadership, 43*, 44–48.

Faugier, J. (2005). Basic instincts. *Nursing Standard, 19*(24), 14–15.

Gardner, H. (1983). *Frames of mind*. New York: Basic Books.

Gardner, H. (1993). *Multiple intelligences the theory in practice*. New York: Basic Books.

Gardner, H. (2006). *Multiple intelligences new horizons*. New York: Basic Books.

Garity, J. (1985). Learning styles basis for creative teaching and learning. *Nurse Educator, 10*(2), 12–16.

Gordon, J. M. (2000). Congruency in defining critical thinking by nurse educators and non-nurse scholars. *Journal of Nursing Education, 39*(8), 340–51.

Goulet, C., & Owen-Smith, P. (2005). Cognitive-affective learning in physical therapy education: From implicit to explicit. *Journal of Physical Therapy Education, 19*(3), 67–72.

Halpern, D. F. (2003). *Thought and knowledge: An introduction to critical thinking* (4th ed.). Mahwah, NJ: Lawrence Erlbaum Associates.

Hodgkinson, G. P., Langan-Fox, J., & Sadler-Smith, E. (2008). Intuition: A fundamental bridging construct in the behavioural sciences. *British Journal of Psychology, 99*, 1–27.

Holland, F. (2007). Bringing the body to life: Using multiple intelligence theory in the classroom. *SportEX dynamics, 14*, 6–8.

Kessler, T. A., & Alverson, E. (2003). Health concerns and learning styles of underserved and uninsured clients at a nurse managed center. *Journal of Community Health Nursing, 20*(2), 81–92.

Kolb, D. A. (1981). Learning styles and disciplinary differences. In Arthur W. Chickering & Associates (Eds.), *The modern American college*. San Francisco: Jossey-Bass.

Kolb, D. A. (1984). *Experiential learning*. Englewood Cliffs, NJ: Prentice Hall.

Krathwohl, D. R., Bloom, B. S., & Masia, B. B. (1964). *Taxonomy of educational objectives: The classification of educational goals. Handbook II: Affective domain.* New York: David McKay.

Kretchmar, J. (2008). *The affective domain.* EBSCO Research Starters. Ipswich, MA: EBSCO Publishing.

Lipman, M. S. (2003). *Thinking in education.* New York: Cambridge University Press.

Marzano, R. J., & Kendall, J. S. (2007). *The new taxonomy of educational objectives* (2nd ed.). Thousand Oaks, CA: Corwin Press

McPeck, J. (1990*). Teaching critical thinking.* New York: Routledge.

Merriam-Webster's Dictionary and Thesaurus. (2007). Springfield, MA: Merriam-Webster.

Miller, M. A., & Babcock, D. E. (1996). *Critical thinking applied to nursing.* St. Louis: Mosby.

Moran, S., Kornhaber, M., & Gardner, H. (2006). Orchestrating multiple intelligences. *Educational Leadership, 64*(1), 22–29.

Noble, K. A., Miller, S. M., & Heckman, J. (2008). The cognitive style of nursing students: Educational implications for teaching and learning. *Journal of Nursing Education, 47*(6), 245–253.

Paul, R. (1990). *Critical thinking: What every person needs to survive in a rapidly changing world.* Rohnert Park, CA: Center for Critical Thinking and Moral Critique.

Rassool, G. H., & Rawaf, S. (2007). Learning style preferences of undergraduate nursing students. *Nursing Standard, 21*(32), 35–41.

Riddell, T. (2007). Critical assumptions: Thinking critically about critical thinking. *Journal of Nursing Education, 46*(3), 121–126.

Ruggiero, V. R. (2007). *The art of thinking* (8th ed). New York: Pearson Education.

Ruth-Sahd, L., & Hendy, H. M. (2005). Predictors of novice nurses' use of intuition to guide patient care decisions. *Journal of Nursing Education, 44*(10), 450–458.

Santrock, J.W. (2008). *A Topical Approach to Life-Span Development* (4th ed.). Boston: McGraw-Hill.

Saylor, C. R. (1990). Reflection and professional education: Art, science, and competency. *Nurse Educator, 15*(2), 8–11.

Scheffer, B. K., & Rubenfeld, M. G. (2000). A consensus statement on critical thinking in nursing. *Journal of Nursing Education, 39*(8), 352–359.

Slavin, R. E. (2009). *Educational Psychology Theory and Practice* (9th ed.). Englewood Cliffs, NJ: Pearson Education.

Sternberg, R. J. (1997). *Thinking styles.* Cambridge, UK: Cambridge University Press.

Tanner, C. A. (2006). Thinking like a nurse: A research-based model of clinical judgment in nursing. *Journal of Nursing Education, 45*(6), 204–211.

Walsh, C. M., & Seldomridge, L. A. (2006). Critical thinking: back to square two. *Journal of Nursing Education, 45*(6), 212–219.

Walthew, P. J. (2004). Conceptions of critical thinking held by nurse educators. *Journal of Nursing Education, 43*(9), 408–411.

Watson, G., & Glaser, E. M. (1980). *Watson-Glaser critical thinking appraisal manual.* New York: Harcourt Brace Jovanovich.

Witkin, H A., & Goodenough, D. R. (1981). *Cognitive styles: Essence and origins.* New York: International Universities Press.

CHAPTER 3

Theories and Principles of Learning

The central task of education is
to implant a will and facility for learning;
it should produce not learned but learning people.
The truly human society is a learning society,
where grandparents, parents, and children are students together.
In a time of drastic change it is the learners who inherit the future.
The learned usually find themselves equipped to live in a world that no longer exists.
—Eric Hoffer, 1973, p. 32.

OBJECTIVES

Upon completion of this chapter you will be able to:

- Apply the following learning theories to selected teaching/learning situations: behaviorism (stimulus-response and operant conditioning), cognitivism (gestalt and information processing), and social cognitive theory.
- Apply designated principles of learning in selected client education situations.

KEY TERMS

attention
behavior change
behaviorism
cognitive/cognitive field gestalt
delayed modeling
information processing
long-term memory
observational learning
operant conditioning

retention
role model
sensory register
stimulus-response
theory
vicarious experience
vicarious punishment
vicarious reinforcement
working memory

INTRODUCTION

This chapter introduces the value of theory and how theories help us understand observations and experiences. We examine the learning theories of behaviorism, cognitivism, and social cognitive theory and how each conceptualizes how people learn.

For each theory, you will learn about how to apply theory to working with clients as learners in a health education context. We also consider learning principles applicable to client education. This knowledge is applied to situations in which nurses are the primary educators and clients are the primary learners.

VALUE OF THEORY

Theory is a way to explain some observed phenomenon. Expressed as abstract thoughts or general subject principles, theories help make sense of the world and of research findings (Merriam-Webster, 2007; Ormrod, 2008). Theories provide the theoretical framework to view the process of learning, the progress of learners, and nurses' role as educators. Although theories help to understand learning, no single theory explains everything about a subject.

Nurses are pragmatic and eclectic thinkers. Nurses freely select ideas from diverse sources and judge something is good if it works. For example, when you observe something, you try to make sense of it by fitting it into your mental and experiential framework. This is most effective when you know something about what is observed

---

BOX 3-1   Reasons for Theories

You need a theory when you:

1. Confront a new situation and what you already know does not apply to that situation.

2. Want to increase your understanding of something relatively familiar.

3. Face a familiar situation but what you already know does not work.

4. Wish to teach what you know to a colleague or client.

5. Question the validity of a cherished belief.

6. Explore new hypotheses.

7. Observe events for which you can find no explanation.

and have had experience with it. When you observe things that are outside your framework; that is, things for which you have neither explanation nor experience, you become curious and begin to seek answers. Current emphasis on using evidence-based research makes us look to the current literature for studies that answer questions. This search for answers is the foundation of theory development. Theory helps to make sense of what you observe; it is a way to view relationships among observed phenomena. Box 3-1 identifies how theory is useful.

THEORIES OF LEARNING

Learning theories provide the theoretical framework to understand how people learn. We want to know how people acquire new knowledge, develop skills, modify attitudes and values, and learn new behaviors. We know that learning is a dynamic, lifelong process that is unique to each individual.

In the context of health education, knowing about learning theories is a way to understand how people learn. Theory-based teaching is an effective way to organize your thinking and conceptualize what you want to convey to clients and team members. Clients experiencing healthcare problems may need to learn new ways to maintain their health or deal with illness or disability. This is the time when clients are motivated to learn about their changing health status. Team members also may need to learn about new illnesses and new procedures. This need for continuing education falls under the nurse's purview as an educator.

Various definitions of learning exist. Common to most definitions of learning is the notion that a change occurs in the learner's behavior, attitudes, or skills (Merriam, Caffarella, & Baumgartner, 2007). The behavioral change is both observable and relatively permanent (Olson & Hergenhahn, 2009). Broadly speaking, learning theories fall into two camps, behaviorism and cognitivism (Ormrod, 2008). Behaviorism focuses on tangible, observable behaviors such as learning to give an injection, changing dietary practices, and safely bathing an infant. Cognitivism focuses on the thought processes as humans learn; for example, seeing a relationship between food intake and blood glucose levels, using memory tricks to recall health instructions, and gaining insight into one's own behavior. Because there are many learning theories within these two camps and different ways to group them, for purposes of this discussion we will look at two theories of behaviorism (stimulus-response and operant conditioning), two theories of cognitivism (gestalt and information processing), and social cognitive theory.

BEHAVIORAL VIEWS OF LEARNING

Behavioral learning theories were among the first to be developed and were the first to be used in the United States educational system. They continue to be pervasive, and when the term *learning theory* is used, it usually refers to the body of knowledge accumulated by researchers in the field of behavioral psychology.

Behavioral theorists have generally accepted several basic assumptions in approaching their research (Ormrod, 2008):

- Humans and animals learn in the same way; consequently, early researchers studied rats and pigeons and applied that to human learning.
- Studying stimuli and response objectifies the learning processes.
- Internal processes such as thoughts, motives, and emotions are unimportant in understanding learning because they are not observable. Later behaviorists stated that motivation and the strength of the stimulus-response associations were important.
- Learning involves changing behavior.
- Organisms are born as blank slates with learning occurring after birth.
- Learning is largely the result of environmental events that condition behavior.
- The most useful theories explain behavior using as few learning principles as possible.

Learning for the behaviorist is focused on an observable change in the learner's behavior and is not concerned with the internal thought processes of the learner. The learner as a research subject is described as an organism rather than a person or human being. Behaviorists believe that the learner's behavior is shaped by elements in the environment that either precede (*stimulus*) the behavior or the consequences that follow it. These preceding events can precipitate the behavior, and the events that follow can have positive or negative consequences on the behavior. These events must occur closely in time so that a bond is formed, called the *principle of contiguity* (Olson & Hergenhahn, 2009). An example of a preceding event is a nurse approaching a child with a clearly visible syringe intending to vaccinate him. The sight of the syringe frightens the child who anticipates pain, starts crying, and clings to his mother for protection. Thereafter the child may be frightened of syringes until he matures and learns differently. An example of a *reinforcing* event is a smile and hug from the child's mother that assures him he is safe and well. The child knows he can find solace and protection from his mother and will seek her out in future frightening situations.

Behavioral theories today encompass a number of individual theories and continue to be widely applied in understanding how people learn. We review the stimulus-response theories of Pavlov, Thorndike, and Gutherie, and Skinner's operant conditioning.

Stimulus-Response

Stimulus-response theories have their origins in the nineteenth century with Ivan Pavlov (1849–1936) and Edward Lee Thorndike (1874–1949), who studied how animals and humans learn. Pavlov was a Russian physiologist who is famous for discovering the principle of classical conditioning in his work with a hungry dog. He discovered that when meat powder was placed in a dog's mouth, the dog automatically salivated *(unconditioned stimulus)*. When a bell was sounded simultaneously with the offering of meat powder, the bell *(conditioned stimulus)*, became paired with the dog's salivation. Eventually the bell by itself stimulated the dog to salivate. If the bell was presented often enough without the accompanying meat powder, eventually the dog stopped salivating. This phenomenon was called *extinction*. Pavlov's experiment is commonly known as *classical conditioning* (Santrock, 2008).

Thorndike did extensive pioneering research in learning, and his work is considered the first modern theory of learning. He noted that the most characteristic method of learning for both animals and humans was trial and error, also called connectionism, or the stimulus-response theory of learning. The organism confronts a problem and selects a response most likely to lead to the goal. Much random behavior occurs until the goal is met. On each successive trial, the random behavior decreases and the goal-directed behavior increases. This forms the basis for the principle of positive reinforcement that Thorndike called the *Law of Effect*. It means that the organism remembers responses that had satisfying effects, which strengthens the connection. If the responses were unsatisfying, the strength of the connection decreases. Thorndike formulated two other laws, the *Law of Exercise* and the *Law of Readiness*. The Law of Exercise states that repeated use of meaningful connections results in substantial learning, whereas lack of use of connections inhibits learning. The Law of Readiness states that learning is enhanced when the organism is ready for the connection; otherwise it is inhibited (Olson & Hergenhahn, 2009).

Edwin Ray Guthrie (1886–1959) built on the work of Thorndike and Pavlov. Guthrie felt that the rules they proposed were unnecessarily complicated; he proposed one law of learning, the *Law of Contiguity* (Olson & Hergenhahn, 2009). He wrote, "A combination of stimuli which has accompanied a movement will on its recurrence tend to be followed by that movement" (Guthrie, 1935, p. 23). It means that events that occur together in time tend to be paired. If, for example, a person did something in a given situation, he tends to repeat that when in that situation again.

Guthrie proclaimed, as do behaviorists today, that a science of psychology must be based on a study of what is observable: behaviors, bodily changes, data that can be detected by an observer and/or a measuring device. All data are admissible except introspection, which can only be reported by the client. Later Guthrie revised his theory to recognize the many stimuli to which the organism is exposed and that associations cannot be formed with all of them. The organism responds selectively to only a small number of stimuli and those are the ones that become associated with the response being made. He restated his law to read "What is being noticed becomes a signal for what is being done" (Guthrie, 1959 as quoted in Olson & Hergenhahn, 2009, p. 207). What captures the organism's attention becomes important along with the association formed.

Operant Conditioning

Burrhus Frederick Skinner (1904–1990) is probably the most familiar of the behaviorists in the United States. He is famous for his Skinner box, an experimenter-controlled cage in which the behavior of animals (rats and pigeons) was studied. Skinner acknowledges two kinds of learning. The first is *respondent behavior*, which occurs in response to a known stimulus, such as the knee jerk in response to the examiner's hammer. The second type of learning, which Skinner believes is more important in human behavior, is an *operant response* and refers to the *consequences* of behavior. When a response is reinforced, whether random or planned, the behavior tends to be repeated; when the consequences are unpleasant, the behavior tends to be suppressed (Slavin, 2009). This statement is a simple way to explain operant learning. Most human behavior is the result of operant learning according to Skinner. The propositions of behavioral theory as it is understood today follow (Olson & Hergenhahn, 2009; Slavin, 2009).

Propositions of Behavioral Theory

1. Behavior that is followed by reinforcement tends to strengthen the behavior. After being taught how to transfer from bed to chair, a client is given smiles and verbal encouragement from the nurse. Praise reinforces the client's behavior and increases the likelihood of further attempts to transfer.
2. Behavior followed by punishment tends to be suppressed. For example, a young man is compliant with his father's commands because he knows that his father will react negatively to his behavior. The son complies because he has learned that rebellion or questioning will result in punishment.

3. Behavior followed by the removal of a negative stimulus tends to increase in strength. Deep breathing relieves tension during an asthma attack and thus decreases the severity of the attack. When clients experience how proper breathing makes a difference, they are motivated to continue this type of breathing.

4. Behavior that tends to recur is in some way being reinforced or is reinforcing itself. An infant crawls and gets into things because it is fun and satisfies the infant's curiosity. Overeating under stressful conditions is reinforcing when it relieves client anxiety.

5. A behavior may serve to reinforce or strengthen another behavior. Schizophrenics can be persuaded to act appropriately for something they value. For example, a client can be given something in exchange for sitting quietly.

6. Irregular and inconsistent reinforcement of a behavior strengthens the continuance of that behavior. Parents who try to resist a whining child's demands but who eventually give in are inadvertently strengthening the whining behavior with the most powerful method known: intermittent reinforcement.

7. Immediate and consistent reinforcement of a behavior strengthens that behavior most rapidly. A breastfeeding baby soon learns that sucking satisfies hunger.

8. Rewards that are specific to and desired by the learner are more powerful than general or routine rewards. A teenage client may respond well to compliments from the nurse, whereas another client may respond better to matching wits with the nurse.

9. Rewards and punishments that are clearly connected to the behavior are more powerful than vague or inconsistent responses. The client who moves in certain ways after surgery quickly learns that certain motions produce pain so those movements are avoided. This principle helps explain why eating disorders are so difficult to change. The pleasure or relief that the overeater experiences outweigh the hazards, because the pleasure is more immediate and the hazards more remote. The effects of overeating do not show on the body or on the scale for days, and the health hazards may not become evident for many years. The connection between overeating and health issues is vague and inconsistent because other variables, such as genetics and exercise, are thought to add to or reduce the health risks.

10. Behavior that receives no response and meets no biologic need tends to extinguish. Children bring home new words that they hear while playing. Some of the words may include language the family does not sanction. Children who experience no response when they try out the new vocabulary tend to lose interest in those words.

Behavior modification is the application of learning theory to modify a behavior by changing the stimulus that elicits it or by changing the consequences that follow it. Classical conditioning emphasizes that whatever came before a behavior (antecedent event) influences that behavior (responding behavior). Operant conditioning stresses that a behavior is influenced by the response that follows. A behavior that is followed by a negative response or no response at all will diminish, whereas a behavior followed by a positive consequence will increase. When both of these theories are applied together, behavior is seen as a result of an antecedent event and that behavior is further influenced by the consequences that follow it. This is illustrated in Figure 3-1.

Implications for Health Education

Decreasing an undesirable behavior involves eliminating or changing the antecedent event that evoked the behavior. Another option is to punish the behavior after it occurs. To increase a desirable behavior, the educator changes the antecedent event to one that is more likely to evoke the desired behavior or reinforces the desired behavior when it occurs or does both actions. An example of controlling antecedent behavior is to advise a client learning weight control: "Shop on a full stomach and use a shopping list." The antecedent event of a full stomach and a shopping list prepared in

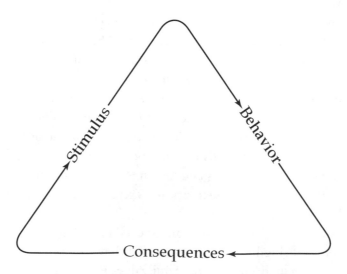

FIGURE 3-1 Stimulus-Behavior-Consequences. To change a behavior you can change the stimulus that elicits it and/or the consequences that follow it.

advance influences shoppers' behavior in the desired direction: wise shopping for wholesome food.

Using behavioral principles, the nurse identifies a client's desired behavior and then creates an environment that stimulates the client to comply by producing this desired response. When the desired behavior occurs, the nurse reinforces it. Immediate reinforcement increases the likelihood that the behavior will recur. Over time, the nurse moves from reinforcing the behavior every time it occurs to an intermittent reinforcement schedule. This gives the new behavior more stability.

Educators have discovered that punishment is not a long-term solution to undesirable behavior. Punishment may indeed suppress it, but if the behavior is meeting some need, that behavior is likely to return as soon as the threat is removed. Another possible consequence of punishment is erratic and unpredictable response. The most effective way to eliminate an undesirable behavior is to find out what need the behavior is meeting, and reinforce a more desirable method of meeting that need. The example used previously was a whining child. It could be applied just as easily to a whining client of any age. Solutions to the problem of client whining include frequent, pleasant, and predictable attention by nurses along with encouragement and assistance.

COGNITIVE VIEWS OF LEARNING

Cognitivism (also known as cognitive psychology) is the predominant theoretical perspective for studying human learning today. Its focus is on the cognitive processes, that is, "how people perceive, interpret, remember and in other ways think about environmental events" (Ormrod, 2008, p. 149). Cognitive theorists study humans, believing that some human learning is unique and differs from how animals learn. Whereas behaviorism focuses on observable behavioral changes, cognitivism expands the understanding of learning to include internal mental processes unique to each person, such as perception, insight, and meaning (Olson & Hergenhahn, 2009; Ormrod, 2008). Cognitive views of learning encompass several perspectives; in this section we focus on Gestalt psychology and information processing theory.

Gestalt or Cognitive Field View of Learning

Three German psychologists, Max Wertheimer (1880–1943), Wolfgang Kohler (1887–1967), and Kurt Koffka (1886–1941) departed from behaviorism and are considered the founders of Gestalt psychology. Later, another German Gestalt psychologist, Kurt Lewin (1890–1947), developed a field theory of human learning. These psychologists insisted that behavior was much more than a conditioned response and that perception and memory can be studied by introspection in addition to external observation. Further, they posit that humans selectively perceive and react to complex patterns of stimuli as wholes, not as disconnected parts. It is the total pattern of stimuli that determines what a person perceives and learns (Olson & Hergenhahn, 2009; Ormrod, 2008).

Gestalt is a German word that means "the configuration or pattern" (Olson & Hergenhahn, 2009), the whole or totality. In the field of Gestalt psychology the concept means that the whole is more than merely the sum of all of its parts. Gestalt psychologists hold that psychological phenomena are irreducible wholes that cannot be derived just from analysis of their parts. If the totality of a particular perception is dissected, the meaning is lost.

Perception refers to the act of becoming aware of something by the use of any of the senses. To perceive means to take notice of, observe, detect, become aware of in one's mind, achieve understanding of, or apprehend. Perception refers to the portion of the world that is grasped mentally through sight, hearing, touch, taste, and smell (Merriam-Webster, 2007).

Our perception of any object is affected by the context in which we become aware of it. Clients who are in a strange hospital and in pain will perceive your messages differently than clients who greet you in their homes. Team members who just heard about another reduction in work force and feel overloaded with responsibilities will perceive your messages differently than those who feel in control of their circumstances. Our perceptions of events are affected by life experiences and interests.

Gestalt and cognitive-field theories of learning take into account both the learner and the learning context and all of the individual's experiences and perceptions. In many circumstances individuals' perceptions are dissimilar, and other possible perceptions are not easily seen. Even individuals who experience the same event at the same time may have different perceptions of that event. Because of the tendency to assume that others perceive events the same way you do, you may not be aware that clients see events differently.

It is possible that you and others may not perceive the same events the same way. An equally important factor to consider is that you may not even be aware of your perceptual differences. It is important to look for clues to these differences and address them. Reconsider the example of the 23-year-old Hispanic woman from Chapter 2 who had given birth to her second child and subsequently experienced kidney failure. On her fifth day of undergoing peritoneal dialysis, the client asked what the doctor had left in her body that the nurses were trying to wash out. She understood neither the treatment nor the reason it was necessary. Had she not asked the question, her misunderstanding would never have been known. This supports how important it is to assess client perceptions.

Lewin stated that each individual exists in an environment also known as a field or life space, affected by many forces. Life space is a psychological field unique to each individual and includes things to which the person reacts; for example, material objects, people, private thoughts, tensions, and goals. He proposes that behavior is the interplay of these forces in the life space at the moment in which the behavior occurs. Analysis begins with examining the environment as a whole. Lewin made it clear that the environment as interpreted by the individual did not necessarily correspond with actual reality. Learning occurs as a result of a change in individual psychological interpretations or changes in the internal needs or motivations of the individual (Knowles, Holton, & Swanson, 2005; Olson & Hergenhahn, 2009).

Jean Piaget (1896–1980), a Swiss psychologist, focused his detailed studies on the thinking process of children (1972). He conducted one-on-one interactions, during which he presented various stimuli to infants and children. He then observed and recorded their responses. The responses led him to believe that thinking and learning are active processes, not merely passive, or trial-and-error responses to stimuli as behaviorists believe. As the children grew old enough to speak, Piaget spoke with the children as he conducted the experiments. He concluded that intellectual development is a gradual process that evolves over time. You will learn more about how children learn in Chapter 5.

Learning is a transactional process in which individuals gain further understanding, new insights, or more developed cognitive structures through interaction. Two ways of learning that Piaget identified were *assimilation* and *accommodation*. Assimilation is a way of learning in which new ideas are incorporated by association with known ideas, concepts, and memories. Individuals may assimilate new ideas into their current beliefs. If the knowledge is different from what they already know, they may respond with the intellectual process known as accommodation, which is more difficult than assimilation. When accommodating new ideas, individuals give up former beliefs or substantially change their frame of reference or they do both. Accommodation may also occur after a person has assimilated so many new concepts that the concepts can no longer be contained in the person's old cognitive structure. A paradigm shift occurs in the aftermath of an accumulation process (Olson & Hergenhahn, 2009). Figure 3-2 illustrates assimilation and accommodation.

Implications for Health Education

Nurses frequently deal with clients who are undergoing life transitions such as birth, death, parenthood, or divorce. It also includes clients who experience alterations in personal integrity such as physical assault, accidental loss of sight or limb, loss of a way of life, or surgical removal of an organ. Such transitions can force clients into

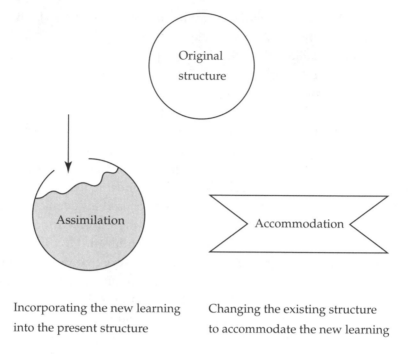

Incorporating the new learning
into the present structure

Changing the existing structure
to accommodate the new learning

FIGURE 3-2   Assimilation and Accommodation.

reconstructing and reorganizing their perceptions of themselves and reality (Edelman & Mandle, 2006; Selder, 1989). When clients struggle with issues such as "Who am I?" and "What is life about?" they are going through the process of accommodation.

The following is an example of the use of Gestalt psychology in teaching children. The nurse involved with doing preoperative teaching of young children arranges for the children and their parents to come to the day-surgery area for a visit. While the children are in the unit, they see a video portraying surgery from a child's perspective. The video tells them:

> You wear green pajamas with a hat and socks to match. You get a shot (ouch) that makes you sleepy, and you ride on a table with wheels. The ceiling and people look funny when you ride flat. When you wake up you will be sore, but you will get more shots that will make the soreness go away.

After the video the children are led to a room with pieces of equipment, drapes, and surgical clothing that they are invited to play with. Dolls set up with various kinds of medical equipment (without real needles) are also within reach so that children can handle and play "operation." The nurse observes the children and listens to their conversations, using their responses as clues to what further teaching might be needed.

The main goal of the Gestalt perspective is to promote understanding and insight. Nurses as educators assess the client's perceptions and design a learning situation that will stimulate interest and understanding. Nurses organize the learning situation to fit the client's developmental stage, previous experiences, and learning ability.

Information Processing View of Learning

Another view of human learning is as a sophisticated form of information processing. This view of learning was inspired by advances in computer science by theorists who hypothesized that human minds performed mental operations like computers (Santrock, 2008). Atkinson and Shiffrin propose a model of information processing with three components focusing on how individuals register sensory information taken in from the environment, how they process information in short-term memory, and how that information is stored and retrieved from long-term memory (Ormrod, 2008; Slavin, 2009).

The first component of the information processing model is the *sensory register*, which receives large amounts of information from the five senses: sight, hearing, touch, smell, and taste. This component decides whether or not to notice or register an external sensory bit of datum, such as an odor, flavor, touch, sound, or visual stimulus. It also decides whether or not to register sensory datum that are internal, for example, an itch, a chill, a peristaltic wave, a headache, or a memory. The information is quickly lost if it is given no further attention. Humans often describe stimuli that they did not notice if they are asked to do so immediately after the stimulus. However, they are unable to do this after a couple of seconds have passed. In addition, people retain less if they are bombarded with too many diverse stimuli at one time (Slavin, 2009).

The second component of information processing model is *short-term memory*, also called *working memory*. This is where the sensory information goes when the individual pays attention to it. It holds thoughts a person is conscious of having at any given moment. The storage capacity of short-term memory appears limited in most individuals, holding approximately five to seven thoughts. As if they were bowling pins, ideas in the mind can be crowded out by the introduction of more items. These thoughts can be related to what the person is feeling, doing, or thinking at the moment, or they can be related to thoughts retrieved from storage in long-term memory that are associated with current stimuli.

For example, a nurse admits a small child for surgery who is tightly clutching a teddy bear. While observing the child's color, breathing ability, alertness, and the parent-child interaction, the nurse remembers the teddy bear from years ago, or that of a daughter or son. Such recollections make the nurse more sensitive to the child at hand. If too many memories impinge on the nurse's consciousness, the memories may detract from the nurse's ability to note and track client data. Another example is a charge nurse giving instructions to a health team member at the change of shift. The team member is struggling with personal issues, including a paraplegic husband at home without a caretaker. Her personal concerns are crowding the space that might store the instructions she is receiving from the charge nurse.

The third component of the information processing model is the *long-term memory*, in which an infinite amount of information is stored for a prolonged period of time. Long-term memory is thought to have a large capacity provided that it has not been damaged by pathology. Stored in long-term memory are images and thoughts about past experiences (episodic memory); facts, knowledge, general information that we have learned, as well as problem-solving and learning strategies (semantic memory); and procedural knowledge such as how to do things such as giving an injection, riding a bike, and general living skills (procedural memory) (Squire, Knowlton, & Musen, 1993).

Implications for Health Education

The nurse's job as an educator from an information processing point of view is to program the client with the new information. It is important to divide learning into steps that are compatible with the client's health, intelligence, and previous learning experiences. The nurse assists the client in acknowledging current beliefs that enhance or inhibit learning. The new information is then translated into a message that the client is able to process.

The information processing model is particularly useful for teaching skills online, such as procedures that must be done in an orderly sequence. As educators, nurses assess educational needs and choose online resources to facilitate learning. This is a useful teaching strategy for individuals who are self-directed, visual, and experienced with computers. Nurses give feedback through discussion forums, e-mail, or phone.

In using the information processing model, it is important for nurses to avoid overloading clients with too much information, especially if the information is new. If a lot of information must be communicated in a short period of time, try grouping the information in categories that make sense. For example, if you are teaching a client newly diagnosed with diabetes, it would be helpful to create groupings of information to aid the client's memory. Grouping information for diabetic clients includes: dietary information, exercise routine, injection procedure and supplies, and signs and symptoms of hyperglycemia and hypoglycemia. Having printed information about each group also facilitates learning. Clients who have concerns should have written instructions to read at home that serves as memory aids. Booklets with illustrations are helpful.

If the client in the preceding example had diabetes for many years and was well informed about the disease, your approach would be different. Assess where the client has gaps in knowledge and provide appropriate instruction. The goal is to complement what the client already knows and facilitate learning where it is needed.

SOCIAL COGNITIVE VIEW OF LEARNING

Albert Bandura developed the social cognitive theory of learning. Born in 1925, he is currently a Professor of Social Science in Psychology at Stanford University. His theory is an outgrowth of the behavioral theories of learning that resulted from his belief that these theories lacked a complete explanation for learning. He incorporated many contributions from cognitive theorists into what is now referred to as observational learning. Bandura believes that people are neither driven by inner forces, nor automatically shaped by external forces; rather, they are creative, active participants in shaping their lives. In other words, people are proactive rather than reactive; they have some control over how they live their lives (Bandura, 1986, 2001).

Bandura's social cognitive theory states that people learn from observing others in a social setting. By observing others, people acquire knowledge and skills, learn social rules and norms, and develop beliefs and attitudes. They observe which behaviors are useful, appropriate, and valued by society and which are not. Social cognitive theory posits that people learn most efficiently from observing others' behavior and less from the consequences of behavior (Skinner's view). In other words, this theory states that people learn primarily by observing the successes and failures of others (Santrock, 2008; Slavin, 2009). It is important to distinguish between learning by observation and the act of imitation. Learning may or may not include imitating the observed behavior.

Models and modeling behavior are important concepts. A model can be anything that conveys information, for example, a person, film, television, picture, or instructions. Models convey messages about behavior. Bandura believes that behavior is the result of the bidirectional interaction of three classes of behavioral determinants: cognitive and personal factors, environmental events, and behavior. The interaction is reciprocal in that each operates interactively as determinants of each other. Behavior is a result of the interacting determinants and cannot be understood by viewing them in isolation. The strength of the influence of each determinant on behavior varies according to the situation. Figure 3-3 illustrates this reciprocal relationship, which Bandura calls *reciprocal determinism* (Bandura, 1986; Olson & Hergenhahn, 2009).

An example helps to understand some cognitive factors in social learning. Emily, a student nurse, observes Nurse X assisting a physician during a diagnostic procedure. The nurse is poorly prepared to assist the physician and does not have knowledge of the procedure or the physician's requirements and needs. Consequently, both Nurse X and the physician are unhappy at the conclusion of the procedure. The next day Emily observes Nurse Y assist a physician with the same procedure. Nurse Y is prepared, organized, and familiar with the physician's requirements and needs. The outcome is better and the physician thanks Nurse Y for her preparedness and efficiency. Later Emily seeks out her instructor and together they discuss both situations. They identify what was effective and ineffective behavior of each nurse's performance. In this example Emily observes both positive and negative modeling and is able to see the differences. Emily verbally rehearses her responsibilities with her instructor. Six months later, Emily is assigned to assist a physician with the same diagnostic procedure. She mentally rehearses her role and responsibilities. The procedure goes

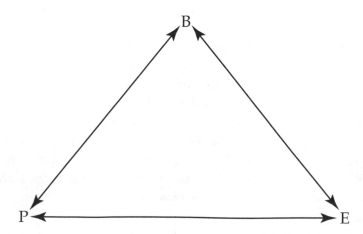

FIGURE 3-3 Reciprocal Determinism. Behavior is the result of the bidirectional interaction of three classes of behavioral determinants: cognitive and personal factors, environmental events, and behavior, called reciprocal determinism. Used with permission, courtesy of Albert Bandura.

smoothly and the participants are satisfied. This shows how modeling can produce successful performance. From this example, the following components of social cognitive learning theory are illustrated (Bandura, 1986; Ormrod, 2008):

- Emily's learning was a mental activity; she learned by observing. She paid attention to what each nurse was doing and made a mental note of what was ineffective (Nurse X) and what was effective (Nurse Y). She learned by observing each nurse and mentally rehearsing effective behavior *(vicarious learning)*.

- Although Emily did not have an opportunity to immediately imitate Nurse Y's behavior, her learning also was verbal when she discussed her observations with her instructor. Together they reviewed what she learned through observation.

- Emily had no opportunity to immediately imitate the desired assisting behavior; however, six months later she remembered what she learned and was able to imitate the behavior *(delayed modeling)*.

- Emily was aware of how unhappy both Nurse X and the physician were at the conclusion of the procedure. Observing their unhappiness, Emily experienced *vicarious punishment (response-punishment contingency)* and did not want to experience the same outcome.

- Emily was aware of how pleased Nurse Y and the physician were at the conclusion of the procedure. Observing their satisfaction, the physician's compliments, with her instructor's positive input, Emily experienced *vicarious reinforcement (response-reinforcement contingency)* and she desired that outcome for herself.

- Emily felt confident and believed in her ability to successfully perform the behavior *(self-efficacy expectation)*. Subsequently when she was in the assisting role again, she fulfilled her expectations of herself and rewarded herself with a mental pat on the back.

Bandura identified four processes that influence observational learning (Bandura, 1986; Olson & Hergenhahn, 2009): attentional processes, retentional processes, behavioral production processes, and motivational processes. *Attentional processes* occur when the learner actively pays attention to what is observed. Models that are similar to the observer in terms of age, gender, respected, and who are competent, powerful, attractive, and have high status are attended to more often. Heroes in various age groups act as models for people of their age groups. *Retentional processes* mean that, for observational learning to be useful, what is learned must be remembered for future use. Learning can be stored verbally in words or in the form of mental pictures or images of modeled behaviors (imaginally). When needed, learning is retrieved, rehearsed, and used long after it is observed. *Behavioral production processes* refer to the person's ability to actually perform what has been learned. Some individuals may be unable to perform or retain information that was learned because of age-related developmental immaturity, illness, or injury. *Motivational processes* include two aspects: First, it refers to the expectation that acting like the model in certain situations will result in reinforcement similar to that received by the model. Second, it serves to motivate a person to use (perform) what has been learned.

Implications for Health Education

Role modeling is a form of observational learning. Nurses learn by observing their professional colleagues. In the same way, clients learn by observing nurses. Clients observe nurses and other healthcare providers and regard them as experts. If they model good health practices, that behavior sends an important message to clients; the converse is also true. Nurses who are overweight or smoke have little credibility when it comes to teaching clients about weight reduction or smoking cessation. The old adage is true: what we do is a stronger message than what we say regardless of how sincerely we present the message. If nurses are to be effective educators, they must model good health practices and behaviors (Rush, Kee, & Rice, 2005; Spencer, 2007).

Table 3-1 summarizes the views of learning discussed in this chapter. Each view has advantages and disadvantages depending on the type of intended learning and on the learner and teacher interaction. When selecting a view, ask yourself the following questions: What is the purpose of the learning? Who initiates the learning? Who evaluates whether or not the learning has been effective?

Educator responsibilities vary depending on the learning view used. In each view, the teacher's role is that of the director (behaviorism), designer (gestaltism), programmer (information processing), or model (social cognitive). The main goal of the learner in each view is to change behavior (behaviorism), understand (gestaltism), register, retain, and recall information (information processing), and observe and imitate (social cognitive). Table 3-1 compares these concepts.

PRINCIPLES OF LEARNING

Principles are the foundation or general laws of teaching and learning derived from research based on consistently observed phenomenon. Learning principles are formulations that are generally true and stable over multiple learning situations (Ormrod, 2008). These principles, summarized in Box 3-2, are derived from research

TABLE 3-1	Views Regarding Thinking, Learning, Teacher, Learner			
Views of:	**Thinking**	**Learning**	**Teacher**	**Learner**
Behaviorist	Covert trial and error	Change in behavior	Directs	Complies
Gestaltist	Knows, perceives	Understands, gains insight	Designs	Participates
Processor	Processes information	Registers, retains, recalls	Programs	Inputs, outputs
Social Cognitivist	Observes, mentally processes	Attends, retains, performs	Models	Imitates

(Slavin, 2009) and informal feedback from over 800 registered nurses over 15 years who were taught clinical teaching methods in a baccalaureate registered nurse program by authors Babcock and Miller (1994). These principles of learning are applicable to health education.

Focusing Intensifies Learning

Individuals vary in ways that help them learn. Some learners depend on eye contact with the teacher; they focus on the teacher's verbalizations and body language. Others make images in their mind of what is being presented. Kinesthetic learners are people who learn through the awareness of body position. Some learners write images on paper or write notes to stay actively involved.

While studying, some learners listen to music to help them concentrate. Others want minimal auditory and visual distractions. Some learners have rituals that help them focus. Examples of rituals include meditation, organizing materials, and preparing a snack. Most learners enhance their ability to retain and recall information by developing a pattern that provides for physical comfort, a heightened level of arousal, and a clear mind.

Repetition Enhances Learning

This approach is where learners repeat the information until they are able to produce it from memory. Sustained practice enforces learning. This is true for memorizing facts as well as for mastering psychomotor skills.

BOX 3-2   Principles of Learning

Principles of Learning

1. Focusing

2. Repetition

3. Learner control

4. Active participation

5. Individual styles

6. Organization

7. Association

8. Imitation

9. Motivation

10. Spacing

11. Recency

12. Primacy

13. Arousal

14. Accurate and prompt feedback

15. Application

16. Personal history

Learner Control Increases Learning

Learners do better when they feel in control of the learning process and are more likely to choose learning methods that worked for them in the past. Past experience demonstrates that nurses are successful adult learners who can verbalize what they need to master new information and skills. Most nurses take responsibility for their learning and do better when educators acknowledge this in both actions and words. This same principle applies to learners of any age. Older learners generally need more time to absorb new information. They are successful when in control of both the pace and the increments of learning.

Active Participation is Necessary for Learning

Learning is an active process. Most people find that the more they are able to involve themselves in learning, the more they are able to learn. Participation in learning means having input into the learning process including the time, place, pace, and increments of learning.

Learning Styles Vary

Some learners find it easier to comprehend verbal discourse, while others comprehend visual cues more easily. Still others seek hands-on experience to grasp the meaning of learning concepts. Many find that a combination of verbal, visual, auditory, and kinesthetic experiences is most effective. Be aware of your preferred learning style because it is the style you are most likely to use when you teach. Assess your clients' learning styles so that you can plan an approach to enhance learning. The skill in facilitating learning is to find an effective match between the clients' learning styles and your teaching approach.

Organization Promotes Learning

Learners often highlight readings, summarize paragraphs, explain their assignments to others, and ask questions. These are ways of actively organizing learning materials. This personal intellectual activity makes the information meaningful and easier to retain. Methods of organization vary, but to be most effective, materials should be organized in a way that fits both the content and the learner. A cognitive task, such as learning historical facts, is facilitated by using chronology. Learning psychomotor skills is enhanced by teaching from the simple to the complex. Affective learning frequently is best organized around the principle of low- to high-risk behaviors from the learner's point of view.

Association Is Necessary to Learning

To retain any new information or skill, learners must be able to associate the new learning with phenomena already within their repertoire of experience. Association provides relevance to learners.

Imitation Is a Method of Learning

Imitating is particularly useful for mastering psychomotor skills, but attitudes and beliefs can also be incorporated if learners observe a respected role model.

Motivation Strengthens Learning

It is easier for learners to grasp facts, learn new skills, and change attitudes when they anticipate gaining benefits from the effort. Past success and the expectation of future success are powerful motivating forces. Educators should perform a needs assessment to understand what motivates clients and use this knowledge to create an atmosphere that sustains motivation and builds confidence.

Spacing New Material Facilitates Learning

It is wiser for educators to present small amounts of new material incrementally rather than larger amounts presented at one time. Learners should be encouraged to read instructional materials to give them exposure to information over time so they have a more thorough understanding. This also provides an opportunity to ask questions of the educators.

Recency Influences Retention

The more recently learners have been exposed to information or have practiced a skill, the greater the possibility that clients will recall it correctly. Retention is the ability to repeat information or grasp or hold onto information or a skill.

Primacy Affects Retention

Learners tend to learn the first few items best; this concept is referred to as primacy. Learners pay more attention to and devote more energy to items presented first. The human mind is capable of retaining a limited number (five to seven) of new bits of information at one time. Once these new bits of information have been associated with other more solidly retained memories, learners are better able to grasp and retain other sets of facts.

Arousal Influences Attention

Arousal is affected by novelty. The human mind is attracted to change and glitches in patterns. Other sources of stimuli besides novelty include sensory intensity, emotional arousal, and other sources of tension. A certain amount of tension enhances learners' ability to focus. This tension is caused by fear, anger, anxiety, curiosity, and amusement. When tense, a client's neurochemistry changes. Chemicals are released that improve circulation, provide sugar to the brain and muscles, and enhance visual acu-

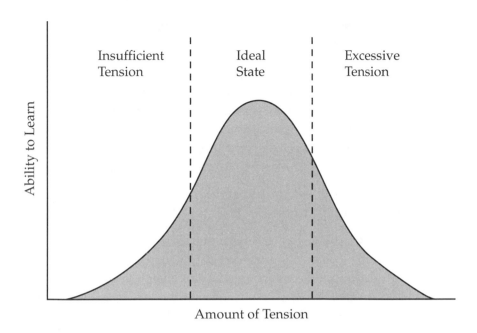

FIGURE 3-4 Arousal and Learning. A moderate amount of tension enhances learning. Too little tension fails to engage learner's attention. Too much tension interferes with learning.

ity. Clients vary in how much tension is ideal for them. This is illustrated in Figure 3-4. For example, too much tension interferes with learning, whereas a moderate level is motivating (Cassady & Johnson, 2002; Stephenson, 2006). With too much tension, clients may become immobilized or restless and engage in behavior that further obstructs learning. Fear of punishment, such as job loss, usually impedes learning and interferes with the ability to apply learning to new situations.

Accurate and Prompt Feedback Enhances Learning

Learners need to know how well they are meeting learning objectives. Self-assessments are helpful; consider how frequently newspapers and magazines publish self-scoring tests and questionnaires. Clients want to know how their attitudes compare with others and their level of knowledge. Feedback is necessary for clients and educators to determine if learning occurred. Prompt feedback reinforces desired behaviors and gives clients feelings of satisfaction when they are successful. Even when correction is necessary, feedback can reduce tension because learners know what is learned and what is still to be mastered.

Application of New Learning in a Variety of Contexts Broadens the Generalization of That Learning

Application of knowledge helps to broaden and generalize learning. An example is practicing crutch walking in a lab setting and then applying the skill in actual practice settings, such as walking up and down steps. Exposure to a particular concept, attitude, or skill in varying situations assists learners to retain new material and develop the ability to apply the material in a wider variety of situations.

The Learner's Biologic, Psychologic, Sociologic, and Cultural Realities Shape the Learner's Perception of the Learning Experience

Health affects energy level and ability to concentrate. Self-esteem and previous experiences with learning affect the willingness to risk, tolerance for temporary failure, and expectations of success. If clients are at a developmental level in which memorization and concrete processing are necessary, educators must respect that. Nurses as educators need to listen and be observant of the signs that learners are handling all they can.

Societal norms and learners' previous experiences with healthcare institutions affect the ability to learn. Clients' attitudes toward learning, their beliefs about personal responsibility for health, and the learning climate are all influenced by their culture. More information about the effect of culture on health education is found in Chapter 8.

BOX 3-3   Evidence-Based Nursing Practice

Hicks, M., McDermott, L. L., Rouhana, N., Schmidt, M., Seymour, M. W., & Sullivan, T. (2008) Nurses' body size and public confidence in ability to provide health education. *Journal of Nursing Scholarship, 40*(4), 349–354.

Purpose: This study examined the relationship between a nurse's body size and perceived confidence in health teaching received from that nurse.

Method: A quasi-experimental posttest-only design was used. Participants were randomly assigned to groups and shown images of a nurse who was either overweight or weight-appropriate and asked to rate their confidence in health teaching received from that nurse. Descriptive statistics, *t*-test for independent samples, and covariate analysis were performed.

Results: A significant difference in confidence was noted between participants who viewed the images. Results indicate that weight-appropriate nurses may inspire more confidence in their health teaching. This replication study confirms the findings of the original study.

SUMMARY

This chapter has examined prominent theories of learning: behaviorism (stimulus-response and operant conditioning), cognitivism (Gestalt and information processing), and social cognitive theory. With each theory, application was made to how nurses as educators could apply that information in a clinical setting when working with clients as learners. Selecting which theory works best for clients and what is taught is your job as the educator. The chapter concluded with a discussion of principles of learning, principles that are broadly applicable in a wide variety of health education situations.

EXERCISES

Exercise I—Integrating Learning Theories and Principles

Purpose: Apply learning theories and principles in preparation for client education.

Directions: Divide into groups and choose which assignment(s) your group will prepare.

Group Assignment A

What learning theories and principles would you apply in each of the following situations? Act out one of the following scenes.

1. You are going to teach home safety/accident prevention to an elderly client after hip replacement surgery before she goes home.
2. As a nurse working in the gynecology clinic, you are to teach breast self-examination to groups of women in the waiting room.
3. As a public health nurse, you are to teach a group of young parents at a day-care center about behavior modification using the propositions of behavioral theory. The objective is to translate the most important concepts into plain English and give practical examples.

Group Assignment B

You are a group of nurse entrepreneurs who have been granted an interview with a TV station program producer. Select two members to collaborate in playing the role of station program producer.

1. Your task is to talk to the TV station program producer into buying your television program package. Prepare the following information:
   a. Identify the target audience. Who are the viewers? Are they in school? If so, which grade level? Are they at the worksite? If so which one(s)? Why did you choose this audience?
   b. What population trends make your program feasible?
   c. Suggest how often your program should be shown. Daily? Monthly? What day? What hour? Provide your rationale.
   d. List the topics you would cover with your target audience.
   e. Identify the sponsors you would approach.
2. Place yourself in the role of the producer. Identify questions and concerns you have. Consider issues such as profit; market acceptability; risk; controversy; sensitivities of various cultural, ethnic, and age groups; and timeliness. Present these concerns to the nurse entrepreneurs.

Group Assignment C

Conduct the following activities on your regular television health program.

1. Your first guest is a self-styled fitness expert or nutritionist who is very popular but whose scientific base you question. Conduct the interview in a way that will promote critical thinking in your audience.
2. Create a commercial break in which you:
   a. Market nurses as health educators, consultants, and care providers.
   b. Advertise a health product/system with which you would like to be associated.
3. Interview a nurse colleague about the changing trends in health care and what that means for the average citizen.

Exercise II—Compare and Contrast Learning Theories

Purpose: Examine behaviorism, cognitivism, and social cognitive theories.

Directions: Divide into small groups of four to five and discuss the theories of learning described in this chapter. Discuss the following questions:

1. How are the theories alike?
2. How are they different?
3. What is the difference between learning, teaching, and health education?
4. Do people think like computers?
5. How have computers influenced your way of thinking?

Exercise III—Reflecting on Self-Learning

Purpose: Reflect on how you learn.

Directions: Form dyads with someone in the class with whom you have not worked with before. Take a few minutes and reflect individually on how you learn and then share with your partner. Listen to how he or she learns. Compare the ways your learning is alike and different.

Exercise IV—Information Processing and Memory

Purpose: Contemplate on the information processing model.

Directions: Form small groups of three or four. Then:

1. For 5 to 10 minutes, think alone about how you memorize lists and new information.
2. Discuss your thoughts and memory aids with others in your group and compare how your memorization strategies are alike and different.
3. Did you learn new strategies that will help you in the future?

Exercise V—Role Modeling

Purpose: Reflect on role models and role modeling.

Direction: Reflect on the following for 5 to 10 minutes and then form small groups and discuss your responses.

1. Who are your present role models in your social life? Who are your present role models in your role as a student?
2. What have you observed them doing that has helped you?
3. What have you observed them doing that you wish to avoid?
4. In what ways are you a role model to others?

SUPPLEMENTAL ONLINE RESOURCES

Journal of Technology Studies. The Theories:
http://tip.psychology.org/theories.html
B.F. Skinner Foundation:
www.bfskinner.org
At Learning-theories.com:
http://www.learning-theories.com/

An Overview of Gestalt Therapy Theory:
http://www.g-gej.org/4-3/theoryoverview.html
Information Processing Theory of Learning:
http://www.sil.org/lingualinks/literacy/ImplementALiteracyProgram/Informa-
    tionProcessingTheoryOfL.htm
Psychology History, Albert Bandura:
http://fates.cns.muskingum.edu/~psych/psycweb/history/bandura.htm
        Personality Theories, Albert Bandura:
http://www.ship.edu/~cgboeree/bandura.html

REFERENCES

Babcock, D. E., & Miller, M. A. (1994). *Client education: Theory and practice*. St. Louis: Mosby.

Bandura, A. (1986). *Social foundations of thought and action: A social cognitive theory*. Englewood Cliffs, NJ: Prentice Hall.

Bandura, A. (2001). Social cognitive theory: An agentic perspective. *Annual Review of Psychology, 52,* 1–26.

Cassady, J. C., & Johnson, R. E. (2002). Cognitive test anxiety and academic performance. *Contemporary Educational Psychology, 27*(2), 270–295.

Edelman, C. L., & Mandle, C. L. (2006). *Health promotion throughout the life span* (6th ed.). St. Louis: Mosby.

Guthrie, E. R. (1935). *The psychology of learning*. New York: Harper & Row.

Guthrie, E. R. (1959). Association by contiguity. In S. Koch (ed.). *Psychology: A study of a science* (Vol. 2). New York: McGraw-Hill.

Hoffer, E. (1973). *Reflections on the human condition*. New York: Harper & Row.

Knowles, M. S., Holton III, E. F., & Swanson, R. A. (2005). *The adult learner* (6th ed.). Burlington, MA: Elsevier.

Merriam, S. B., Caffarella, R. S., & Baumgartner, L. M. (2007). *Learning in adulthood* (3rd ed.). San Francisco: Jossey-Bass.

Merriam-Webster's dictionary and thesaurus. (2007). Springfield, MA: Merriam-Webster.

Olson, M. H., & Hergenhahn, B. R. (2009). *An introduction to theories of learning* (8th ed.). Englewood Cliffs, NJ: Pearson Education.

Ormrod, J. E. (2008). *Human learning* (5th ed.). Englewood Cliffs, NJ: Pearson Education.

Piaget, J. (1972). Intellectual evolution from adolescence to adulthood. *Human Development, 15*(1), 1–12.

Rush, K. L., Kee, C. C., & Rice, M. (2005). Nurses as imperfect role models for health promotion. *Western Journal of Nursing Research, 27*(2), 166–187.

Santrock, J. W. (2008). *A topical approach to life-span development* (4th ed.). Boston: McGraw-Hill.

Selder, F. (1989). Life transition theory: The resolution of uncertainty. *Nursing and Health Care, 10*(8), 437–451.

Slavin, R. E. (2009). *Educational psychology theory and practice* (9th ed.). Upper Saddle River, NJ: Pearson Education.

Spencer, C. (2007). Should nurses model healthy behaviour? *Kai Tiaki Nursing New Zealand, 13*(7), 14–15.

Squire, L. R., Knowlton, B., & Musen, G. (1993). The structure and organization of memory. *Annual Review of Psychology, 44*, 453–495.

Stephenson, P. I. (2006). Before the teaching begins: Managing patient anxiety prior to providing education. *Clinical Journal of Oncology Nursing, 10*(2), 241–245.

PART III

Assessment for Health Education

CHAPTER 4

Learner and Setting Assessment

All behavior is communication
And
All communication affects behavior.
—Stuart, G. W., 2005, p. 24

OBJECTIVES

Upon completion of this chapter you will be able to:

- Explain how your perceptions and those of the client affect teaching and learning.
- Identify three aspects of readiness to learn.
- Describe how the theories of learning relate to motivation to learn.
- Explain how you will apply Maslow's hierarchy of needs to a teaching and learning situation.
- Describe how the client's level of wellness affects teaching and learning: acute illness, convalescence, chronic illness, and full health.
- Describe how socioeconomic factors and educational level affect health education.
- Identify four types of client communication challenges that affect teaching and learning.
- Describe the ideal teaching and learning environment in terms of: space; temperature; visual, auditory, and olfactory stimuli; equipment; resources; furniture arrangement; physical comfort; and time.
- Compare and contrast the effect of the following environmental settings on teaching and learning: hospital, long-term care facility, private home, school, worksite, and community.
- Apply the CCCC/AOL Quick Teaching Assessment Tool and the Assessment Tool for Teaching Groups.

KEY TERMS

communication patterns	experiential readiness
teaching/learning environment	hierarchy of needs
cultural competence	level of wellness
culture	motivation
developmental readiness	socioeconomic factors
ethnicity	values
ethnocentrism	

INTRODUCTION

In this chapter we examine factors to consider when assessing the client and the learning environment in preparation for health education. First we look at the client's readiness to learn. This includes the client's and educator's perceptions affecting learning. Then we focus on the client's motivation to learn, level of wellness, socioeconomic factors, and educational level. Generational differences are identified and communication challenges discussed. Psychological and physical factors affecting the teaching and learning environment are described and clarified. The chapter concludes by describing assessment factors in different settings, such as the hospital, long-term care facility, private home, school, worksite, and community where teaching and learning occur.

ASSESSMENT OF LEARNERS

In preparing for health teaching, the nurse as educator must first assess factors that influence the learner's response to health education. Assessment is the first phase of the nursing process, an essential step before developing a teaching plan. The assessment of clients in a variety of settings should take into consideration multiple factors. Figure 4-1 illustrates the factors that comprise the assessment and analysis stage of health education.

Perception

Assessment of the educator's and client's personal perceptions is critical when preparing for health teaching. Perception is the ability to receive stimuli through the senses of sight, hearing, taste, touch, and smell, and to give meaning to those sensations. Perceptions are the parts of the universe to which we attend and result from our biologic, psychologic, sociologic, and cultural history. The following example illustrates how perceptions can affect client learning.

Christine was an 18-year-old homeless client seen at an urban clinic. Her chief complaint was dysuria and frequency of urination with a history of smoking marijuana and taking stimulants and depressants. She was diagnosed with a urinary tract infection and was prescribed antibiotics. The nurse instructed her on how to take the medication and emphasized the importance of taking it all. Christine had difficulty understanding why she could not stop taking the medication when her symptoms were relieved. She wanted to know what would happen if she failed to take the prescribed medication, and verbalized that she might be harmed by taking it all. To

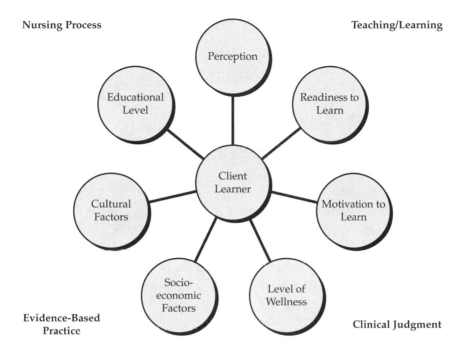

FIGURE 4-1 Assessment and analysis factors in preparation for health education.

Christine, the antibiotic represented a quick fix, and she could not see the need for medication when she felt better. Even though taking street drugs was a regular "safe" part of her life, she distrusted the healthcare system and did not see the need for taking all the medication. The nurse's knowledge influenced her perceptions of the need for the medication, whereas Christine based her perceptions on fear of the healthcare system and her experience of taking street drugs for a desired effect. It was important for the nurse to be aware of Christine's perceptions as she prepared a teaching plan.

As a health professional, your perceptions are shaped by personal history, nursing knowledge, and the amount of meaningful clinical and teaching experience you have accumulated. The ability to perceive a client's situation in preparation for teaching will grow as you expand your repertoire of life experiences and nursing skills. The development of empathy and the ability to put your self in the "shoes of another" is achieved by purposefully gaining experiences that expand life perceptions. This may involve selecting service learning experiences that offer the chance to broaden life experiences and deepen your understanding of the human condition.

Perceptions of clients not only shape the way you view them, but also influence clients' self-perceptions. Clients and team members tend to perceive themselves in response to your reaction to them. What you know about their biologic, psychosocial, and cultural characteristics will greatly influence how you perceive them. Be alert to the fact that it is easier to hear messages that already fit your belief system and that come from people whom you like and respect. To illustrate this, consider how you might react differently to clients perceived as mentally challenged or smart, unmotivated or motivated, hopeless or hopeful, uncooperative or cooperative, and ignorant or informed. It is important to validate perceptions before acting upon them.

Nurses' emotional states also affect their perceptual fields. When you are feeling confident and self-actualized, you are better able to be perceptive of client assessment data. When tired or rushed, you may become distracted, which can cause you to perceive information selectively. This may contribute to the nurse as educator failing to perceive important client data needed to develop the teaching plan. Table 4-1 identifies variables that affect listening perception by the client and the nurse as educator.

TABLE 4-1   Variables That Affect Listening Perception

Listening is Enhanced	Listening is Diminished
When a person is motivated to listen.	When a person is not motivated to listen.
When the listener is attentive.	When the listener is inattentive or distracted.
When the speaker is perceived as trustworthy.	When a speaker is perceived as not trustworthy.
When the speaker is perceived as knowledgeable.	When the speaker is perceived as uninformed.
When an idea or speaker is important to the listener.	When an idea or speaker is not important to the listener.
When the message fits the listener's beliefs.	When the message conflicts with the listener's beliefs.
When the message makes sense to the listener.	When the message does not make sense to the listener.

Readiness to Learn

Readiness to learn is based on the client or team member's willingness and ability to engage in a given learning activity. It includes an aroused interest or curiosity to learn, the learner's experiential background, and physiologic/developmental maturation. Readiness to learn is most intense when the learner's life situation creates the desire or necessity to acquire new knowledge, attitudes, and skills. It is important to assess readiness to learn as it greatly impacts the learning situation.

The nurse as educator assesses clients' readiness to learn by listening to them talk about their concerns and the questions they ask (Whyte, Watson, & McIntosh, 2006). Clients often express their health concerns and ask questions while the nurse is administering medications, performing nursing procedures, or delivering nursing care. This is an unplanned opportunity to note the client's openness and readiness for informal health education. Team members also indicate their interest in learning while on the job and engaged in client care activities.

To assess learner readiness, first ask learners what they want to know or explain the learning needs that you have observed. Ask for background information and history of the issue. After completing an assessment of their understanding, determine if you can build on what they already know. Inaccuracies or misunderstandings that could affect health status should be immediately and politely corrected. Ask whether they are interested in learning new material. Do they verbalize willingness to take the time to learn? Do they see themselves as playing a role in the learning process? Do they consider themselves instrumental in their own healing? What is their attitude about making life changes? Do they believe that they will receive support to make changes from friends, family, and co-workers? Will their culture be a supportive or inhibiting factor in learning new behaviors? What is their perception of healthcare professionals? Readiness to learn can be assessed and classified according to learners' verbalizations. Table 4-2 reviews the levels of readiness for health education. The guide can be readily adapted to individual client situations and addresses a client's cognitive skills, desire to learn, and psychomotor abilities.

Levels of readiness to learn are adaptable to fit a wide variety of teaching and learning situations. For example, Bonner *et al.* (2002) developed an educational intervention to improve asthma management and used four levels to assess clients' readiness to manage asthma. Educational interventions are indicated at each level. The four readiness levels, based on family attitudes and behaviors about the diagnosis of asthma, are: Level 1: asthma symptom avoidance, no recognition of asthma as a chronic disease. Level 2: asthma acceptance, acknowledges asthma symptoms when

TABLE 4-2	Levels of Readiness for Health Education
Level 1	Client verbalizes no interest in health education and avoids the topic. Client holds the health team responsible for their health. Client lacks physiologic and/or developmental abilities required for learning.
Level 2	Client verbalizes some interest in health education but is easily distracted and unable to stay on the topic. Client is willing to follow some health team directions. Client has limited physiologic and/or development abilities.
Level 3	Client verbalizes more interest in health education and is able to stay on topic for brief periods of time. Client seeks and follows health team directions. Client has the requisite physiologic and/or developmental skills.
Level 4	Client verbalizes great interest in health education and asks many questions. Client follows health team directions and assumes responsibility for own health. Client has full physiologic and developmental ability to learn.

they occur. Level 3: asthma compliance, uses preventive pharmacotherapy but considers fluctuations as treatment failures. Level 4: asthma self-regulation, applies asthma actions plans when symptoms change. The authors reported successful educational interventions based on this readiness to learn model.

Motivation to Learn

Motivation is "an internal state that arouses, directs, and sustains human behavior" (Glynn, Aultman, & Owens, 2005, p. 150). It is important to assess an individual's motivation before providing health education. Glynn *et al.* (2005) identified four theoretical orientations to motivation: behavioral, humanistic, cognitive, and social. Behavioral, cognitive, and social were discussed in Chapter 3 as components of learning theories. Recall the propositions of behavioral theory. Behavior that is reinforced tends to recur, whereas behavior that is ignored or punished tends to be suppressed. When certain behaviors are repeatedly reinforced, individuals are motivated to continue behaving in that manner. When these behaviors are health promoting, the nurse can continue to reinforce them. When these behaviors are not healthy, then the nurse is confronted with a challenge to teach the client new, health-promoting behaviors.

In the cognitive view of learning, the individual's goals, plans, and expectations are important. Clients who are undergoing life changes and health problems are often in the process of reconstructing and reorganizing their perceptions of themselves and reality. The nurse's role is to assist clients to change their cognitive view to a more appropriate and healthful one. In the social cognitive orientation to motivation, individuals learn new behaviors by observing others, called role models. To model new behaviors, clients must believe that they are capable of performing the new behaviors successfully. This is called the *self-efficacy expectation* in social cognitive theory.

Abraham Maslow, a prominent figure in the humanistic movement, proposed a theory of human motivation based on a hierarchy of needs. His theory has been widely adopted in nursing education (Maslow, 1954, 1987). His concept of self-actualization refers to human motivation to achieve personal growth and self-determination. Maslow's hierarchy has five levels of human needs that people tend to satisfy in sequence, beginning with the physiologic needs. See Table 4-3 to illustrate how these needs apply to health education.

In Maslow's hierarchy, the needs at each level must be at least partially met before needs are satisfied at the next higher level. Maslow distinguishes between deficiency needs and growth needs. Deficiency needs are things people lack and that need to be met by others or events in the environment. They are critical to physical and psychological well-being. They include the first four levels of the hierarchy: physiologic, safety and security, love and belonging, and self-esteem. Once these needs have been satisfied, the individual is motivated to seek out new experiences that involve self-actualization, which Maslow called growth needs. Motivation to meet growth needs is intrinsic and comes from within the individual. Needs are rarely completely satisfied. Maslow believed people strive toward self-actualization, a condition that is made possible when the individual's deficiency needs have been satisfied (Ormrod, 2008; Slavin, 2009). Your role, as an educator, is to assess which needs are the most important to the client to ascertain her or his motivation.

The last motivation model we discuss is the ARCS model. It is a useful, easily applicable model to assess motivation when involved in a specific learning activity. Developed by Keller (1987, 2008), it identifies four conditions essential for sustaining motivation in a learning situation. The acronym comes from the letter of each category: attention, relevance, confidence, and satisfaction. *Attention* addresses arousing the client's curiosity and capacity to participate in learning. *Relevance* addresses whether or not the educational activity is meaningful to the client. *Confidence* addresses whether or not the client believes she or he is capable of learning the material. *Satisfaction* addresses the emotional response the client has toward the learning experience, whether it was positive or negative.

TABLE 4-3 Maslow's Hierarchy of Needs Applied to Health Education	
Maslow's Hierarchy of Needs	**Application to Health Education**
Physiologic needs (oxygen, food, hydration, warmth, exercise, and sleep)	Clients who are tired, hungry, in pain, or critically ill have little motivation to focus on health education. Postpone teaching until a more appropriate time.
Safety and security needs	Clients who do not feel safe and secure are not open to health education. Inform them about routines and procedures.
Love and belonging needs	Clients who do not feel accepted by the health team are not open to health education. Accept and welcome them to health education opportunities.
Self-esteem needs (feeling respected, valued, and appreciated)	Clients who do not feel respected, valued, or appreciated are not receptive to health education. Listen and appreciate their viewpoint and address their learning needs.
Self-actualization (achieving one's potential)	Clients who focus on lower level needs will not achieve their full potential. Help them achieve their full potential by focusing on higher level needs to improve their lives.

Source: Maslow, 1987.

Level of Wellness

Clients' readiness for health education is related to their health status, and health education must be appropriate to their level of wellness. Level of wellness refers to the health status of individuals at any point in time. Health is a dynamic state and can be conceptualized on a bipolar continuum with high level of wellness at one end and acute and preventable illnesses at the opposite end. Individuals move freely along the continuum depending on their current health status and their willingness to engage in health-promoting activities. The Wellness/Illness Functional Continuum was introduced in Chapter 1 and could be used as a tool to assess clients' perception of level of wellness. Listed under Supplemental Online Resources at the Health and Lifestyle Awareness Web site, you will find a tool that may be helpful to assess clients' perceptions of level of wellness. The assessment tool covers the areas of physical health, mental and emotional health, and social health.

The level of wellness of acutely and chronically ill clients may change daily as they respond to medical and nursing care. These clients have the potential for achieving a higher level of wellness. It is important to remember that the highest level of wellness is individual to each client (Zuluaga, 2000). Nurses as educators need to be aware of how an individual client's level of wellness affects the teaching plan.

Acutely ill clients are concerned with physical survival. Clients are frequently in pain, confused, anxious, and fearful. They can receive medications that cloud their thinking. Medications can also interact, causing problems. Clients at this level are not receptive to formal teaching. They benefit from information that will ease their fears and help them maintain orientation to their condition, surroundings, and time of day. Nursing interventions and teaching that make them more comfortable are welcome. In the case of very ill individuals, the family may be the client who is receptive to teaching.

Clients who are recovering are more receptive to health education than those who are acutely ill. These clients are found in subacute or home care shortly after the acute illness stage. Public health nurses encounter clients who are still acutely ill when sent home. These clients and their families need much support, supervision, and teaching. Families need instruction in how to give care and perform procedures that were previously done by skilled nurses and physicians. Recovering clients and their families are likely to be interested and motivated learners. They are usually motivated to learn whatever is necessary to resume normal life as soon as possible. In general, it is believed that clients recover more quickly in their own homes, surrounded by familiar support systems.

Chronically ill clients vary in their openness to receiving health education depending on their acceptance of the reality of their illness. Some clients with long-term illnesses may have researched their disease and have increased understanding of diagnosis and treatment. These clients want to be active participants in their care and expect a collaborative relationship with health professionals. The nurse is a resource person and care manager.

When chronic illnesses wax and wane, clients may become weary and discouraged. It reduces physical and psychic energy. The nurse as educator's role in such situations will be one of listener and collaborator for learning. Together the nurse and client experiment with adaptations designed to make the best of the client's abilities and energies. Clients are likely to be more motivated when their aggravating symptoms subside.

The nurse as educator also encounters clients who are physically well and interested in preventing illness and maintaining their health. Today many clients realize that the way they conduct their lives is directly related to their health, longevity, and well-being. You will encounter potential clients among visiting friends and relatives of clients in the hospital, their homes, free-standing surgical and medical clinics, and workshops and classrooms. You will also encounter them in your neighborhood. Figure 4-2 illustrates how a client's needs and learning ability change depending on

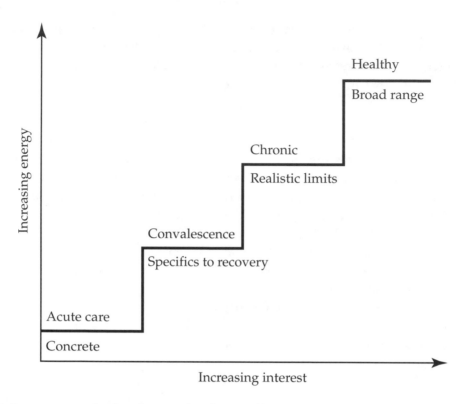

FIGURE 4-2   Levels of Wellness Related to Healthcare Needs. A client's energy and readiness to learn increases as his or her level of wellness increases. Courtesy Maureen Sullivan, RN, BS. Used with permission.

the level of wellness related to healthcare needs. When a client is acutely ill and has little energy, learning needs are very limited and concrete. During recovery, clients are interested in what they can do to promote their own recovery and return to optimum health. Those with chronic illnesses are greatly affected by the reality and constraints of their illness. Those in good health are open to a wide range of health education (O'Brien, 2007).

Socioeconomic Factors

Nurses as educators need to consider socioeconomic factors when planning for health education. Consider the client's living situation, availability of family support, financial status, health insurance or lack thereof, employment status, and the nature of the illness itself in your planning.

Clients living alone need to be more independent in meeting their healthcare needs than clients living with supportive families and significant others. Clients living alone need realistic options suitable for their living situation. For example, a client living alone without neighbor or family support who is in need of a dressing change must be taught how to do so safely and independently. A client living with supportive family members may wish to have a family member taught how to do the dressing change. Homeless clients and those living in shelters present additional health education challenges (Busen & Engebretson, 2008). A difference in health perception is illustrated when nursing students serving in a homeless shelter were puzzled when they observed a 5-year-old child rolling an apple around on the floor. When the student spoke with the child's mother, she explained that her child had never seen an apple before and thought it was a toy. Regardless of the living situation, health education must be appropriate to the client's actual situation.

Clients' financial resources influence health status and health education. Middle- and high-income clients who are employed and have health insurance are able to purchase necessary services and supplies. Researchers have found that those with sufficient financial resources have a lower mortality when compared with those with limited resources. Lower-income clients have access to lower-quality services and housing, fewer social supports, higher stress, and more limited access to health care (Krueger, Rogers, Hummer, LeClere, & Huie, 2003). Box 4-1 provides the nurse with the basic information needed to offer financially appropriate health suggestions.

Nurses as educators need to be more sensitive, creative, and adaptable in meeting the health education needs of clients with limited financial resources. Nurses should be aware that decreasing the number of prescriptions, not taking prescribed medications, and skipping doctor visits are common behaviors of clients with limited financial resources (Brown, 2008; Roberts-Grey, 2008). Part of your assessment is to verify whether clients are taking all their medications and then to teach them the importance of taking them as prescribed. A trusting nurse/client relationship will encourage the client to discuss her or his needs so that the education can be appropriate.

BOX 4-1 Rapid Socioeconomic Assessment Tool

- What is your occupation?

- Is your monthly income sufficient to meet your expenses?

- Do you have health insurance?

- Do you have unmet financial needs related to health care?

In addition to socioeconomic factors affecting illness, clients' illnesses can impinge on their socioeconomic well-being. Individuals who are obese or suffering the effects of AIDS or Hepatitis C may find that their diagnosis is a barrier to employment, health insurance, social freedom, and other sources of socioeconomic support. Illnesses that family and friends perceive to be contagious can impinge on clients' socioeconomic well-being and lead to social isolation.

Cultural Factors

Culture is defined as "the totality of socially transmitted behavior, patterns, arts, beliefs, values, customs, lifeways, and all other products of human work and thought characteristic of a population of people that guides their world view and decision-making" (Purnell, 2003, p. 5). *Cultural factors* include beliefs, values, moral principles, habits, dress, language, rules for behavior, economics, politics, dietary practices, and health care (Burchum, 2002). Not only do cultural factors relate to race and ethnicity, but also to behaviors and beliefs characteristic of particular social, ethnic, disabled, age, and gender groups. Cultural factors are important to take into consideration when providing health education. The United States is increasingly multicultural and often described as a melting pot (Racher & Annis, 2007). Minorities are projected to become the majority in 2042 and 54% of the population by 2050 per US Census Bureau projections prepared in 2008. Every region in the United States has a culturally diverse population. For nurses to be effective educators, it is important to assess cultural factors that will affect teaching and learning. Each person attributes his or her beliefs, values, and customs to cultural factors, and all nurses are affected by the culture of nursing and the health delivery system. Within cultures there are many similarities and differences. Not all members of a single group hold the same worldview or values (Burchum, 2002). Believing that your culture is superior to all others is called *ethnocentrism*. It is a barrier to critical thinking because it devalues the beliefs and values of people from other cultures and contributes to many social ills embodied in the practices of prejudice, discrimination, and racism (Kulwicki, 2009; Miller & Babcock, 1996).

How nurses view health promotion, prevent illness, treat disease, and care for the dying is determined by their culture (DeRosa & Kochurka, 2006). Nurses should strive to understand a client's cultural background and provide culturally congruent health education in cross-cultural situations. *Culturally congruent health education* is providing education that is meaningful and useful for individuals, families, groups, and communities, as well as for team members. It is identifying what is important to

---

BOX 4-2   Cultural Assessment for Health Education

1. Do you identify with a particular ethnic or cultural group?

2. Are you an immigrant or first or second generation in this country?

3. What do you believe is the cause of your health problem?

4. What do you believe makes you healthy?

5. What do you believe makes you sick?

6. What remedies have you used to treat your health problems?

7. What is your religious affiliation?

8. Do you engage in any religious practices that you believe affect your health?

9. Do you read and write in English or do you prefer another language?

10. What foods do you prefer and what foods do you avoid?

11. Do you have sufficient income (money) to meet your needs?

12. Do you have family or friends who are available to support you if you need help?

---

the client, the client's values, and how the client sees his or her present health situation (Cutilli, 2006). Culture is discussed in greater depth in Chapter 8.

As a busy educator, you will need to do an initial cultural assessment that covers the pertinent cultural factors related to teaching and learning. The questions in Box 4-2 will guide you as you work with culturally diverse clients. Answers to these questions will give direction to selecting teaching content, help you identify teaching strategies, and give you information to determine what instructional materials you will share with the client. More in-depth cultural assessment tools are presented in Chapter 8.

Educational Level

Approximately 30 million people older than 16 years in the United States read at the level of the average elementary school child, according to ProLiteracy Worldwide, Inc.; and 14% of the adult population cannot read a newspaper story written at the eighth grade level. Health literacy is a concern in working with clients who need supplemental written material but are unable to read at a level sufficient to under-stand. Health literacy has profound implications for nurses as educators as they communicate with clients and provide health education reading materials. You will learn how to evaluate health education materials for readability in Chapter 11.

The vocabulary that clients use is to some extent a measure of their health literacy and educational level. Those with large vocabularies are more apt to comprehend what you are saying. Clients with less education are less likely to comprehend the more abstract and technical language you might inadvertently use. Concrete answers and examples are more likely to be meaningful to those with less education. Clients' vocabulary impacts the type of health education materials that you provide, such as booklets and pamphlets (Seligman *et al.*, 2007).

As you interact with clients, assess their knowledge about health and illness. Such an assessment provides clues that can guide health education activities. The client's level of education is often related to knowledge about health and illness. In general, the higher the level of education, the more likely the client is to engage in health-promoting behaviors such as exercise, proper diet, and smoking cessation (Kimbro, Bzostek, Goldman, & Rodriguez, 2008). This observation is not necessarily true for specific health problems. For example, the advantage of having more education does not seem to have an impact on adult clients who are obese. Research reports that obesity is increasing at a faster rate for those with more than a high school education than those with less than a high school education (Himes & Reynolds, 2005).

Clients who research health problems may have comprehensive knowledge of their illnesses. Nurses report this phenomenon more often in this era of increased availability of information on the Internet and the vast availability of materials and publications from libraries and healthcare providers. Clients are often articulate and well informed about the latest treatments for disease and are eager to collaborate with healthcare providers.

Because health literacy is so important in health education, we have included an easy-to-administer tool to assess health literacy called the Newest Vital Sign (NVS) published by the Partnership for Clear Health Communications. The tool takes approximately 3 minutes to administer and involves clients reading a nutrition label and then answering six questions. Four or more questions answered correctly indicate adequate literacy. The tool is also available in Spanish (Figures 4-3 and 4-4).

Assessing health literacy is also a concern when teaching team members. The concern is not for those who have years of formal educational preparation, but rather for team members in support roles such as nursing assistants. Team members may have limited knowledge of health and illness and often possess inaccurate informa-

Nutrition Facts

Serving Size	1/2 cup
Servings per container	4

Amount per serving
Calories 250   Fat Cal 120

	%DV
Total Fat 13g	20%
Sat Fat 9g	40%
Cholesterol 28mg	12%
Sodium 55mg	2%
Total Carbohydrate 30g	12%
Dietary Fiber 2g	
Sugars 23g	
Protein 4g	8%

* Percent Daily Values (DV) are based on a 2,000 calorie diet. Your daily values may be higher or lower depending on your calorie needs.

Ingredients: Cream, Skim Milk, Liquid Sugar, Water, Egg Yolks, Brown Sugar, Milkfat, Peanut Oil, Sugar, Butter, Salt, Carrageenan, Vanilla Extract.

FIGURE 4-3 Newest Vital Sign.
Reprinted with permission from "Quick Assessment of Literacy in Primary Care: The Newest Vital Sign," December, 2005, *Annals of Family Medicine*. Copyright 2005 American Academy of Family Physicians. All Rights Reserved.

tion. They benefit from in-service activities that advance their understanding of their employment responsibilities. When preparing educational activities for team members, it is helpful to know what kind of theoretical and experiential preparation they have for their respective roles. This will help you plan educational activities that build on their current level of knowledge. If clients or team members are from a different

	ANSWER CORRECT?	
	YES	NO

READ TO SUBJECT: This information is on the back of a container of a pint of ice cream.

QUESTIONS

1. If you eat the entire container, how many calories will you eat?

    Answer ☐ 1,000 is the only correct answer   ————   ————

2. If you are allowed to eat 60 g of carbohydrates as a snack, how much ice cream could you have?

    Answer Any of the following is correct: ————   ————
            ☐ 1 cup (or any amount up to 1 cup)
            ☐ Half the container

            Note: If patient answers "2 servings," ask "How much ice cream would that be if you were to measure it into a bowl?"

3. Your doctor advises you to reduce the amount of saturated fat in your diet. You usually have 42 g of saturated fat each day, which includes 1 serving of ice cream. If you stop eating ice cream, how many grams of saturated fat would you be consuming each day?

    Answer 33 is the only correct answer   ————   ————

4. If you usually eat 2500 calories in a day, what percentage of your daily value of calories will you be eating if you eat one serving?

    Answer 10% is the only correct answer   ————   ————

Pretend that you are allergic to the following substances: Penicillin, peanuts, latex gloves, and bee stings.

5. Is it safe for you to eat this ice cream?

    Answer ☐ No   ————   ————

6. (Ask only if the patient responds "no" to question 5): Why not?

    Answer Because it has peanut oil.   ————   ————

                        Total Correct   ————

Figure 4-4 Newest Vital Sign Scoring Sheet.
Reprinted with permission from "Quick Assessment of Literacy in Primary Care: The Newest Vital Sign," December, 2005, *Annals of Family Medicine*. Copyright 2005 American Academy of Family Physicians. All Rights Reserved.

BOX 4-3   Evidence-Based Research: Newest Vital Sign

Weiss *et al.* (2005). Quick assessment of literacy in primary care: The newest vital sign. *Annals of Family Medicine, 3*(6), 514–522.

Purpose: The purpose of this research was to develop a quick and accurate screening test for limited literacy available in English and Spanish.

Method: To create the tool, candidate items for the new instrument and the Test of Functional Health Literacy in Adults (TOFHLA) were administered to 250 English-speaking and 250 Spanish-speaking primary care patients. Statistical tests were used to determine which of the candidate test items from the new instrument best correlated with results of the TOFHLA.

Results: The final instrument, the Newest Vital Sign (NVS) is a nutrition label that is accompanied by six questions and requires 3 minutes for administration. It is reliable in English and Spanish and correlates with the TOFHLA. NVS is suitable for use as a quick screening for limited literacy in primary healthcare settings.

The NVS is available online only at: http://www.annfammed.org/cgi/content/full/3/6/514/DC1 and http://www.newestvitalsign.org/nvs-resources.aspx

---

culture or have limited English-speaking ability, this can affect their vocabulary and communication skills, a topic discussed further in Chapter 8.

Health literacy and educational level are only approximations of what an individual client or team member can grasp. As educators, nurses must monitor the feedback from clients as they engage them in educational activities to determine their effectiveness. Also keep in mind that emotions may influence clients' ability to understand. For example, clients and their families have repeatedly reported to us that their anxiety level and other concerns interfered with their ability to comprehend material that would be quite understandable under normal circumstances.

ASSESSMENT OF GENERATIONAL DIFFERENCES

Nurses as educators must consider the age of the client as an important assessment factor when preparing health education offerings to adult learners. It is important to be aware of potential factors that can impede or promote learning. When building a teaching plan it is helpful to consider fundamental generational differences beyond learners' control to choose effective teaching methods and strategies. Table 4-4 examines the psychological and generational differences among the Silent, Boomer, Generation X, and Millennial generations. This is not intended to describe an individual, but rather to understand a cohort of learners.

TABLE 4-4   Generational Differences

	Silent 1925–1945	Boomer 1946–1964	Gen X 1965–1980	Millennial 1981–2000
Years				
Other names	Veterans Traditionalists	Consciousness generation "Me" generation	"Lost" generation "Latchkey" "Slacker" Generation	Generation Y Echo Boom Generation Next
Family life	Earliest to marry and have children Divorce common Large number of women entered the workforce	Religious and spiritually oriented Health conscious Defer childbirth until later in life Attentive to children "helicopter" parents	Adult oriented at an early age Less parental supervision than earlier generations Little peer interaction in childhood Balance work and family	Children considered special and eagerly anticipated Families with fewer children Balance work and family
Work	Many entered the "helping" professions Hard work is good Respect authority Sacrifice Duty before fun Adhere to the rules	Workaholics Career focused Work efficiently Personal fulfillment Desire quality Will question authority	First to seek balance between work/life Self-reliant Want structure and direction Skeptical Challenge others Work is a difficult challenge	Financially oriented More discretionary income than any previous group Multitasking Tolerant Goal oriented
Learning preferences and interactive style	Like traditional structure Will not contradict instructor in public Do not like being singled out in discussions Prefer to practice alone May not ask questions in discussions May struggle with technology Prefer learning individually	Enjoy working creatively and independently Sensitive to criticism May have significant professional experience Like interaction, discussion, and group work May dislike authoritarian teachers Prefer learning as part of a team	Self-reliant Like frequent feedback May lack interpersonal skills Largest segment of online learners Often impatient, but adaptable and informal Technologically capable Value autonomy Prefer an informal learning approach	Team-oriented, like group work Multitask and technological experts Goal and achievement oriented Require more structure and mentoring Enjoy active learning Prefer participative learning

Communication style	Formal Memo	In person	Direct Immediate	E-mail Voice mail
Teaching strategies	Emphasize important points in the teaching plan	Give time to practice skills	May resist group work outside of a formal class	Present information and activities in steps
	Use font large enough to see writing and read handouts	Use font large enough to see for older learners	Give individual attention	Use up-to-date technology and resources
	Fastest growing group learning to use the Internet	May not like role-playing exercises	Prefer information in short lectures (15–20 minutes)	Make learning relevant to real-life situations
	Encourage periodic movement while teaching	Enjoy most team projects	Like working in small groups to review information	Encourage creativity and be creative in presentations
		Like being group leaders	Prefer graphics that are visually appealing and reflect the culture	Give supplemental reading and instructional materials
		Like well-organized materials with headings	Want to have explanation for learning and skill acquisition	

Modified from Baker College Effective Teaching and Learning Department (2004), *Generational comparison chart, Teaching across generations* and Campbell, J., & Brooks, C. (2008, November 10). Tools for effective teaching. PowerPoint lecture presented at Palm Beach Atlantic University, School of Nursing. Retrieved on July 22, 2009 from: https://cache.trustedpartner.com/docs/library/000223/Transforming%20Behaviors%20Conference%20Materials/Effective%20Teaching%20Stategies_J%20Campbell_C%20Brooks_11_21_08.pdf

COMMUNICATION CHALLENGES DURING ASSESSMENT

To assess clients accurately, you must be skilled at communication. Communication is both verbal and nonverbal. It facilitates health education or hinders it. Words convey a variety of meanings and can be misinterpreted, especially by members of different cultural groups. In addition, never assume that all clients from one ethnic group hold the same beliefs. Nurses can overcome these problems by asking clients how they interpreted the message. Nonverbal communication (body cues, tone of voice, facial expression, and space between communicants) all send a message. Nurses who answer clients' or team members' questions but appear to be in a hurry will stifle communication (Horowitz, 2006; Stuart, 2005).

Communication difficulties become challenges for nurses to overcome as they provide health education. The sources of these challenges come from clients as well as nurses (Pohl, 1981). This section addresses common communication problems affecting the teaching and learning process and suggests solutions.

Hearing Impairment

Approximately 28 million Americans are deaf or hard of hearing (Lucas, Schiller, & Benson, 2004, as cited in Lieu, Sadler, Fullerton, & Stohlman, 2007). The prevalence of hearing trouble (defined as a little trouble, a lot of trouble, or deaf) among noninstitutionalized civilian adults aged 18 and older in the United States increases with age. Eighteen percent of adults ages 45–64, 32% of adults ages 65–74, and 49% of adults older than 75 years of age are affected (Lethbridge-Cejku, Rose, & Vickerie, 2006). Clients with long-standing hearing deficits inform nurses of what modes of communication work best for them. During the initial assessment, nurses can identify the various ways clients communicate. Clients or family members can provide this information, but family members should not be used as interpreters if confidentiality is a concern (Lieu *et al.*, 2007). To quickly assess a client's hearing, talk to the client in a normal tone of voice and note her or his reaction. If the client answers appropriately, you will know the client's hearing is sufficient for teaching and learning. Another assessment strategy is to cover your mouth and ask a question, again in a normal tone of voice. The client with a hearing impairment will not hear to answer you.

Check to see if the client wears a hearing aid. If so, make sure it is turned on and that the batteries are working. Creating other means of sound augmentation, such as cupping your hands around the client's ears or using the stethoscope in reverse, are other options.

When working with hearing impaired clients, position yourself close on the same level, and face the client so that they know you are communicating with them. The client should be able to see your face and read your lips. Avoid standing in an area with a background glare, as that interferes with the client's ability to read your lips. Remember to enunciate clearly and slowly. Clients who are proficient lip readers discern less than half of what you say and depend on the context and guesses to determine your meaning (Lieu *et al.*, 2007).

Clients who rely on American Sign Language (ASL) require the assistance of a qualified sign language interpreter. This is considered a reasonable accommodation the healthcare institution is required to offer under the Americans with Disabilities Act. Communication tools, such as flash cards, pencils and pads, and a laptop computer are all helpful to clients who know how to write and have the strength to do it. If using the written mode, remember to choose simple words and phrases and write legibly (Lieu *et al.*, 2007). The most important point is that you find a way to elicit responses that help you assess the client's hearing abilities and comprehension.

Vision Impairment

More than 21 million noninstitutionalized civilian adults aged 18 and older in the United States experience vision trouble (defined as trouble seeing even with glasses or contact lenses). The prevalence of visual impairment increases with age particularly among those over 75. Eleven percent of adults ages 45–64, 14% of adults ages 65–74, and 20% of adults age 75 years and older are affected (Lethbridge-Cejku, Rose, and Vickerie, 2006; Ryskulova *et al.*, 2008). As clients live longer, visual impairment is an important consideration for nurses providing health education. To quickly assess a client's vision, give the client a magazine or newspaper and have him or her read aloud a paragraph. As the client does so, note the distance between the paper and the client's face. Holding the paper more than 14 inches away may indicate presbyopia, or hyperopia (farsightedness). This gives you a sense of the client's visual capabilities and consequently how to adapt your teaching plan.

People who have been blind for some time develop other senses, particularly hearing, to compensate. Their acute listening skills make being shouted at a painful experience, and it does not aid their comprehension. Clients who are blind are unable to make use of body language or lip reading. If you are accustomed to expressing yourself with your hands and shaking your head, be alert to the fact that such clues are unavailable to blind clients. We recommend that you learn to use more verbal descriptions and psychomotor learning strategies that might not be necessary with a sighted client.

The blind often discern whether a door is open or closed by the sound in the room. A door halfway ajar, however, can be deceiving as well as dangerous. We recommend that you close doors or open them all the way. It is also courteous to announce your presence and your purpose; for example, "My name is Fred Jones, and I'm your nurse for today. I'm going to teach you about . . . , then later we'll review. . . . Tell me what you are most interested in learning."

Speech Impairment

Speech impairment concerns clients who have pathologic impairment in their ability to communicate. The type of impairment is related to the location and type of brain lesion. There are other forms of speech impairment related to a psychological etiology, but our reference here is to clients with brain pathology resulting in dysphasia. Dysphasia is impairment of speech consisting of lack of coordination and failure to arrange words in the proper order. If a client has a form of dysphasia as an aftermath of stroke, consult with the psychologist and neurologist to determine the best way to deal with the speech impairment. One client may understand your words and not be able to answer. Another may not understand your words but can interpret your pantomime, drawings, flash cards, or objects. Shouting is not helpful in communicating with clients who are speech impaired. In Chapter 8 we address communication with clients who speak little or no English.

Nurses as Educators' Contribution to Communication Challenges

The final communication problem we address is the one that nurses might inadvertently create. Mumbling, using technical jargon, or talking when you should be listening interferes with effective communication. Learn to recognize signs of poor client communication: confused facial expression, lack of attention, and questions that indicate a lack of understanding.

Suggestions to reduce this barrier include the art of active listening and observing. While listening and watching body language, nurses develop sensitivity to other communication clues (Burger, 2009). Listening is an active, not a passive, process. Listening is an essential skill required of effective nurses in the educator role. Nurses may not agree with everything a client or team member says, but it is important to listen and respect the individual. Give complete attention to the learner and do not be preoccupied with your own thoughts. As educators, it is easy to think we should do the talking, but it is just as important to listen (Stuart, 2005).

ASSESSMENT OF THE TEACHING AND LEARNING ENVIRONMENT

The teaching and learning environment is composed of the psychological environment and physical environment in which teaching and learning takes place. It is the nurse's responsibility to establish the psychological and physical environment to maximize learning.

Psychological Environment

As educators, nurses create the emotional tone for the learning environment. A positive, enthusiastic tone does much to make clients comfortable and helps to create a therapeutic environment. If the nurse is stressed, clients pick up this perception and may assume that it is related to them. Conversely, if the nurse enjoys teaching and shows enthusiasm, that perception is conveyed as well.

Showing respect for learners and valuing their questions and input are all part of creating a positive teaching and learning environment. The nurse's attitude should be nonjudgmental. However, that does not mean the nurse agrees with or condones the client's beliefs and statements. Respect is accepting and valuing the client. The nurse has a responsibility to correct misinformation (Stuart, 2005).

Physical Environment

As educators, nurses are responsible for assessing the physical environment and making it as conducive to learning as possible (Hall, 2009). The physical environment includes: space; temperature; visual, auditory, and olfactory stimuli; equipment; resources; furniture arrangement; physical comfort; and sufficient time for learning.

Space is needed so that you can get maximum display and use of your instructional materials. This is true whether you are speaking to an individual, a family, or a group in a living room or auditorium. Examine the space for sight and sound barriers. Pillars will make it difficult for clients to see you. Poorly placed partitions may act as sound barriers that will prevent sound from getting through.

Temperatures that are too hot or too cold interfere with learning. Clients distracted by heat spend their time fanning themselves, or if cold, by clutching their arms instead of listening to you.

Visual stimuli are distracting and interfere with vision. Do not place yourself in front of a sunny window. The glare behind you turns you into a shadowy figure. Your audience will be squinting and wanting to look elsewhere. Try to pick a spot where you can control the appearance of the learning situation. If you cannot control all of the stimuli, look for ways to control the area in which you intend to teach. In the hospital you may draw the curtain around the client's bed. One way to modify sound in a client's room is to hang a sign on the door:

> "Client teaching in progress.
> Please return in . . . minutes. Thank you."

If your client is a family, you may be able to cordon off a corner of the waiting room. In a dining area of an extended care facility, you may be able to use moveable privacy screens to provide privacy. Auditory stimuli may or may not be under your control. Choose a quiet place and turn off your cell phone. Olfactory stimuli are distracting and can be deflected by a fan. You could try cutting a lemon or putting a drop of cinnamon oil on a nearby heated surface, such as a light fixture or use a room deodorizer.

Availability of equipment and teaching resources influence your options. Find out what equipment, expertise, and resources are available in the hospital or community to enhance teaching. Observe where the electrical outlets are if you will need them. If needed, arrange the room to give access to the outlets.

Arrange furniture in a way that is conducive to learning. Be sure to take into account the learning objectives and teaching strategies. Do you plan to have the clients interact with each other? Do you wish a relative to see everything you are doing for the client? Do you plan to make a presentation to a group or have a guest lecturer? Nurses should be involved in designing the spaces where teaching occurs.

Physical comfort is an important variable in enhancing the teaching and learning environment. Teach clients after the morning routine when they are comfortable and relaxed. You will find that your clients learn better when they are sufficiently medicated to not be distracted by pain but not too sleepy to pay attention. Lighting and temperature also affect comfort. You will want the lighting to be bright enough to allow lip readers to see your face but not so strong that it creates glare.

Time is a factor to take into consideration. Be sure you have sufficient time to teach. If time is limited, be selective about what you teach, focusing on only the most important topics. Do not make your teaching session too long. A mistake we have seen busy nurses make is trying to include too much information too quickly into the time available.

TEACHING AND LEARNING SETTINGS

The teaching and learning settings that we consider here include the hospital, long-term care facility, private home, school, worksite, and community settings. Each has unique characteristics that affect the way health education is delivered.

Hospital

The value of health education is supported by hospitals. Although the quantity and quality are frequently affected by policies and administrative support, the importance of health education in acute care settings is reflected in role expectations and job descriptions. The mission and philosophy of many hospitals reflects the importance of client education. Hospital administrators are now required to meet the Joint Commission standards by providing necessary support and resources for patient teaching. Every hospital has an education department that focuses on client and staff education. They are responsible for discharge planning and case management for clients and competency training for staff. Hospitalized clients have teaching needs that revolve around acute illness and discharge planning. Some hospitals also offer classes for the community related to health promotion.

Long-Term Care Facility

Long-term care facilities include nursing homes, assisted-living homes, and other facilities that care for clients over a prolonged period of time. Long-term care includes a wide range of services that are provided over an extended period of time to clients who need help to perform normal activities of daily living because of a variety of health problems. Services within long-term care include rehabilitative therapies, skilled nursing care, palliative care, and social services, as well as supervision and a wide range of supportive personal care provided by family caregivers and/or home healthcare agencies. Most long-term care facilities also have education departments.

Goals of long-term care include training to help clients adjust to or overcome limitations. Like hospitals, health education in long-term care facilities can occur individually or in groups. Effective educational programs can prevent minor illness or injury from progressing to the point of needing professional intervention. Increased client awareness through education can also result in earlier detection of problems and timelier outpatient intervention, thus decreasing hospitalizations. Lastly, clients with chronic illnesses who have been empowered through health education programs generally have better coping skills and are usually less reliant on healthcare providers.

Private Home

According to some estimates, approximately 80% of all health problems could be treated at home (Brown-Spath & Associates, 2001). This statistic brings out the importance of addressing health education in the private home. Home visits for elderly clients have been found to have direct benefits when measured in terms of morbidity and admission to long-term institutional care. Remember that in the client's home, you are a guest and not in charge, as you are when the client is in a healthcare institution. Clients are discharged from acute care settings with increasingly complex treatment and learning needs. Families are expected to learn skills and information that, only a decade ago, were reserved for healthcare personnel.

Clients often find it easier to learn in familiar surroundings. During home health nursing it will be easier for you to be realistic in your teaching because you can see the reality of the client's environment. Family dynamics that may enhance or impede recovery will be more evident in the home, which means you will be more likely to be realistic in teaching the family as well as the client.

School

School is an ideal site for health education because it is a focal point for reducing health risk behaviors and improving the heath status of youth. Based on the potential to reach a large number of youth, schools are logical sites for interventions that help them develop skills, change health behaviors, and empower them to take responsibilities for their own health. Some of the most effective health education efforts for youth incorporate peer support. Although most schools require health education, teachers are often not comfortable with sensitive subjects and need the contributions of school nurses in addressing certain topics.

If you are teaching a class, you will want to find out more information about the group of students. Ask about the culture of the classroom. What ages are the children? Are they accustomed to discipline and to giving polite attention? Are they able to sit and listen? What are the learning style preferences? What health education tools are already available? This is important information for the teaching plan.

Schools are often good settings for teaching and learning, with multiple audiovisual aids. Teaching disease prevention and providing anticipatory guidance are excellent topics. Nurses are informed role models to address today's concerns about how to avoid communicable diseases and substance abuse and teach behaviors that promote healthful living. Learn the age of the group you will speak to and address age-appropriate topics. Health education desirably begins in grade schools.

Worksite

Worksite settings are beneficial to managers, employees, and the community. Nurses in worksite settings are effective providers of health education. These educational programs provide an opportunity to support health while reducing healthcare costs, increasing worker productivity, and decreasing absenteeism. Interventions in the workplace may target behavioral change, the development of policies to facilitate a healthier, safer workplace, and environmental support to maintain behavioral change.

Concerns that nurses in worksite settings can address include consultation about cost-effective insurance plans, infection and accident control, and health promotion and maintenance programs. These nurses can also conduct physical assessments, teach prevention to employees, provide screening services, produce health newsletters, and inform employers about major health hazards in the setting. The political system at the worksite greatly affects the ability of the nurse as an educator to be effective. Self-help groups for alcoholism, smoking cessation, stress management, prevention of accidents, and safety precautions are all worthy topics for consideration.

Community

Health education in the community focuses on health problems identified as a priority by the public health department or other community agency responsible for community health planning. The focus of nurses as educators in public health is to provide direct care through a process of evaluation and assessment of the needs of individuals in the context of their population group. Regardless of the environment within the community where nurses work, the health education process can be used to establish partnerships with their clients providing education and counseling to promote self-management. Nurses as educators work with other providers of care to plan, develop, and support systems and programs in the community that emphasize health promotion, disease prevention, and access to care.

Community assessment focuses on populations rather than individuals. Those individuals who make up a population share one or more personal or environmental characteristics. A population can be categorized as a population at risk or a population of interest (Keller, Strohschein, & Briske, 2008). A population at risk shares an identified risk factor or risk exposure that threatens its health. For example, all individuals who smoke are at risk for developing respiratory and cardiovascular health problems.

A population of interest is basically healthy but could improve its health and prevent illness from developing. Examples include making home visits to new mothers to encourage breastfeeding or working with adolescents to prevent sexually transmitted diseases by offering programs in the public schools. Other populations of interest may be needs-based such as maternal-infant or cancer survivors; age-based such as adolescents, older adults (65 and older); gender-based such as men and/or women; and ethnic-group-based such as African American, Hispanic American, Asian American, and American Indian.

ASSESSMENT TOOLS FOR TEACHING INDIVIDUALS AND GROUPS

Box 4-4 is an assessment tool for nurses who find themselves in a teachable moment with clients. It is for those unplanned opportunities that arise in the course of nursing practice when the nurse needs a tool for guidance. It is a quick teaching assessment guide that is useful in a variety of settings in which the teaching is informal and spontaneous. For example, the guide can be useful for nurses at the bedside, in a client's home, a clinic, a school, at the worksite, and in a doctor's office. Practicing nurses are busy; it is not always possible to conduct a thorough assessment as outlined in this chapter. The tool addresses client *Concerns*, *Client* knowledge, then moves to *Create* a teaching plan, *Carry Out* a teaching plan and for each area requires the nurse to *Ask*, *Observe*, and *Listen* (CCCC/AOL Assessment Tool for Teaching Individuals). The purpose of this tool is to guide nurses as educators in quickly assessing and teaching a client when health education is indicated.

Table 4-5 is an assessment tool for nurses who are planning health education for a group of people. Interested groups may be found in hospitals, long-term care facilities, schools, worksites, and community settings. We recommend that the nurse review teaching priorities, goals, objectives, and content with a representative at the facility before the presentation. Careful assessment of the educational needs and communication with a representative at the facility will help bring about a successful educational offering.

An example of using this tool is a situation in which a nurse gives a presentation on preventing back injuries to a group of registered nurses. With the facility's support the nurse surveys the registered nurses to determine their perceptions and knowledge of the topic. The nurse reviews the literature for evidence-based research related to

---

BOX 4-4   CCCC/AOL Assessment Tool for Teaching Individuals

*Assess Client Concerns

Ask: What are your concerns?

Observe: Nonverbal behavior.

Listen: Spoken and unspoken words.

*Assess Client Knowledge

Ask: What do you understand about condition?

Observe: Nonverbal behavior.

Listen: Determine accuracy of knowledge and teaching needs.

*Create Teaching Plan

Ask self: What type and amount of information is needed?

Observe: Context of client situation.

Listen: Reflect on appropriateness of teaching plan.

*Carry Out Teaching Plan

Ask: What is your understanding of what I have explained?

Observe: Nonverbal cues to understanding/not understanding, return demonstration.

Listen: Client feedback, evaluate teaching effectiveness, determine additional educational needs.

---

the topic and develops a teaching plan that includes learning objectives, content, and teaching strategies.

The next step in the assessment process is to determine the facility's support and approval for the educational offering. The nurse seeks facility support throughout the assessment process. This tool can be used for nurses planning educational programs in clinics, community centers, schools, worksite settings, and for civic groups. Health education is appropriate in any place in which there is an educational need. The tool applies to groups of students, clients, employees, and health team members in a multitude of settings.

TABLE 4-5 Assessment Tool for Teaching Groups	
Assessment Steps	**Action Steps**
1. Identify the educational need	1. Obtain group members' perceptions and knowledge base through surveys and focus groups. 2. Examine and clarify educational needs
2. Identify group characteristics	1. Size 2. Educational level 3. Pertinent cultural aspects 4. Other demographic characteristics
3. Identify current evidence-based practice research	1. Review the literature for evidence-based research on the topic. 2. Evaluate the current EBP research applicable to the educational need.
4. Identify goals, objectives, and content	1. Formulate goals and objectives based on the educational need. 2. Prepare a content outline.
5. Determine facility support	1. Does the facility agree with the educational need? 2. Does the facility support the content you are proposing in the educational offering? 3. Will the facility provide space and resources for the educational offering? 4. Are facilities and resources available to hold the class? 5. Does the facility have a plan to ensure that group members can participate in the educational offering?

SUMMARY

This chapter covered a multitude of factors that nurses as educators must take into consideration when planning for health education, be it with individuals, families, groups/communities, or health team members. The assessment of clients and their teaching and learning needs are greatly influenced by your perception of their ability to learn. We provide tools to assess readiness to learn, motivation to learn, level of wellness related to healthcare needs, socioeconomic factors, cultural factors, and health literacy. Clients who are members of different generations require special recognition about how their lived experiences affect teaching and learning.

Communication is an essential component in client assessment. Clients with hearing, vision, and speech impairment require special adaptations. Nurses also might inadvertently create communication problems. Nurses as educators are expected to create a positive teaching and learning psychological and physical environment. Teaching and learning occurs in a variety of settings, each of which has unique characteristics that impact learning. Settings discussed included the hospital, long-term care facility, private home, school, worksite, and the community. The CCCC/AOL Quick Teaching Assessment Tool and the Assessment Tool for Teaching Groups provide guidance to the nurse as educator in planning health education.

EXERCISES

Exercise I—Perception in Assessment

Purpose: Examine how your interpretations of what you see and hear affect your interactions with clients.

Directions:

1. Share one example in which the client's perception of his or her health status was significantly different from yours.
2. Describe a situation in which it was easy to relate to a client. What factors in you and the client made it easy to relate?
3. Describe a situation in which it was difficult to relate to a client. What factors in you and the client made it difficult relate?
4. How did this affect your assessment of the client's learning needs?

Exercise II—Assessing Readiness to Learn

Purpose: Apply the knowledge of readiness to learn to clients.

Directions:

1. In small groups, differentiate among experiential readiness, emotional readiness, and physiologic and developmental readiness.
2. Give an example of each.
3. How will you apply this knowledge to teaching a client about diabetes care?

Exercise III—Assessing Levels of Wellness

Purpose: Examine how a client's level of wellness affects readiness to learn.

Directions:

1. Working alone, assess your own level of wellness using the Wellness/Illness Functional Continuum found in Chapter 1. Plot the continuum for each factor to determine strengths and weaknesses. Give yourself a score between 0 and 10.
2. Give an example of teaching content that would be appropriate for each of the needs you have identified.

Exercise IV—Critical Thinking and Health Education

Purpose: Apply critical thinking to health education in a variety of situations.

Directions: Form small groups of three to four members and assign each group one of these examples. After a discussion period, return to the whole class and share the solutions generated by each group.

1. You are concerned about clients being discharged early from the surgical unit before they have dealt with any of the stages of emotional adjustment to trauma, and you have grave doubts about the effectiveness of the teaching you are expected to do. Identify a real situation and work on creative ways to assess clients and achieve reasonable educational goals.
2. You are working with an unemployed, homeless client who lives on the streets and needs daily insulin injections. He is mildly retarded but seems motivated to help himself. Provide creative, workable solutions for this client.
3. You are a home health nurse visiting a client with slowly advancing dementia who lives alone, has no family and few neighbors. She insists on living in her home. You find very little food in her cupboards and spoiled food in the refrigerator. What creative solutions can you find to help this client?

Exercise V—Teaching and Learning Settings

Purpose: Assess the impact of teaching and learning settings on health education.

Directions: You are preparing to teach clients the importance of eating a healthy diet to include the food categories and daily nutritional requirements needed to maintain health. Discuss how your teaching approach will change in the following settings:

1. Hospital, convalescent, and nursing home
2. Client's private home
3. High school

4. Worksite setting
5. Community setting

Exercise VI—Apply the CCCC/AOL Assessment Tool for Teaching Individuals and the Assessment Tool for Teaching Groups

Purpose: Apply the assessment tools for teaching individuals and groups.

Directions: Divide the class into at least two groups and assign one group to discuss how they will apply the CCCC/AOL Assessment Tool for Teaching Individuals. Assign the other group to discuss how they will apply the Assessment Tool for Teaching Groups. Allow approximately 15 minutes. Reconvene the class and let each group report on their discussion.

SUPPLEMENTAL ONLINE RESOURCES

Exploring Psychology, readiness to learn:
http://www.dushkin.com/connectext/psy/ch03/readiness.mhtml
Student motivation theory:
http://www.kidsource.com/kidsource/content2/Student_motivatation.html
Student motivation to learn, an overview:
http://chiron.valdosta.edu/whuitt/col/motivation/motivate.html
Maslow's theory of motivation and human needs:
http://home.earthlink.net/~denmartin/maslow.html
Health and Lifestyle Awareness: What is your level of wellness? http://www.
    d11.org/doi/healthpe/documents/Health%20Awareness%20Scale.doc
ProLiteracy, improving lives and communities:
www.proliteracy.org
Patient education, Oncology Nursing Society:
http://www.ons.org/patientEd/
MedlinePlus, hearing disorders and deafness:
http://www.nlm.nih.gov/medlineplus/hearingdisordersanddeafness.html
MedlinePlus, vision impairment and blindness:
http://www.nlm.nih.gov/medlineplus/visionimpairmentandblindness.html

REFERENCES

Baker College Effective Teaching and Learning Department (2004). Appendix A: Generational comparison chart and Appendix B: Classroom implications chart. Retrieved on February 8, 2009 from http://www.mcc.edu/pdf/pdo/teaching_across_gen.pdf

Brown-Spath & Associates (2001). Evaluating the long-term impact of patient education. Retrieved on February 8, 2009 from http://www.brownspath.com

Bonner, S., Zimmerman, B. J., Evans, D., Irigoyen, M., Resnick, D., and Mellins, R. B. (2002). An individualized intervention to improve asthma management among urban Latino and African-American families. *Journal of Asthma, 39*(2), 167–179.

Brown, S. B. (2008). A dangerous bind for American workers. *Hospitals and Health Networks, 82*(11), 54.

Burchum, J. L. R. (2002). Cultural competence: An evolutionary perspective. *Nursing Forum, 37*(4), 5–15.

Burger, J. (2009). Communication. In Potter, P. A., & Perry, A. G. *Fundamentals of Nursing* (7th ed.) (pp. 339–360). St. Louis: Mosby Elsevier.

Busen, N. H., & Engebretson, J. C. (2008). Facilitating risk reduction among homeless and street-involved youth. *Journal of the American Academy of Nurse Practitioners, 20*(2008), 567–575.

Campbell, J., & Brooks, C. (2008). Tools for effective teaching. PowerPoint lecture presented at Palm Beach Atlantic University School of Nursing. Retrieved on July 22, 2009 from https://cache.trustedpartner.com/docs/library/000223/Transforming%20Behaviors%20Conference%20Materials/Effective%20Teaching%20Stategies_J%20Campbell_C%20Brooks_11_21_08.pdf

Cutilli, C. C. (2006). Do your patients understand? *Orthopaedic Nursing, 25*(3), 218–224.

DeRosa, N., & Kochurka, K. (2006). Implement culturally competent healthcare in your workplace. *Nursing Management, 37*(10), 18–26.

Glynn, S. M., Aultman, L. P., & Owens, A. M. (2005). Motivation to learn in general education programs. *The Journal of General Education, 54*(2), 150–170.

Hall, A. M. (2009). Client education. In Potter, P. A., & Perry, A. G., *Fundamentals of Nursing* (7th ed.) (pp. 361–383). St. Louis: Mosby Elsevier.

Himes, C. L., & Reynolds, S. L. (2005). The changing relationship between obesity and educational status. *Gender Issues, 22*, 45–57.

Horowitz, J. A. (2006). The therapeutic relationship. In Edelman, C. L., & Mandle, C. L. (Eds.). *Health Promotion Throughout the Life Span* (6th ed.) (pp. 77–99). St. Louis: Mosby Elsevier.

Keller, J. M. (1987). Development and use of the ARCS model of instructional design. *Journal of Instructional Development, 10*(3), 2–10.

Keller, J. M. (2008). First principles of motivation to learn and e3-learning. *Distance Education, 29*(2), 175–185.

Keller, L. O., Strohschein, S., & Briske, L. (2008). Population-based public health nursing practice: The intervention wheel. In Stanhope, M., & Lancaster, J. *Public Health Nursing: Population-centered Health Care in the Community* (7th ed.) (pp. 187–214). St. Louis: Mosby Elsevier.

Kimbro, R.T., Bzostek, S., Goldman, N., & Rodriguez, G. (2008). Race, ethnicity, and the education gradient in health. *Health Affairs, 27*(2), 361–372.

Krueger, P. M., Rogers, R. G., Hummer, R. A., LeClere, F. B., & Huie, S. A. B. (2003). Socioeconomic status and age: The effect of income sources and portfolios on U.S. adult mortality. *Sociological Forum, 18*(3), 465–481.

Kulwicki, A. (2009). Culture and ethnicity. In Potter, P. A., & Perry, A. *Fundamentals of Nursing* (7th ed.) (pp. 106–120). St. Louis: Mosby Elsevier.

Lethbridge-Cejku, M., Rose, D., Vickerie, J. (2006). Summary health statistics for U.S. Adults: National Health Inverview Survey, 2004. National Center for Health Statistics. Vital Health Stat 10(228).

Lieu, C. C., Sadler, G. R., Fullerton, J. T., & Stohlmann, P. D. (2007). Communication strategies for nurses interacting with patients who are deaf. *Dermatology Nursing, 19*(6), 541–551.

Lucas, J. W., Schiller, J. S., & Benson, V. (2004). Summary health statistics for U.S. adults: National Health Interview Survey, 2001. *Vital Health Statistics, 10*(218), 1–134. As cited in Lieu, C. C., Sadler, G. R., Fullerton, J. T., & Stohlmann, P. D. (2007). Communication strategies for nurses interacting with patients who are deaf. *Dermatology Nursing, 19*(6), 541–551.

Maslow, A. H. (1954). *Motivation and personality.* New York: Harper & Row.

Maslow, A. H. (1987). *Motivation and personality* (3rd ed.). New York: Harper & Row.

Miller, M. A., & Babcock, D. E. (1996). *Critical thinking applied to nursing.* St. Louis: Mosby.

O'Brien, P. G. (2007). Patient and Family Teaching. In Lewis, S.L., Heitkemper, M. M., Dirksen, S. R., O'Brien, P. G., & Bucher, L. *Medical-Surgical Nursing* (7th ed.). (pp. 53–65). St. Louis, MO: Mosby Elsevier.

Ormrod, J. E. (2008). *Human learning* (5th ed.). Upper Saddle River, NJ: Pearson Education.

Pohl, M. L. (1981). *The teaching function of the nursing practitioner.* Dubuque, IA: Wm. C. Brown.

Purnell, L. D. (2003). Transcultural diversity and health care. In Purnell, L. D., & Paulanka, B. J. (Eds.). *Transcultural health care: A culturally competent approach* (pp. 1–18). Philadelphia: F. A. Davis.

Racher, F. E., & Annis, R. C. (2007). Respecting culture and honoring diversity in community practice. *Research and Theory for Nursing Practice: An International Journal, 21*(4), 255–270.

Roberts-Grey, G. (2008). Got coverage? *Essence, 39*(7), 160–164.

Ryskulova, A., Turczyn, K., Makuc, D. M., Cotch, M. F., Klein, R. J., & Janiszewski, R. (2008). Self-reported age-related eye diseases and visual impairment in the United States: Results of the 2002 National Health Interview Survey. *American Journal of Public Health, 98*(3), 454–461.

Seligman, H. K., Wallace, A. S., DeWalt, D. A., Schillinger, D., Arnold, C. L., Shilliday, B. B., Delgadillo, A., Bengal, N., & Davis, T. C. (2007). Facilitating Behavior change with low-literacy patient education materials. *American Journal of Health Behavior, 31*(Suppl 1), S69–S78.

Slavin, R. E. (2009). *Educational psychology theory and practice* (9th ed.). Upper Saddle River, NJ: Pearson Education.

Stuart, G. W. (2005). Therapeutic nurse-patient relationship. In Stuart, G. W., & Laraia, M. T. (Eds.), *Principles and Practices of Psychiatric Nursing* (8th ed.) (pp. 15–49). St. Louis: Mosby Elsevier.

U.S. Census Bureau: State and County Quickfacts, Retrieved January 10, 2009, from http://quickfacts. census.gov/qfd/states/00000.html and http://www.census.gov/PressRelease/www/releases/ archives/population/012496.html

Weiss, B. D., Mays, M. Z., Martz, W., Castro, K. M., DeWalt, D. A., Pignome, M. P. M. J., & Hale, F. A. (2005). Quick assessment of literacy in primary care: The newest vital sign. *Annals of Family Medicine, 3*(6), 514–522.

Whyte, R. E., Watson, H. E., & McIntosh, J. (2006). Nurses' opportunistic interventions with patients in relation to smoking. *Journal of Advanced Nursing, 55*(5), 568–577.

Zuluaga, B. H. (2000). Implementation of the Zuluaga-Raysmith (Z-R) Model for assessment of perceived basic human needs in home health clients and caregivers. *Public Health Nursing, 17*(5), 317–324.

CHAPTER 5

The Child Learner

Creating a world that is truly fit for children does not imply simply the absence of war. It means having the confidence that our children would not die of measles or malaria. It means having access to clean water and proper sanitation. It means having primary schools nearby that educate children, free of charge. It means changing the world with children, ensuring their right to participate, and that their views are heard and considered. It means building a world fit for children, where every child can grow to adulthood in health, peace and dignity.
—Bellamy, C., 2002
Former Executive Director of the United Nations Children Fund (UNICEF)

OBJECTIVES

Upon completion of this chapter you will be able to:
- Describe the biologic changes, psychosocial stages, and developmental tasks characteristic of newborns through adolescents.
- List health education topics for newborn through adolescent clients related to biologic changes, psychosocial stages, and developmental tasks.
- Define pedagogy and apply it to teaching newborns through adolescents.
- Describe five steps that nurses as educators take to streamline the process of providing efficient yet personalized healthcare teaching to children in a variety of settings.
- List ways that nurses as educators work with families, are involved in the community, and work with healthcare teams.

KEY TERMS

autonomy versus shame and doubt	pedagogy
centering	preoperational stage
developmental task	psychosocial stages
formal operations	reflex
identity versus role confusion	reinforcer
industry versus inferiority	schema
irreversibility	sensorimotor stage
medical play	separation anxiety
operant conditioning	transductive reasoning
parallel play	trust versus mistrust

INTRODUCTION

Understanding development of children, including biologic characteristics, psychosocial stages, and developmental tasks, is fundamental to effective client education. A developmental task is a set of skills and competencies peculiar to each developmental stage that children must accomplish or master to deal effectively with their environment (Wong, Hockenberry-Eaton, Wilson, Winkelstein, & Schwartz, 2008). Young clients react differently depending on their developmental stage. Differences in development not only affect clients' reactions to their condition, but also their responses to and motivation for carrying out treatment recommendations. As the educator, you need to take into account the client's developmental stage based on an understanding of the health issues faced at that stage. Another important aspect of effectively teaching children is to know how children learn at different stages. This chapter describes child development in five major stages: the infant (0–1), the toddler (1–3), the preschooler (3–4), the school age child (5–12), and the adolescent (13–19). It looks at the concept of pedagogy and children's styles of learning at various stages. Your role as the educator is examined in working with pediatric clients within families, groups, communities, and health team members.

BIOLOGIC CHARACTERISTICS, PSYCHOSOCIAL STAGES, AND DEVELOPMENTAL TASKS

Children grow, develop, and learn throughout their lives from birth and infancy to adulthood. Development of the child learner refers to change or growth that occurs in a child during the life span from birth to adolescence. A *developmental task* represents our culture's definition of "normal" development at different points in the life span (Perkins, 1997). A child's development is measured through biologic characteristics, psychosocial stages, and developmental milestones or tasks. Although there are universally accepted assumptions about human development, no two children are alike. Children differ in physical, cognitive, social, and emotional growth patterns. They also differ in their genetic background and the ways they interact with and respond to their environment. Psychosocial stages emphasize the development of healthy personality traits (Erikson, 1963). Developmental changes normally occur in an orderly sequence, in predictable patterns that are age related; however, there are differences in the rate or timing of the changes from one child to another. It is important to have an understanding of the sequence of development to respond to the learning needs of young clients and their parents. It is also important to be aware that regression in development may occur with stress and illness.

Infants (Birth to One Year)

Biologic Characteristics

Infants at birth have reflexes as their sole physical ability. A reflex is an automatic body response to a stimulus that is involuntary; that is, the infant has no control over the response. Many reflexes disappear within a few weeks or months after birth. The presence of reflexes at birth is an indication of normal brain and nerve development. If reflexes are not present or if the reflexes continue past the time they should disappear, this is considered an abnormal finding and the infant should be seen by a healthcare provider for further evaluation (Wong *et al.*, 2008). Table 5-1 reviews the major infant reflexes and when they normally disappear.

There are a number of growth landmarks and physical changes that occur as infants grow in the first year. Weight gain of infants is particularly important. A newborn generally weighs between 6 and 9 pounds. A baby's size is influenced by a variety of factors, including parents' size, gender, birth order, mother's health and nutrition, life style choices during pregnancy, and medical problems. Babies often lose a few ounces in the first week after birth, but regain the weight by the second week. By the end of the first month, newborns will generally have gained about 15 ounces. Between the ages of 1 and 3 months, a newborn generally gains about 6 ounces per week. Between the ages of 4 and 7 months, weight gain is about 1½ to 2 pounds per months. This rate typically slows a bit around 6 months of age, to between 1 and ¼ pound per month. By 8 months the baby usually weighs around 2½ times the birth weight. Between the ages of 8 and 12 months, weight gain is steady but at a slower pace. By the first birthday, an infant should weigh around three times the birth weight.

Psychosocial Stages

Erikson's theory of psychosocial development (1963) focuses on how children socialize and how this affects their sense of self. According to the theory, successful completion of each stage results in a healthy personality and successful interactions with others. Failure to successfully complete a stage can result in a reduced ability to progress; however, stages can be resolved successfully at a later time. Of the nine stages identified by Erikson, five relate to children (Table 5-2). The task in infancy is the development of *trust versus mistrust*. From the time of birth to 1 year, infants begin to learn to trust others based on the consistency of the responses of their caregivers. If trust develops successfully, the child gains confidence and security in the world around him, and is able to feel secure in future relationships. Unsuccessful

TABLE 5-1	Common Infant Reflexes
Reflex	**Response**
Blinking	In response to a puff of air, the infant closes both eyes. Disappears as the neurologic system matures within the first year.
Babinski	In response to stroking the side of its foot, the infant twists its foot inward and fans out its toes. Disappears at about 1 year.
Grasping	In response to an object pressed against its palm, the infant attempts to grasp the object. Disappears at 5 to 6 months.
Moro	In response to surprise movement or loud noise, the infant startles with the legs and head extending while the arms jerk up and out with the palms up and thumbs flexed. Disappears at 3 to 6 months.
Rooting	In response to stroking its cheek, the infant turns its head toward the touch and attempts to suck. Disappears at about 4 months.
Stepping	In response to holding the infant so that its feet barely touch a surface, the infant "makes stepping movements." Disappears at about 10 to 15 months.
Sucking	In response to inserting a finger or nipple into its mouth, the infant begins sucking. Voluntary movement occurs at around 2 months.
Glabellar	In response to tapping the forehead, the infant blinks. Disappears as the neurologic system matures within the first year.
Plantar	In response to touching the ball of the foot, the infant curls its toes under. Disappears at 9 to 12 months.
Tonic neck	In response to turning his head to one side, this reflex causes a relaxed baby to straighten his arm on that side and bend his other arm in the fencing position. Disappears at 4 to 9 months.

Adapted from Wong et al. (2008).

completion of this stage can result in an inability to trust, fear, anger, and a sense of insecurity about the world. It may result in anxiety, and a feeling of mistrust in the world around him or her.

The most important social task for the infant is the development of attachment to the primary caretaker, most often the child's mother. This forms the basis for attachment, which is the cornerstone of emotional development. Separation anxiety is another attachment behavior of infants characterized by the infant showing distress

TABLE 5-2   Erikson's Stages of Psychosocial Development

Stage	Description
Trust versus mistrust Age birth to 1 year	• Learns to trust others based on caregiver response. • If trust develops, gains confidence and trust; is able to feel secure when threatened. • Unsuccessful completion results in inability to trust, and fear of the world.
Autonomy versus shame and doubt Age 1 to 3	• Asserts independence, walks away from mother, makes choices. • If encouraged, becomes confident and secure in own abilities. • If criticized, overly controlled, or not given the opportunity to assert self, may feel inadequate, become overly dependent, lack self-esteem, and feel shame or doubt.
Initiative versus guilt Age 3 to 6	• Asserts self more frequently. • Plans activities, makes up games, and initiates activities with others. • Develops a sense of initiative, feels secure in ability to lead others and make decisions. • If discouraged through criticism or control, develops a sense of guilt; will remain a follower and lack self-initiative.
Industry versus inferiority Age 6 to puberty	• Develops pride in accomplishments. • Initiates and completes projects, feels good about achievements. • Teachers play an increased role in development. • If encouraged and reinforced, feels industrious and confident about achieving goals. • If discouraged, feels inferior, doubts abilities, and may not reach potential.
Identity versus role confusion Puberty to adolescence	• Transition from childhood to adulthood. • More independent, looks to the future: career, relationships, families, housing, etc. • Explores possibilities and forms own identity based on outcomes of explorations. • Can be hindered, resulting in a sense of confusion about self and role in the world. ("I don't know what I want to be when I grow up.")

Adapted from Erikson (1963).

by crying when a familiar caregiver leaves (Wong et al., 2008). The first signs of separation anxiety appear at about 6 months of age and are clearly evident by 9 months of age. Separation anxiety is the strongest by 15 months of age and then begins to gradually weaken.

Developmental Tasks

Infant developmental tasks for this age group include the areas of motor development and cognitive development. Motor development follows cephalocaudal and proximodistal patterns, so that motor skills become refined first from the center and upper body and later from the extremities and lower body (Wong et al., 2008). Physical development is orderly and occurs in predictable sequence. The motor sequence of new movements for infants involves the following approximate sequence:

- Lack of head and trunk control—first few months after birth
- Lifts chin while lying flat—1 month
- Raises chest while lying flat—2 months
- Grasps rattle—fourth month
- Sits with support—fourth month
- Rolls over—fifth month
- Sits upright in a high chair—fourth to sixth month
- Sits without assistance—eighth month
- Crawling—ninth month
- Stand with help—10th month
- Walk with help—12th month
- Stands alone—14th month
- Walk alone without support or help—15th month
- Walks up stairs with help and runs clumsily—18th month

The ages for each motor skill milestone are averages; the rates of physical and motor developments differ among infants depending on a variety of factors, including heredity, the amount of activity the infant participates in, and the amount of attention the infant receives.

Cognitive development refers to intellectual or mental development. It includes the activities of thinking, perception, memory, problem solving, language, and speech. Jean Piaget's theory of cognitive development in the 1920s challenged the then-prevalent thinking that children think like adults. Piaget's theory (1952) is based on the idea that the developing infant builds cognitive structures, or schemes, to understand and respond to physical experiences within the environment. Piaget

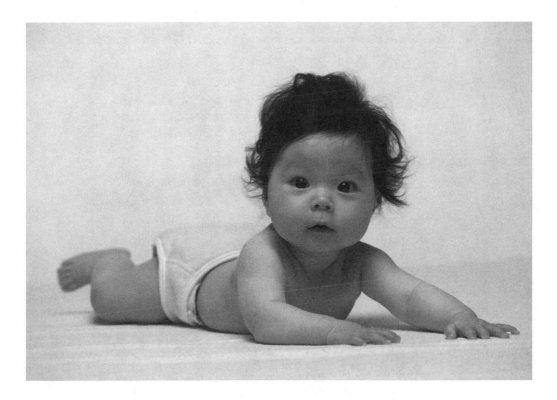

FIGURE 5-1 Infants develop at different rates.
Source: © Photodisc

posits that an infant's cognitive structure increases in complexity with development, moving from displaying reflexes such as sucking and grasping to highly complex mental activities such as speech. Piaget's four stages of cognitive development are included in Table 5-3. The infant is in the *sensorimotor stage*, in which infants begin to understand the information entering their senses and are able to interact with the world. During this stage, the infant learns to manipulate objects, although he or she will fail to understand the permanency of these objects if they are not within the infant's current sensory perception. Object permanence develops toward the end of the first year.

The most intensive period of speech and language development occurs during the first 3 years of life when the brain is developing and maturing. These skills appear to develop best when the infant is exposed to sounds, sights, and the speech and language of others. The beginning signs of communication occur during the first few days of life when an infant learns that crying will bring food, comfort, and compan-

TABLE 5-3 Piaget's Stages of Cognitive Development		
Stage	**Age**	**Characteristics of Stage**
Sensorimotor	0–2	The child: • Learns by doing: looking, touching, and viewing. • Learns through physical interaction with the environment. • Builds a set of concepts about reality and how it works. • Has a primitive understanding of cause and effect relationships. • Develops object permanence at about 9 months.
Preoperational	2–7	The child: • Is not able to conceptualize abstractly and needs concrete physical situations. • Uses language and symbols, including letters and numbers. • Is egocentric. • Conservation marks the end of the preoperational stage and the beginning of concrete operations.
Concrete operations	7–11	The child: • Starts to conceptualize, creating logical structures that explain physical experiences. • Demonstrates conservation, reversibility, serial ordering, and a mature understanding of cause-and-effect relationships. • Begins abstract problem solving and continues with concrete thinking.
Formal operations	12+	The child: • Begins to develop an abstract view of the world. • Is able to apply reversibility and conservation to both real and imagined situations. • Demonstrates abstract thinking, including logic, deductive reasoning, comparison, and classification. • Has increased understanding of the world and the idea of cause and effect. Can develop theories about the world.

Adapted from Piaget (1963).

ionship. The newborn also begins to recognize important environmental sounds such as the mother's voice. As they grow, infants sort out the speech sounds or phonemes that compose the words of their language. Most infants recognize the basic sounds of their native language (NIDCD, 2009). Table 5-4 reviews the developmental milestones of speech development of the infant.

TABLE 5-4 Language Development: First Year	
Age	**Infant Response**
Birth to 5 months	• Reacts to sounds • Turns head toward the sound • Cries, coos, laughs • Makes noise when talked to • Looks at faces
6 to 11 months	• Understands "no" • Says "da-da" and "ma-ma" • Tries to communicate by making gestures • Tries to imitate sounds

Adapted from National Institute on Deafness and Other Communication Disorders (2009).

Toddlers (One to Three Years)

Biologic Characteristics

During the toddler period, weight gain slows to about 4 to 6 pounds per year as the activity level increases. The physical appearance of the toddler includes a protuberant abdomen, accentuated lumbar lordosis (inward curvature of the spine), and a characteristic gait in which feet are placed wide apart and the child appears to walk flat footed. Birth weight quadruples by the age of 2½. A steady growth in height of 2 to 4 inches a year is expected. During this time the child perfects the gross and fine motor skills that emerged during the first year by developing balance, coordination, stability, and an improved ability to manipulate objects. Emotional and physical readiness for toilet training begins at around 18 months.

Psychosocial Stages

Toddlers are in Erikson's stage, *autonomy versus shame and doubt.* From the ages of birth to 1 year, children begin to learn the ability to trust others based on the consistency of the responses of their caregivers. Toddlers strive to develop a sense of autonomy within the boundaries of a trusting parental relationship. If trust develops successfully, the child gains confidence and security in the world around him. He is then better able to develop affectionate and trusting relationships with family members and with adults outside the family. Unsuccessful completion of this stage can result in an inability to trust, and therefore a sense of fear about the world.

Developmental Tasks

Toddlers are in Piaget's *preoperational stage* of cognitive development. A hallmark of this stage is egocentrism, or the tendency of children to recognize their environment only in terms of their own point of view. They think that parents and others share their thoughts. The toddler applies new knowledge of language and begins to use symbols to represent objects, such as pretending a broom is a horse. They may experiment with objects in their minds; first predicting what will happen if they do something to an object, then transforming their plans into action. To some degree, mental prediction and planning replace overt trial-and-error as growing toddlers experiment and attempt to solve problems. The toddler is now better able to think about things and events that are not present. Language development is proceeding rapidly in the toddler, but the ability to understand language is greater than the ability to express it, which creates frustration. Table 5-5 reviews the milestones for language development at this stage.

Preschool (Three to Four Years)

Biologic Characteristics

The preschooler has a steady growth rate of approximately 4 pounds of weight and 2 inches of height per year. The body lengthens and the protuberant abdomen disappears. In terms of physical abilities the 3-year-old can kick a ball, jump in place, build a tower of nine cubes, copy a circle, put on most clothing and shoes, and eat without assistance. By the age of 4 the child can climb a ladder, throw a ball overhand, hold a pencil, cut and paste, wash and dry hands, brush teeth, and ride a bike with training wheels. Most basic gross motor abilities have emerged. Existing skills are practiced and perfected, and the child develops mastery in applying motor skills to increasingly challenging and complex situations.

Psychosocial Stages

The preschooler moves through two of Erikson's stages of psychosocial development; the stage of *autonomy versus shame and doubt*, and the stage of *initiative versus guilt*. After developing basic trust, the child goes on to begin to plan activities, make up games, and initiate activities with others. If given this opportunity, the preschooler develops a sense of initiative, and feels secure in the ability to lead others and make decisions. If this tendency is not encouraged, either through criticism or control, the child develops a sense of guilt. The child may feel like an annoyance to others, and therefore remains a follower, lacking in self-initiative.

TABLE 5-5 Language Development: Toddler Years	
Age	**Toddler Response**
12–17 months	• Attends to a book or a toy for a few minutes. • Follows simple directions. • Answers simple questions nonverbally. • Points to objects, pictures, or family members. • Says two to three words to label a person or object (pronunciation may not be clear). • Tries to imitate simple words.
18–23 months	• Enjoys being read to. • Follows simple commands without gestures. • Points to simple body parts. • Understands simple verbs. • Makes animal sounds. • Starts to combine words such as "more mild."
2–3 years	• Knows about 50 words at 24 months. • Knows some spatial concepts such as "in," and "on." • Knows pronouns such as "you," "me," and "her." • Knows descriptive words such as "big," and "happy." • Says around 40 words at 24 months. • Speech is becoming more accurate but may still leave off ending sounds. Strangers may not be able to understand much of what is said. • Answers simple questions. • Begins to use more pronouns such as "you" and "I." • Speaks in two- to three-word phrases. • Uses question inflection to ask for something (e.g., "my ball?"). • Begins to use plurals such as "shoes" or "socks" and regular past tense verbs such as "jumped."

Adapted from National Institute on Deafness and Other Communication Disorders (2009).

At 2 years and up the preschooler develops rudimentary relationships with other children, which are usually characterized by parallel play; that is, play in the presence of rather than in interaction with other children. As the child progresses, social relationships increase outside the family and interactive and cooperative play skills with peers are expanded. The preschooler also begins to imitate and practice social roles. Concepts of right and wrong are learned as the child begins to understand the nature of rules, which causes the child to experience guilt when doing wrong.

Developmental Tasks

Preschoolers are in Piaget's *preoperational* cognitive stage. A concrete thought process is evident in this stage by what Piaget calls transductive reasoning, which describes how the preschooler cannot think from the general to the particular or from the particular to the general. Piaget also describes the concept of centering as lacking in the preschooler's thinking. The child cannot consider more than one factor at a time when solving a problem, or connect a reversible operation to the original act. This is called irreversibility. Piaget described preschool-age children as preoperational because they do not yet use logic. They understand the world through magical thinking

TABLE 5-6 Language Development: Preschool Years	
Age	**Preschooler Response**
3–4 years	• Groups objects together such as food and clothes.
	• Identifies colors.
	• Uses most speech sounds but may distort some of the more difficult sounds such as *l, r, s, sh, ch, y, v, z,* and *th*. These sounds may not be fully mastered until age 7 or 8.
	• Uses consonants in the beginning, middle, and end of words. Some of the more difficult consonants may be distorted, but attempts to say them.
	• Strangers are able to understand much of what is said.
	• Able to describe the use of objects such as "fork," "car," etc.
	• Has fun with language. Enjoys poems and recognizes language absurdities such as, "Is that an elephant on your head?"
	• Expresses ideas and feelings, rather than just talking about the world around him or her.
	• Uses verbs that end in -ing, such as walking, talking.
	• Answers simple questions such as, "What do you do when you are hungry?"
	• Repeats sentences.

Adapted from National Institute on Deafness and Other Communication Disorders (2009).

and have difficulty distinguishing between wishes and what really happens. They believe that thoughts and strong feelings can make things happen.

A major accomplishment in the preschool stage is the perfection of language skills and the use of language to communicate with others. During the preschool years language progression depends on aptitude, the opportunity for using language, the quality and quantity of language used at home, and the child's range of experiences using language to communicate. It is also at this stage that grammar and syntax are refined and the vocabulary increases rapidly (Table 5-6).

School Age (Five to Twelve Years)

Biologic Characteristics

The school age child gains an average of 6 pounds and grows approximately 2 inches per year. Growth is marked by spurts and times of little growth as dictated by genetics. During these years boys and girls are of similar size, but school age children tend to be concerned about their rate of growth and what their height and weight will be. The child practices, refines, and masters complex gross and fine motor skills. Examples of gross motor skills for school age children include balancing on one foot, tandem walking, hopping on one foot, pedaling a bicycle, and bathing self. Fine motor skills for this age group include drawing a person with three to six parts, cutting with a knife, tying a bow, drawing a diamond, and having good eye–hand coordination. This is also a time when the school age child begins to lose baby teeth and the permanent teeth emerge.

Psychosocial Stages

School age children are in Erikson's stage of *industry versus inferiority*. In this stage children begin to develop a sense of pride in their accomplishments. They initiate projects, see them through to completion, and feel good about what they have achieved. During this time, teachers play an increased role in the child's development. If children are encouraged and reinforced for their initiative, they begin to feel industrious and confident in their ability to achieve goals. If this initiative is not encouraged, if it is restricted by parents or teacher, then the child will begin to feel inferior, doubting his or her abilities and may not reach full potential. Relationships with people outside the family become more important to the school age child. They develop friendships and participate in peer group activities. The child imitates, learns, and adopts age-appropriate social roles, including those that are gender specific. The child develops an understanding of rules that can be relied on to dictate proper social

FIGURE 5-2   The school age child learns to solve problems.
Source: © Pavel Siamionau/Dreamstime.com

behavior and govern social relationships and activities. The child develops a sense of self as an individual with awareness of likes and dislikes and with special areas of skill. Introspection is possible at this age.

Developmental Tasks

School age children are in Piaget's stage of *concrete operations.* During this stage, accommodation (ability to modify schema to fit the world) increases. The child develops an ability to think abstractly and make rational judgments about concrete or observable phenomena, that in the past the child needed to physically manipulate in order to understand. Some specific skills that develop at this time are the ability to classify items and put them in a series, recognize logical relationships among elements in a serial order, and understand that the quantity, length, or number of items is unrelated to the arrangement or appearance of the object or items (conservation). The school age child can take into account multiple aspects of a problem to solve it. He or she understands that numbers or objects can be changed and then returned to their original state (reversibility). The child moves, in this stage, toward more cooperative interactions and develops the ability to understand other people's perspectives (Figure 5-2).

School age children generally enter this developmental stage with the ability to understand and speak a language. School focuses on learning to read and write. Success in school depends on three things: the child having the visual ability to read, the auditory ability to perceive language spoken to him or her, and the fine motor skills for handwriting.

Adolescent (Thirteen to Nineteen Years)

Biologic Characteristics

Adolescence is a time of accelerated physical growth in weight and height when 15% to 20% of adult height and 50% of adult weight is achieved. This is also the time of onset of puberty, or sexual maturity, which signals the ability to reproduce. Females usually begin puberty 2 years earlier than males and experience their growth spurt earlier. Physiologic changes in puberty include development of secondary sex characteristics. In females the first sign of puberty is often breast development. Other signs are the growth of hair in the pubic area and armpits. Menarche, the onset of menses in girls, usually happens later in puberty, at around 13 years of age. In males puberty usually begins with the testicles and penis getting larger. Then hair grows in the pubic area and armpits. Muscles grow, the voice deepens, nocturnal emissions begin, and facial hair develops as puberty continues. Even though the physical changes are usually sequential in nature and are mediated through the hormonal regulatory system, there are individual variations for onset and duration of puberty. Some adolescents may begin puberty earlier than normal, a condition called *precocious puberty*. Others may have delayed puberty, meaning the process begins later than normal.

Psychosocial Stages

The adolescent is in Erikson's stage of *identity versus role confusion*. This is a period of transition from childhood to adulthood. Adolescents want more independence, and begin to look to the future in terms of career and future relationships. Social relationships center on their peer group, with decreased time spent with family. Group values often guide their individual behavior, and acceptance by peers becomes a critical part of self-esteem. Adolescents explore possibilities and begin to form their own identities based on the outcome of their explorations. Identity is defined as a coherent conception of the self, made up of committed goals, values, and beliefs. This sense of who they are can be hindered, which can result in a sense of confusion about themselves and their role in the world. Toward the end of this stage, identity becomes more individualized and the adolescent develops a more stable sense of self that is separate from either family or peer group.

Developmental Tasks

Piaget's stage of *formal operations* describes the adolescent's cognitive development. This stage brings cognition to its final form. Adolescents no longer require concrete objects to make rational judgments. Abstract, theoretical, philosophical, and scientific reasoning become possible. At this time they also develop an understanding of long-term cause and effect. Adolescents question, reinterpret, and revise their previous knowledge base. At this point they are capable of hypothetical and deductive reasoning. There are many possible options for teaching adolescents because they can consider options from different perspectives. It is common for them to challenge current thinking and have a sense of idealism about the world as they move toward a formal thinking process.

Language development is largely complete by adolescence. Language at this stage exhibits evidence of reflective and abstract thought with increasingly complex grammatical construction of speech and writing. Adolescents have the ability to define and discuss abstractions such as health, love, and peace. They are also aware that words can have multiple meanings. The use of slang is common. This is considered to be an opportune time developmentally to learn other languages.

IMPLICATIONS FOR HEALTH EDUCATION

It is critical to understand child development to provide effective health education to children, their parents, and caregivers. Knowledge of child development enables you to prepare teaching plans based on realistic child expectations, and increases the chances of adherence and success in promoting, retaining, and restoring health. As an educator, your knowledge and understanding of cognitive and perceptual behavior serves as a guide in counseling. Use this knowledge to influence behavior by listening to parental concerns, respecting values, and modeling behaviors that support overall health of the child. As the child grows and is able to independently communicate, use understanding of growth and development to interact with the child in ways that acknowledge his or her verbal and physical abilities and encourage self-reliance.

TABLE 5-7   Teaching Implications for Various Developmental Stages

Age	Psychosocial (Erikson)	Cognitive (Piaget)	Language	Teaching Implications
Infancy	*Trust vs. mistrust.* 5–6 weeks: responsive smile to families' faces and voices. Emotionally symbiotic with main caretaker. Individual temperament emerges in earliest weeks of life. Needs balance of rest, exercise, nutrition, love, strokes. Cuddliness varies.	Sensorimotor: Basic reflex habits (i.e., sucking nipple within 2 wks). Higher levels later: 2–3 mos. looks for sounds. 8–9 mos. object permanence. Thinks in pictures.	Prelanguage sounds. Inner language: recognizes objects. Audicreceptive: recognizes spoken words.	Teach parents/caregivers. Calibrate for their anxiety when child is very ill. Anticipatory guidance re: growth and development, safety, and stimulation (talk and touch).
Early Childhood 2–3 years	*Autonomy vs. shame and doubt.* "No!" Frustrated by personal and external limits. Egocentric. Needs: to explore safely, to succeed.	Sensorimotor: still thinks in pictures. Starts development of object formation, representation, extension.	Single, 3-word sentences: nouns, verbs and adjectives: "ball, carry, soft." Age 3, time: "yesterday."	Needs: Safe play space, love, security. Find out routines, special words. Comfort toy. Give positive simple command. Read or make up relevant picture books. Most teaching through parent.
3–6 years	*Initiative vs. guilt.* Fears: unknown, separation, strangers, disapproval, pain, punishment, own aggression, Roles: male, female	Sensorimotor: expanding imagination and concepts.	Rapid growth. By 5 years has usual speech patterns.	Encourage play. Use it to assess child and to teach. Give simple explanations: "You will smell icky perfume." See ... hear ... feel. Make tape and picture books, objects. Use timing: Tell child soon enough to allow processing but not to get panicky. Allow only one stall. Positive commands: "You hold Bandaid."

(continues)

TABLE 5-7   Teaching Implications for Various Developmental Stages (continued)

Age	Psychosocial (Erikson)	Cognitive (Piaget)	Language	Teaching Implications
Late childhood 6–12 years	*Industry vs. inferiority.* Makes things. Peer influence is important. Developing parents and ego states.	Concrete operations. Inductive reasoning. Memory. Conscience teachable in many cultures.	Good command of language: Can use it to tell stories, ask questions, argue, tease.	Assess child's reading ability. Likes mechanical explanations. Help child gain content by participating in his/her own care and procedures. Can pay attention to teaching. Can do own hygiene, choose good food, recognize signs of illness.
Adolescence	*Identity vs. role confusion.* New and more mature relationships. Sexual identity. Changing body. Becoming emotionally independent from parents. Preparing for adult responsibilities, career, love. Workable value system. Social responsibilities. Mood swings and ambivalence. Fears "loss of face."	Formal operations. "One's thinking takes wings." (Paget)	Depends on IQ, culture, socioeconomic group. Slang	Ask for meaning of slang. Use peers to teach and persuade. Protect "face" privacy. Expect mood swings. Be honest and straightforward. Try to read between the lines of what a teenager is trying to say or does not say.

Adapted from Babcock, D. E., & Miller, M. A. (1994). *Client education: Theory and practice.* St. Louis: Mosby.

Use age-specific strategies to prepare teaching plans. Infants expand their gross and fine motor skills by being encouraged to reach and grasp and move toward objects. An example of this would be toys safely placed in the crib that are black and white or brightly colored to attract attention and stimulate movement. Younger children, toddlers through preschool, have language skills that require concrete examples to help them understand information. A younger child will respond well to being told "We always wash our hands before meals." An older child will want more explanation, to which the nurse can respond by discussing that this prevents germs that can make you sick. As the child's gross and fine motor skills develop, it is helpful to supplement explanation with objects that the child can manipulate. When teaching about how to take blood pressure, having the child hold and examine the blood pressure cuff lets him or her gain familiarity with the equipment and gives a sense of mastery and trust. The preschool child enjoys pretend play, which is when the child remembers past experiences and replays them (Graca, Fowler, & Rosenstock, 2009). By pretending, the child is able to share fears and concerns and can gain a sense of mastery over the environment. Use this time to clear up misconceptions that are common in this age group because of magical thinking. Older children enjoy activities that involve peers and are repetitive and entertaining. Games, including those on the computer, are fun and create a sense of mastery. Table 5-7 summarizes psychosocial, cognitive, language, and teaching implications.

Promote and Retain Health

The focus of promoting health is on prevention of illness, whereas the focus of retaining health is on maintaining the present health status, assuming it is satisfactory. Table 5-8 lists suggested topics to promote and retain health appropriate for children at various stages of development. These suggestions are not all-inclusive and need to be adapted to the circumstances of the individual client.

Restore Health

Restoration of health for children refers to working with children with an acute or chronic illness or disability. The purpose of health education at this time is to help clients understand the nature of their health problem, the treatment regimen, and the limitations imposed by the health problem, disability, or injury. This may involve not only working with the client, but also with family members. Table 5-9 explains the approach used by nurses as educators when teaching different age groups. The developmental stage is taken into account and both the parent and the child are viewed as clients.

TABLE 5-8   Suggested Topics to Promote and Retain Health

Nursing Assessment	Health Education Topics
Infant	• Promotion of infant/parent bonding • Infant nutrition: breastfeeding, formula feeding, introduction of solid food and weaning • Developmental milestones • Elimination patterns • Activity and exercise through stimulation and play • Sleep needs • Injury prevention • Sensory stimulation to promote cognitive and social development • Vaccinations
Toddler	• Nutritional needs and preferences • Toilet training • Appropriate toys and activities • Rituals and security objects • Need for autonomy, temper tantrums • Parental frustration • Safety issues, injury prevention • Vaccinations
Preschooler	• Nutritional needs and preferences • Dental care • Appropriate play activities and exercise • Choosing television shows • Managing bedtime concerns • Imaginary friends and magical thinking • Vision and hearing screenings • Gender identification • Injury prevention • Health screenings
School age	• Understanding of health • Balanced nutrition, prevention of obesity • Nocturnal enuresis, encopresis and shy bladder • Sports activities, TV, video, and computer games • Developing socialization skills • Sleep walking, sleep talking, night fears • Health screenings • Attention-deficit hyperactivity disorder (ADHD) • Questions about sex • Coping strategies • Accident prevention

(continues)

TABLE 5-8	Suggested Topics to Promote and Retain Health *(continued)*
Nursing Assessment	**Health Education Topics**
Adolescent	• Physical changes: puberty • Common health issues: acne, scoliosis • Diet and exercise: prevention of obesity and eating disorders • Sexual behavior, contraception • Sexually transmitted diseases • Body image issues • Substance abuse: alcohol and drugs • Injury and violence prevention • Health screening • Vaccinations

TABLE 5-9	Teaching Approach with Different Age Groups	
Age Group	**Clients/Parents**	**Nursing Approach**
Infant (0–1)	Child	• Observe the infant's physical condition: weight and appearance. • Observe child/caregiver interaction: look for bonding behaviors.

	Parent	• Establish rapport.
		• Use good listening skills to identify parent's concerns.
		• Address parental anxiety and stress with calm demeanor.
		• Assess parental educational level, literacy level, cultural influences.
		• Encourage enjoyment of infants.
		• Discuss balance of work and home life.
		• Share knowledge of:
		  Community resources.
		  Developmental milestone.
		  Importance of play for development.
		  Preventive teaching.
		  Infant safety.
		  Nutrition.
		  Health screenings and vaccinations schedule.

(continues)

TABLE 5-9	Teaching Approach with Different Age Groups *(continued)*	
Age Group	**Clients/Parents**	**Nursing Approach**
Toddler (1–2)	Child	• Assess the quality of the parent/child relationship. • Observe the physical status and growth of the child. • Talk and interact with the child on their level to initiate a relationship.
	Parent	• Establish rapport. • Listen to parental concerns and encourage questions. • Determine parental knowledge and literacy level and cultural influences. • Be sensitive to signs of frustration with child's behavior. • Provide appropriate teaching tools and resources. • Share knowledge of: Community resources. Developmental milestone. Importance of play for development. Safety. Techniques of discipline and limit setting. Toilet training.
Preschooler (3–4)	Child	• Talk and interact with the child on his or her level to establish a relationship. • Observe the child at play; listen to vocalizations and observe imaginary play. • Observe the physical status and growth of the child. • Teach children about procedures to be performed. • Keep explanations simple. • Allow children to express their fears.
	Parent	• Establish rapport. • Listen to parental concerns and encourage questions. • Determine parental knowledge, literacy level, and cultural influences. • Teach parents ways to respond to their child's questions. • Provide appropriate teaching tools and resources. • Share knowledge of: Normal developmental milestones. Child's sexual curiosity. Imaginary play and magical thinking. Safety.

(continues)

Age Group	Clients/Parents	Nursing Approach
School age (5–12)	Child	• Observe the physical status and growth of the child. • Develop rapport with the child by introducing yourself and asking about his or her interests and friends. • Ask the child about his or her health and encourage questions. • Explain procedures or teaching in clear, logical ways. • Include child in the patient education process. • Use appropriate tools and resources.
	Parent	• Establish rapport. • Listen to parental concerns and encourage questions. • Determine parental knowledge and literacy level. • Help parents to foster child independence and praise accomplishments. • Give parents tools for teaching. • Share knowledge of: Normal developmental milestones. School adjustment. Enuresis, encopresis. Sleepwalking, sleep talking. Learning disabilities. Obesity, nutritional teaching. Dental health. Safety, accidents, drowning, bicycles. Drugs, alcohol, smoking, sexual activity. Health screening; vision, hearing. Use of television, computer, cell phones, and video games.
Adolescence (13–19)	Child	• Focus on establishing rapport based on openness and trust. • Ask about bodily changes and sexual adjustment. • Ask about family support and facilitate the family relationship. • Ask about peer group and social, cultural influences. • Ask about health concerns and answer questions. • Advocate for the adolescent client. • Be mindful of modesty and privacy issues. • Use empathetic understanding; no lecturing. • Provide appropriate teaching tools and resources.

TABLE 5-9 Teaching Approach with Different Age Groups *(continued)*

(continues)

TABLE 5-9	Teaching Approach with Different Age Groups *(continued)*	
Age Group	**Clients/Parents**	**Nursing Approach**
		• Share knowledge about: Physical change in puberty. Sexual issues and contraception. Body image and eating disorders. Health issues and safety. Body piercing and tattooing. Scoliosis, acne.
	Parent	• Establish rapport.
		• Listen to parental concerns and encourage questions.
		• Determine parental knowledge, literacy level and cultural influences.
		• Assist parents in understanding adolescent behavior.
		• Encourage limit setting and fostering of adolescent independence.
		• Help parents redefine their role in this transition phase.

Adapted from Falvo, D. R. (2004). *Effective patient education: A guide to increased compliance.* Sudbury, MA: Jones and Bartlett.

ORIENTATION TO LEARNING

Learning in Children

Most theorists believe that learning is something that occurs as the result of certain experiences that precede changes in behavior (Olsen & Hergenhahn, 2009). The experiences that precede learning are interactions with the environment. Athey (2007) and Piaget (1963) agree that children's interactions with their environment leads to mental actions through which they construct ideas or schema about what they are encountering. As they come across objects, situations, people, and ideas, they adjust and structure their knowledge to try to make sense of their experiences. Using this cognitive learning process they build a framework for thinking and learning. Children's direct experiences and interactions with things and people around them are central to their learning (David, Goouch, Powell, & Abbott, 2003).

    B. F. Skinner (1968) posits that learning is a change in overt behavior that occurs in response to events or stimuli that occur in the environment. Reinforcement is the key element in Skinner's theory of classical conditioning. A *reinforcer* is anything that strengthens the desired response. It could be a smile, verbal praise, a good grade, or a feeling of increased accomplishment. Skinner also identifies negative reinforcers, which result in the increased frequency of a response when it is withdrawn (different from adverse stimuli or punishment, which results in reduced responses). Babies generally respond well to operant conditioning, which is a process of gradually shaping the infant's behavior. An example of this is an infant who learns that smiling elicits positive parental attention, which in turn causes the infant to smile at his or her parents more (Skinner, 1968). Babies generally respond well to operant conditioning. Cognitive and behavioral theories are applied to teaching in Table 5-10.

Learning Styles in Children

Learning occurs as children respond to environmental, social, emotional, and physical stimuli when trying to understand new information. Learning styles are the way

TABLE 5-10   Application of Cognitive and Behavior Learning Theories for Children

Learning Theory	Principles	Teaching Application
Cognitive theories of learning	Jean Piaget's Cognitive-Development Theory	1. Children will provide different explanations of reality at different stages of cognitive development. 2. Cognitive development is facilitated by providing activities or situations that engage learners and require adaptation. 3. Learning materials and activities should involve the appropriate level of motor or mental operations for a child of given age; avoid asking students to perform tasks that are beyond their current cognitive capabilities. 4. Use teaching methods that actively involve students and present challenges.
Behavioral theory of learning	B. F. Skinner's Operant Conditioning Theory	1. Behavior that is positively reinforced will reoccur; intermittent reinforcement is particularly effective. 2. Information should be presented in small amounts so that responses can be reinforced ("shaping"). 3. Reinforcements will generalize across similar stimuli ("stimulus generalization") producing secondary conditioning.

Application of Cognitive and Behavior Learning Theories for Children adapted from Kearsley (1994 to 2009).

the individual process information. Learning styles refer to three perceptual pathways or modalities of learning: visual (sight), kinesthetic (body, sensation, motion), and auditory (sound). The visual modality occurs when information is received best through visual stimulation (reading, pictures, movies, etc.). Approximately 40% of secondary students are visual learners. The kinesthetic modality occurs when information is received best via touch and hands-on activities (computer assisted instruction, models, field-trips, etc.). Approximately 50% of secondary students are kinesthetic learners. The auditory modality occurs when information is best obtained by hearing (being read to aloud, listening to songs, puppet show, reciting songs or poems, etc.). Approximately 10% of secondary students are auditory learners (Carbo, Dunn, & Dunn, 1986). There is no right or wrong learning style. Most children show a preference for one style, as do nurses and parents. It is not unusual for the nurse and parents to prefer learning styles different from that of the child. To work effectively with children it is important for you to understand your own, the child's, and possibly the parents preferred learning styles. This understanding helps to produce more efficient, productive learning opportunities for children. Including activities that use other styles can be helpful in expanding children's areas of interest and ability to learn.

The Role of Play in Learning

Jones and Reynolds (1992) state that "young children learn the most important things, not by being told but by constructing knowledge for themselves in interaction with the physical world and with other children—and the way they do this is by playing" (p. 1). In play, children expand their understanding of themselves and others, their knowledge of the physical world, and their ability to communicate with peers and adults. Children experience play through all the developmental stages. Infants and toddlers engage in activities that stimulate their senses and develop motor skills. Preschoolers play with other children, develop and refine motor skills, and use basic academic skills such as counting, reading, and writing. School age children play formal and informal games with their peers such as hopscotch, jump rope, board, card, and computer games. Through these activities they enhance their coordination and physical abilities, refine their social skills, and build concepts such as cooperation and competition. In adolescence play is more organized and structured as the need for orderly thinking is expressed through games with rules and in organized sports.

Play is so important that its significance in children's lives is recognized by the United Nations as a specific right (United Nations, 1989). The Association for Child Education International (ACEI, 2005) issued a position paper outlining the following beliefs about the importance of play in children's development. The ACEI stated that:

- Play is a dynamic, active, and constructive behavior and is an essential and integral part of all children's healthy growth, development, and learning across all ages, domains, and cultures.
- Play enhances learning and development for children of all ages, cultures, and domains.
- The forms and functions of children's play must be considered in the context of our knowledge about age-related play behaviors. Knowledge about how children play at different ages should guide the practice of all adults who work with children.
- Play is a powerful, natural behavior contributing to children's learning and development and that no program of adult instruction can substitute for children's own observations, activities, and direct knowledge.

The nurse as educator uses this knowledge of the importance of play to support child learning. Graca et al. (2009) describe *medical play* as developmentally appropriate activities that provide insight into how the child is coping with healthcare events and can be used as a tool in successful teaching. Medical play allows opportunities to deal with both the physical and emotional stressors of health care as well as act as a mechanism to increase understanding. An example of using medical play is rehearsing activities before surgery. The child can manipulate equipment such as an oxygen mask and rehearse what it is like to have the mask in place. The nurse as educator uses knowledge of developmental milestones to choose play strategies that fit the child's need (Figure 5-3).

Practices That Encourage Child Learning

As an educator, you assume a big part in creating the climate and conditions that best promote children's learning. Involvement in learning is built on the confidence and trust that come from good relationships. First, build rapport with the child. It is important to promote self-esteem, confidence, and trust to create an environment conducive to learning. It is also important to involve children both physically and mentally in the learning process (David et al., 2003). Children should be encouraged to explore their world through movement using all their senses to find out what they can do, what things are like, and what things mean. It is through this exploration that they achieve understanding and form ideas from sensory experiences. Learning strategies should include these types of activities.

Provide support to cultivate, sustain, and extend children's explorations and recognize their accomplishments. You should also be aware that part of the active

FIGURE 5-3   Children explore the world through play.
Source: © Artyom Yefimov/Dreamstime.com

learning process is to allow children to make decisions and have control and independence as part of the learning process. Allowing children to decide what and how they are to do things increases their engagement in the learning process (David et al., 2003). This does not mean that children are left on their own to decide what and how they will learn, but it does means that the nurse can create situations for them to make decisions and then support them as they engage in learning activities. Making decisions helps children to become managers of their own learning.

Another important aspect of active learning is to personalize the learning process. This means to build on what the child is familiar with, knows, and can do. Getting to know the child and his or her parents helps you understand how to stimulate and sustain the child's involvement and effort in learning (David et al., 2003). The pace and character of children's learning differs from one child to another, as they have different interests, skills, and knowledge built on their experiences. This means that children learn the same thing in different ways, or learn the same thing at different times in their development. The range and character of learning activities should be planned to address these kinds of differences in a way that enables all children to find something that is relevant and that will engage and sustain their interest. Some children need additional support to become fully involved in learning activities.

It is important for you to consider how learning activities are presented. The context with which children experience things has a considerable effect on their willingness to become involved and their ability to connect with the ideas that are presented (David et al., 2003). Children want to understand the situation or circumstances in which they learn, so explanations should be simple and clear. When they find things that they already know about, and can latch on to, they have a base from which to explore new things. A final important factor that you should consider is the importance of maintaining good working relationships with parents. Strong parental relationships provide essential information about the child's learning at home and help to provide insight into the things with which each child is familiar.

PEDAGOGY

Pedagogy is derived from the Greek word "paid," meaning child, plus "agogos," meaning leading, and is defined as the art and science of teaching children (Hiemstra & Sisco, 1990). In the pedagogic model, the teacher has full responsibility for facilitating learning, including what will be learned, when it will be learned, and whether the material has been learned. Pedagogy is also sometimes referred to as the correct use of teaching strategies, and is described as being a didactic and traditional approach to teaching children. As the educator, you will use pedagogic principles when teaching young clients. One-to-one teaching with the child facilitates individual learning needs, provides for child and family interaction with the nurse, and protects confidentiality. Group teaching may be appropriate when the child can benefit from learning with others. Discussions and demonstrations often work well in groups.

Implications for Health Education

Health education occurs in a variety of situations, including clinics, hospitals, schools, colleges/universities, and community settings. Some situations offer the opportunity for advance planning, developing learning objectives, and arranging multiple teaching sessions. This more formal teaching situation is discussed in depth in Chapters 9 through 13. More often there is no time for a formal teaching approach in the practice area. Woodring (2000) emphasizes that "economic realities require nurses to use both their time with patients and their teaching opportunities more efficiently" (p. 505). Nurses are often placed in the position of needing to maximize the use of time to teach the child and family. There is also an expectation that the child and family have learned the information that is presented and that the learning will be evidenced by positive health outcomes (Woodring, 2000).

There are five steps that nurses as educators can take to streamline the process of providing efficient yet personalized healthcare teaching in a variety of settings. At the core of the teaching process remains the nurse/client relationship as described in the Client Education Model (see Figure 1-1). The first step in building a trusting nurse/client relationship is to clarify the perceptions of the client and family about the health issue by asking questions. Questions regarding client perceptions are drawn from the Health Belief Model (see Table 1-3). For example, What is the need for care? What do you know about the problem? What is the seriousness of the condition? What impact is it having on your life? What are your goals for effective treatment? What are potential barriers to treatment? Careful attention to the answers to these questions and observations of the client as he or she responds help to establish the need for health education and begin the process of building trust. It is important to be attentive to the client's cultural background as the nurse analyzes client responses.

A second step is consideration of the assessment factors that influence learning. It is important to asses the child's physical, psychosocial, and language development. It is also helpful to determine family support for treatment. Tools are available to assess learning styles and literacy level of both child and parent (Davis, Nur, & Ruru, 1994; James & Galbraith, 1984). Assessment factors will weigh heavily when planning learning activities later. It is possible that how the child and family members learn may be discerned simply by observing their responses to activities that occur within the usual care situation, but assessment tools provide an efficient and quick way to gather this information.

As an educator, you will draw on assessment data to establish mutual learning objectives that form the basis of the teaching plan as part of step three. The learning objectives should be reviewed briefly with the child and family to answer questions and determine if all learning needs are identified. You select teaching content appropriate to achieving the learning objectives, and highlight the *must know* information by separating information into small sections as part of the teaching plan. It is important to consider current evidence-based practices as part of the plan.

Selection of teaching strategies and instructional materials to carry out the teaching plan is an important fourth step. Use assessment data to choose strategies and materials that accommodate learners' needs and abilities. It is important to take into account clients' cognitive stage, physical abilities, and language skills when planning activities. Reading capability and comprehension of the child and parent will help determine what instructional materials are appropriate. Learning materials should be age specific, interesting, and reflect the needs of the child. Remember that cultural context of materials should be carefully considered as well. Brochures, pocket-sized flip charts, pamphlets, videos, and comic books depicting children of the client's race and ethnicity are suggestions for educational materials (Ebbinghaus & Bahrainwala, 2003). Samples of educational materials from pharmaceutical companies can be useful when return demonstrations are used.

The fifth step is the implementation of the teaching plan. Select a conducive learning environment to meet the learning objectives of the teaching plan. Explanations should be simple and concrete with instructional materials that enhance understanding of the content. Speak slowly and clearly without interfering extraneous noise. It is particularly important that you create an atmosphere that captures the child's interest. This may entail being adaptable and willing to offer the child options during the course of the teaching session. Pay close attention to body language that indicates distraction or lack of interest. It is particularly concerning if the child or parent does not ask questions. This is a clue that changes are needed in the teaching approach (Woodring, 2000). It is important for you to focus on the ultimate goal of the teaching session: child learning and not on maintaining a stubborn insistence on following the teaching plan. A good way to determine how the teaching session went is to ask the young client and or parent to summarize what has been learned at the conclusion of the session. In this way you may correct any misconceptions related to essential content. Questions such as, "Tell me in your own words how you plan to . . . ?" are helpful to evaluate understanding.

Summative evaluation is the final sixth step of the process, and not only evaluates content knowledge, but also allows the client to give the nurse feedback about what he or she liked or disliked about the whole teaching/learning experience. Client evaluation may include return demonstration, short quizzes, or checklists. Evaluation of the learning experience includes asking the child and family about factors such as the setting, teaching strategies, instructional materials, pace of learning activities, and the nurse/client interactions. Ideally you will see the child and family over time to assess long-term learning and provide reinforcement of essential content. This may involve scheduling follow-up teaching sessions, creating action plans for school use, and initiating a visiting nurse referral to provide ongoing education and support. Figure 5-4 summarizes the steps of the health education process taken with children.

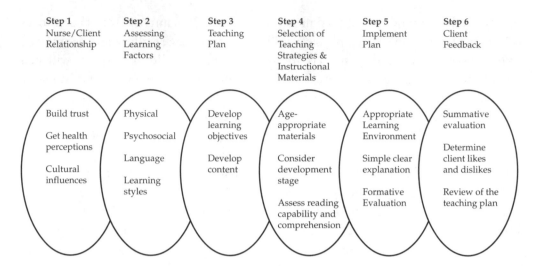

Step 1	Step 2	Step 3	Step 4	Step 5	Step 6
Nurse/Client Relationship	Assessing Learning Factors	Teaching Plan	Selection of Teaching Strategies & Instructional Materials	Implement Plan	Client Feedback

FIGURE 5-4   Health Education Process for Children.

WORKING WITH FAMILIES

Families have considerable influence on children's health practices and the success of health education. As an educator, you must consider the family as part of the unit of care when addressing the health education needs of children. Preparing teaching plans for child clients without considering the family may result in less than adequate adherence to the treatment recommendations.

A family is a "group of individuals with a continuing legal, genetic and/or emotional relationship. Society relies on the family group to provide for the economic and protective needs of individuals, especially children and the elderly" (American Academy of Family Physicians, 2003). Society's definition of family is rapidly expanding and has come to include single parents, biracial couples, blended families, unrelated individuals living cooperatively, and homosexual couples, among others.

It is important to determine who the immediate members of the family are, what roles they play within the structure of the family, their expectations about health care, and the nature of the relationships among family members. Not all families function the same way, so the nurse should assess this information by talking with clients and observing family interactions. Child health issues disrupt family functioning. The extent of disruption is dependent on the seriousness of the illness, the family's level of functioning before the illness, socioeconomic considerations, and the extent to which the illness disrupts family functioning.

Once aware of how the family operates, the nurse can work to address their health education needs. The most effective client education is that which is compatible with the family's frame of reference, and with which the client/family feels most comfortable. The nurse should asses the family's response to health teaching because the group's reaction can have a significant influence on the child and parents' motivation to continue and cooperate with recommended treatment.

WORKING WITH GROUPS AND COMMUNITIES

Nurses serve many different roles within the community. Public health nurses and school nurses assist children and families to take action to improve their health status. Often this takes the form of teaching parents and children about healthy life style choices. Public health nurses assist people in incorporating improved health behavior in their everyday lives. Ensuring children's health is critical not only for reducing child morbidity and mortality, but also for increasing the likelihood of a healthier adult life. The primary goal of child health education in the community is to prevent major causes of disease, illness, and death during childhood. Health prevention teaching covers the topics of accidental injuries, infections, learning problems, and behavioral problems. The nurse may also work within the school settings to develop action plans to support learning objectives.

Public health nurses educate clients concerning issues such as environmental risks, problems related to low family income, and psychological stress. Early detection and treatment of disease and disability requires screening, counseling, and interventions for high-risk populations. For children birth to age 10, screening includes measurement of height and weight, blood pressure, hearing, and vision. Counseling, or anticipatory guidance, relates to injury prevention, diet and exercise, substance use, and dental health. The nurse explains the importance of immunizations for children, which include diphtheria-tetanus-pertussis (DTaP), oral poliovirus, measles-mumps-rubella (MMR), H. influenza type B, hepatitis B, and varicella. For children older than age 10, additional screening recommendations include Pap smear and Chlamydia screening for sexually active females and assessment of problem drinking for adolescents. Counseling with this age group covers sexual behaviors, smoking, drinking, and other drug use. Immunizations for this age group include tetanus-diphtheria booster for those aged 11 to 16. Hepatitis B and varicella vaccines should be given to those who did not receive them at earlier ages. High-risk populations include those who engage in high-risk sexual behavior or drug use and those with certain medical conditions.

Often the nurse will inform families about services available to them. The nurse needs to be knowledgeable about community programs. Among the services that community programs provide are: health services for low-income families, supplemental nutritional programs, child care services, safe-houses for domestic violence, pediatric vaccine programs, and health education classes. One such nutrition program is the Women, Infants and Children Program (WIC). WIC provides federal grants to states for supplemental foods, healthcare referrals, and nutrition education for low-income pregnant, breastfeeding, and non breastfeeding postpartum women. It also provides help for infants and children up to age 5 who are found to be at nutritional risk. Another government service is Medicaid, which provides medical assistance for low-income families, mainly woman and children. SCHIP is insurance that is available for children not covered under Medicaid. A child must be younger than 19 in a family that is 200% below the poverty level. It is important for you to become familiar with services that can support health education, and evaluate funding requirements for which the family might be eligible.

WORKING WITH HEALTH TEAM MEMBERS

The nurse as educator works with a multidisciplinary healthcare team in many settings. Each member of the team brings skills that contribute to the overall health of the child. Ideally the team collaborates to develop individualized and comprehensive treatment plans that serve as the foundation for health education. Team members should

---

BOX 5-1   Evidence-Based Nursing Practice

Boweman, K. G., & Ruchala, P. L. (2006). A comparison of the postpartum learning needs of adolescent mothers and their mothers. *Journal of Obstetric, Gynecologic, and Neonatal Nursing, 35*(2), 250–256.

Purpose: This study described postpartum learning needs of adolescent mothers and their mothers, and compared the differences between the learning needs of the two groups.

Method: A descriptive cross-sectional survey design was used to assess the postpartum learning needs of a convenience sample of 100 women (50 mother/daughter pairs) in three Midwestern hospitals over 1 year.

Results: There were three group differences; emotional changes, resumption of sexual activity, and birth control. Results indicate that nurses may need to use different teaching strategies for adolescent mothers about resumption of sexual activity; however, teaching strategies for other topics may be the same.

include the child, family, primary care physician, specialty physicians if necessary, the nurse (nurse practitioner, home care nurse), and other healthcare professionals depending on the need. Other team members could include a social worker, patient care coordinator, pharmacist, dietitian, respiratory therapist, occupational therapist, physical therapist, speech pathologist, radiologist, psychiatrist/psychologist, school teacher, and the school nurse. It is important to view the child and family as an equal partner in the process of developing teaching plans. This type of client education is a family-centered and community-based approach (Box 5-1).

SUMMARY

This chapter reviewed the biologic characteristics, psychosocial stages, and developmental tasks of infants, toddlers, preschool, school age, and adolescent children. Implications for health education were given for each age group. Orientation to learning in children involves how children learn, learning styles in children, and the role of play in learning. Specific teaching practices are used to promote child learning. Pedagogic concepts assist you as the educator in preparing teaching plans. Working with families, groups, communities, and health team members brings together the importance of a multidisciplinary, holistic community-based approach to health education for children.

EXERCISES

Exercise I—Deepen Sensitivity to Child Clients and Their Families

Purpose: Practice application of child learning theory.

Directions: Visit a preschool and gather a group of 6 to 10 preschoolers.

1. You are teaching a health education class to a group of preschoolers. Compose a health promotion song with gestures, using the tune of a popular nursery song or popular song; for example, Safety the Snowman (to the tune of Frosty the Snowman).
2. Use props you have on hand to enhance the meaning of the song (e.g., bicycle helmets, street signs, etc.).
3. Share the songs with members of the class.
4. Discuss how you think the children learned the information.

Exercise II—Pretend Play

Purpose: Practice applying theory found this chapter with children.

Directions: Role-play a Baby Doll Clinic. Involve a nurse, children, and their dolls in a preschool setting.

1. Have the "mothers" come and see the nurse by walking into the (pretend) clinic or making an appointment on the (pretend) phone.
2. Have the nurse notice concern for the doll's health and ask what the mother wants (doll check-up or illness).
3. Have the nurse perform an examination, treatment, or give advice.
4. Ask a health or safety question about the doll.
5. Use real equipment or pretend you are using equipment.
6. Discuss what you have learned doing this exercise with your peers.

Exercise III—Helping Children with Chronic Illness

Purpose: Use knowledge of child development and learning strategies.

Directions: In small groups:

1. Describe an adolescent with a long-term chronic illness. Include information such as age, developmental needs, amount of regression, and how the illness interferes with normal developmental tasks.
2. Design substitute experiences that would enhance the child's chances for meeting appropriate developmental needs.

Exercise IV—Group Teaching with Children

Purpose: Apply child learning theory to working in groups.

Directions: Role-play the following teaching/learning scenario with school age children:

1. You are working with a group of fifth or sixth graders discussing a topic of your choice.
2. Choose topics such as peer pressure, drugs, sex, abuse, eating disorders, or bullying.
3. Lead the children in role playing and discussing a difficult situation.

4. Offer suggestions to address the problems that the children present; for example, how to develop refusal skills to drugs, or how to seek help for bullying.
5. Discuss what you have learned doing this exercise with your peers.

SUPPLEMENTAL ONLINE RESOURCES

Erikson's Stages of Psychosocial Development:
http://psychology.about.com/od/theoriesofpersonality/a/psychosocial.htm
Child and Teen Health:
http://health.nih.gov/category/ChildTeenHealth
Oxford Brooks University, theories of learning:
http://www.brookes.ac.uk/services/ocsd/2_learntch/theories.html
Save Kids USA:
http://www.usa.safekids.org/
Life Stages and Specific Populations:
http://www.cdc.gov/LifeStages/
Baby Steps: Learn the Signs, Act Early:
http://www.cdc.gov/CDCtv/BabySteps/
Robert Wood Johnson Information about Children State by State:
http://www.commissiononhealth.org/StateByStateData.aspx
Motivation theory:
http://ezinearticles.com/?Motivation-Theory&id=410700
National Council on Patient Information and Education:
http://www.talkaboutrx.org/

REFERENCES

American Academy of Family Physicians. (2003). Definition of Family. Retrieved on June 18, 2009 from http://www.aafp.org/online/en/home/policy/policies/f/familydefinitionof.html

Athey, C. (2007). *Extending thought in young children: A parent teacher partnership* (2nd ed.). London: Paul Chaptman Educational Publishing.

Bellamy, C. (2002) Opening Plenary Statement to Special Session of the General Assembly on Children. Retrieved on June 20, 2009 from http://www.unicef.org/media/media_9532.html

Carbo, M, Dunn, R., & Dunn, K. (1986). *Teaching students to read through their individual learning styles.* Englewood Cliffs, NJ: Prentice-Hall.

David, T., Goouch, D., Powell, S., & Abbott, L. (2003). *Birth to three matters: A review of the literature.* Research Report 444. London: DfES. Retrieved on July 22, 2009 from http://www.dcsf.gov.uk/research/data/uploadfiles/RR444.pdf

Davis, E. C., Nur, H., & Ruru, S. A. (1994). Helping teachers and students understand learning styles. *English Teaching Forum, 32*(3), 12–15.

Ebbinghaus, S., & Bahrainwala, A. H. (2003). Asthma management by an inpatient asthma care team. *Pediatric Nursing, 29*(3), 177–183.

Erikson, E. (1963). *Childhood and society* (2nd ed.). New York: W.W. Norton.

Falvo, D. R. (2004). *Effective patient education: A guide to increased compliance.* Sudbury, MA: Jones and Bartlett.

Graca, S., Fowler, K., & Rosenstock A. (2009). Play—an educational tool in health care. In Lowenstein, A., Foord-May, L., & Romano, J. C. *Teaching strategies for health education and health promotion: Working with patients, families and communities.* Sudbury, MA: Jones and Bartlett.

Hiemstra, R., & Sisco, B. (1990). *Individualizing instruction.* San Francisco: Jossey-Bass.

James, W., & Galbraith, M. (1984). Perceptual learning styles: Implications and techniques for the practitioner. *Lifelong Learning, 8*(4), 23.

Jones, E., & Reynolds, G. (1992). *The play's the thing: Teachers' roles in children's play.* New York: Teachers College Press.

Kearsley, G. (1994 to 2009). Explorations in Learning and Instruction: The Theory Into Practice Database. Retrieved on June 18, 2009 from http://tip.psychology.org/

National Institute on Deafness and Other Communication Disorders (NIDCD). (2009). Speech and Language Developmental Milestones. Part of NIH retrieved on June 20, 2009 from http://www.nidcd.nih.gov/health/voice/speechandlanguage.asp#mychild

Olsen, M. H., & Hergenhahn, B. R. (2009). *An introduction to theories of learning* (8th ed.). Upper Saddle River, NJ: Pearson Prentice-Hall.

Perkins, D. J. (1997). Fact Sheet FCS 2118, a series of the Department of Family, Youth and Community Sciences, Florida Cooperative Extension Service, Institute of Food and Agricultural Sciences, University of Florida. Retrieved on June 20, 2009 from http://edis.ifas.ufl.edu/HE820#FOOTNOTE_2

Piaget, J. (1952). *The origins of intelligence in children.* New York: International Universities Press.

Piaget, J. (1963, 2001). *The psychology of intelligence.* New York: Routledge.

Skinner, B. F. (1968). *The technology of teaching.* New York: Appleton-Century-Crofts.

The Association for Child Education International (ACEI) (2005). *Resolution for play.* Resolutions presented and accepted by ACEI members at the Annual Business Meeting on March 25, 2005. Retrieved on June 20, 2009 from http://www.acei.org/05resolutions.htm

United Nations. Convention on the Rights of the Child, G.A. res. 44/25, annex, 44 U.N. GAOR Supp. (No. 49) at 167, U.N. Doc. A/44/49 (1989). Entered into force Sept. 2, 1990. Retrieved on June 20, 2009 from http://www1.umn.edu/humanrts/instree/k2crc.htm

Woodring, B. C. (2000). If you have taught—have the child and family learned? *Pediatric Nursing, 26*(5), 505–509.

Wong, D. L., Hockenberry-Eaton, M., Wilson, D., Winkelstein, M. L., & Schwartz, P. (2008). *Wong's essentials of pediatric nursing* (6th ed.). St. Louis: Mosby Elsevier.

CHAPTER 6

The Adult Learner

A technological transformation during the past decade
has eliminated the boundaries between
formal and informal learning.
As we adapt to a knowledge-driven society,
a cultural transformation is occurring.
Lifelong learning is an essential goal of education
as a means to improve the quality of life
for an individual, a culture, or a society.
—Derrick, M. G., 2003, p. 5

OBJECTIVES

Upon completion of this chapter you will be able to:

- Describe the biologic changes, psychosocial stages, and developmental tasks characteristic of early and middle adulthood.
- List health education topics for clients in early and middle adulthood related to biologic changes, psychosocial stages, and developmental tasks.
- Distinguish among goal, activity, and learning-oriented learners and state which category best fits your motivation.
- Distinguish between pedagogy and andragogy.
- Describe how adult and child learners are alike and different in two of the assumptions of andragogy.
- Apply andragogic theory to teaching adult learners.
- Identify teaching and learning implications of working with individuals, families, groups/communities, and health team members.

KEY TERMS

activity-oriented learner	intrinsic motivation
andragogy	learning-oriented learner
developmental task	pedagogy
extrinsic motivation	psychosocial stage
goal-oriented learner	

INTRODUCTION

This chapter continues the discussion of the previous chapter on child learners and progresses to learning in adulthood, dividing this period into early and middle adulthood. Learning and development are lifelong processes with identifiable features, including biologic characteristics, psychosocial stages, and developmental tasks. Learning and development are multidimensional and unique for each client with implications for those who are seeking to promote, retain, and restore health.

Nurses work with clients of all ages with different learning needs and at different stages of development. This information is important because it affects what you teach as well as how you teach it. The first section of this chapter examines the biologic characteristics, psychosocial stages, developmental tasks, and their implications for nurses as educators. Andragogy, a theory of adult learning, and its underlying assumptions are examined. We describe how andragogy differs from pedagogy, the theory of how children learn.

BIOLOGIC CHARACTERISTICS, PSYCHOSOCIAL STAGES, AND DEVELOPMENTAL TASKS

Adulthood is divided into two periods: early and middle. This division is made because the biologic characteristics, psychosocial stages, and developmental tasks that accompany these periods are distinct. Figure 6-1 illustrates the overlapping influence of these factors.

Early Adulthood (Early Twenties Through the Thirties)

Biologic Characteristics

Clients complete their physical growth and experience peak functioning of the musculoskeletal system in their twenties. Laboratory findings are generally within normal limits. The health status of men and women is generally uneventful unless severe illness or injury occurs. Women have additional health concerns during pregnancy and lactation. The occurrence of chronic disease is unusual but can occur in this period (Ruchala, 2009; Santrock, 2008).

Psychosocial Stages

Chapter 5 introduced Erikson's (1963) psychosocial stages for the early years, and we resume that discussion here for the early and middle adult. Recall that during puberty

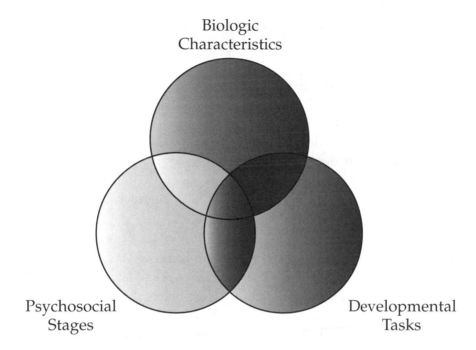

Biologic
Characteristics

Psychosocial
Stages

Developmental
Tasks

FIGURE 6-1   Factors Influencing Development Across the Lifespan.

the psychosocial stage was *identity versus role confusion*, from which a sense of identity develops. As young adults continue to mature, they move into Erikson's next stage, *intimacy versus isolation*, a stage characterized by an increasing ability to love and care about others. They seek meaningful friendships and intimacy with others (Balakas, 2009). It is also at this stage that young adults clarify their values, understand themselves and others better, and develop a philosophy of life (Knowles, 1990). It is the longest of Erikson's psychosocial stages covering the years from 40 to 65.

Developmental Tasks

Becoming economically independent, establishing a career, and developing job-related skills are important tasks during this time. Making new friends and selecting a mate or significant other, starting a family, and rearing children are common tasks. Learning to get along with others at work, one's mate, and friends are other tasks. Dealing with ethnic and gender factors, changing role expectations in the United States, and the need for two-career families are stressors that influence these tasks (Santrock, 2008).

Middle Adulthood (Forties to Late Sixties)

Biologic Characteristics

Clients in this stage begin to experience gradual physical changes, the rate of which can vary widely among individuals. Changes are influenced by genetic and life style factors. Clients tend to gain weight, skin begins to wrinkle and loosen, hair turns gray, muscle mass and strength decline, blood pressure and cholesterol levels may increase. Vision and hearing acuity decreases, women experience menopause, and men experience climacteric, which is similar to menopause. Cognitive functioning remains intact unless affected by illness or injury (Ruchala, 2009; Santrock, 2008).

Psychosocial Stages

Erikson's (1963) stage for this period is *generativity versus self-absorption and stagnation* with a focus on helping the younger generation develop and lead useful lives. Generativity refers to the concern mature adults have for guiding the next generation. It includes being productive and creative. If they have children, parents may help them choose a suitable career. Cultural interests increase, as does social involvement and leadership responsibilities in organizations and the community (Knowles, 1990; Santrock, 2008).

Developmental Tasks

Clients are learning advanced job skills, often supervising others. Some are dealing with unemployment. If so, clients may be looking for new careers or educational opportunities to acquire new skills (Knowles, 1990). Cultural interests increase, as does social involvement with others. As children leave home, spouses must readjust their marital relationship. If divorce occurs, further life style adjustments are needed. Stay-at-home mothers may return to the job market. These clients may have living parents who require time and financial attention. Because adults in this stage are still involved with raising their children and caring for aging parents, they are called the sandwich generation (Knowles, 1990; Santrock, 2008).

Implications for Health Education

How does this information help you become more sensitive and effective in your role as an educator? We look at how this information helps you to promote, retain, and restore the health of your clients.

Promote and Retain Health

The focus of promoting health is on prevention, whereas the focus of retaining health is on maintaining one's present health status, assuming it is satisfactory. With this in mind, Table 6-1 lists suggested topics to promote and retain health appropriate for adult learners (Ruchala, 2009). These suggestions are not all-inclusive and will need to be adapted to the circumstances of the individual client.

TABLE 6-1 Suggested Topics to Promote and Retain Health	
Nursing Assessment	**Health Education Topics**
General health habits	• Eating nutritious diet with dietary changes to control weight • Practicing regular oral hygiene and dental care • Obtaining adequate sleep • Knowing benefits of an exercise program • Managing physical stress • Coping with mental stress, e.g., depression • Minimizing risks of disease for which there is a family history, e.g., diabetes mellitus, cardiovascular disease
General living conditions	• Avoiding exposure to hazardous cleaning supplies • Maintaining home safety for elderly and children (slip-resistant rugs, night lights, nonskid adhesive textured strips in tub, shower, handrails on steps, grab bars in bathrooms, electrical outlets, etc.) • Maintaining cleanliness in the home • Managing family stress/abuse
Medications	• Using prescription medications properly • Minimizing use of caffeine, tobacco, alcohol • Avoiding/dangers of illicit drugs • Promoting medication safety with children in the home
Sexual habits	• Preventing sexually transmitted diseases • Knowing mode of STD transmission • Knowing partner's sexual history and practices • Practicing safe sexual practices • Recognizing STD symptoms

(continues)

TABLE 6-1 Suggested Topics to Promote and Retain Health *(continued)*	
Nursing Assessment	**Health Education Topics**
Pregnancy/children	• Knowing about family planning • Addressing pregnancy and lactation issues • Knowing child growth and developmental stages • Obtaining immunizations • Parenting skills
Worksite/employment	• Maintaining safe occupational environment • Avoiding exposure to hazardous substances • Minimizing economic stress • Minimizing job stress
Disease prevention	• Getting routine health screening, blood pressure checks • Knowing serum cholesterol levels • Performing monthly skin checks • Obtaining monthly breast exam/annual mammogram • Performing monthly male genitalia exam • Obtaining annual flu shots • Getting regular physical and screening exams

Restore Health

Restoration of health for individuals in adulthood refers to addressing the needs of those who are experiencing an acute or chronic illness or disability. The purpose of health education at this time is designed to help clients understand the nature of their health problem, the treatment regimen, and the limitations imposed by the health problem, disability, or injury. This may involve not only working with clients, but also with family members. Table 6-2 suggests suitable topics related to the restoration of health (Ruchala, 2009). These suggestions are not all-inclusive and need to be adapted to the circumstances of the individual client.

TABLE 6-2 Suggested Topics to Restore Health	
Nursing Assessment	**Health Education Topics**
Acute illness	• Knowing nature and cause of the health problem or disability • Common conditions: upper respiratory infections, urinary tract infections, minor surgery, substance abuse • Understanding diagnostic tests • Supporting/explaining treatment regimen • Knowing hospital/clinic environment and routines • Preventing spread of communicable illness • Dealing with life style changes • Supporting continued physician supervision
Chronic illness	• Knowing nature and cause of the health problem or disability • Possible conditions: multiple sclerosis, rheumatoid arthritis, hypertension, diabetes mellitus, AIDS, cancer, substance abuse • Understanding diagnostic tests • Using physical, occupational, speech therapies • Managing exacerbations/remissions • Preventing complications • Adapting to life style changes • Making environmental adaptations • Using self-help devices • Supporting/explaining treatment regimen • Supporting continued provider supervision
Disability	• Knowing strengths/limitations of disability • Managing activities of daily living • Building on abilities
Accidents	• Adapting to nature of injury and impact on function • Managing activities of daily living • Building on abilities • Addressing rehabilitation issues • Preventing accidents/injury • Providing safe home environment (slip-resistant rugs, night lights, nonskid adhesive textured strips in tub, shower, handrails on steps, grab bars in bathrooms, etc.)

ORIENTATION TO LEARNING

Houle (1961, 1980) found that adults continue learning for a variety of reasons. He identified three categories that describe adults' general orientation to learning: goal-oriented learners, activity-oriented learners, and learning-oriented learners.

Goal-Oriented Learners

Goal-oriented learners use their educational endeavors to accomplish clear and identifiable objectives. They often wait until their middle twenties to make a start on their education and sometimes much later. Their educational activities tend to occur in episodes, each beginning with the realization of a need or an interest to expand their skills and knowledge. Houle (1961, 1980) found that learning was a recurring pattern in their lives. These learners were not restricted to an academic setting or to any one institution or topic. They sought courses of instruction or other forms of learning when they became aware of a need. Exploration on the Internet, attending night courses, and enrolling in workshops were ways to add to their level of expertise.

Activity-Oriented Learners

Activity-oriented learners select activities that are likely to meet their need for human contact. They are "course takers" and "group joiners." The course content or purpose of the organization is secondary to their social needs. These learners often begin their educational activities when their need to reach out to others becomes pressing. For example, divorce adjustment groups attract people attempting to fill specific needs. A young mother joins a La Leche group to fulfill her need for socialization as well as for support and information to breastfeed successfully. A divorced man takes a class in astronomy to talk to other people and ease his loneliness.

When setting up health education programs for adult learners, it is helpful to assess their interests via a survey. Although many adults indicate specific interests, a substantial number just want something to do and seek out classes for social reasons. You should become aware of community support groups and consider this category of learning activities whenever social isolation and loneliness is encountered. Newspapers periodically print lists of self-help and special interest groups. You should include such lists in your resource files and maintain connections in the community.

Learning-Oriented Learners

Learning-oriented individuals seek knowledge for its own sake. Often they have been engrossed in learning all of their lives and are avid readers. These individuals see themselves as lifelong learners and investigate everything of interest. They join groups, classes, and organizations they anticipate will be educational. An example of this is a learner who joins a books discussion group at the local library. When these learners travel, they prepare for trips by engaging in activities that make the trips more informative. They read about their destination in books, periodicals, on the Internet, or they might take a language course.

Figure 6-2 summarizes Houle's (1961, 1980) three orientations to learning. Most people find that they fit into each of the categories at different times in their lives. People find that they emphasize one category more often than others. Houle concluded that most adults engage in continuing education every year, which are planned by learners themselves. He also noted that people do not have to fit into only one

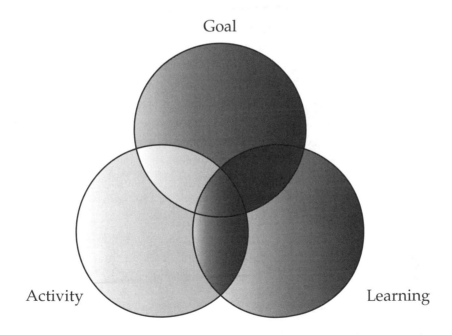

FIGURE 6-2 Primary Orientations to Learning. Individuals learn for different reasons; three primary orientations to learning are goal, activity, and learning.

category. His generalizations were meant to clarify motivations rather than to confine people to categories.

ANDRAGOGY

Adults learn differently than children; to explain this process, Malcolm Knowles (1990) developed a theory of learning called andragogy. His theory is about the art and science of how adults learn. Knowles' theory has its roots in the work of Abraham Maslow and Carl Rogers, who were concerned with self-actualization of the individual and a pragmatic philosophy that values knowledge gained from experience rather than formal authority (Knowles, Holton, & Swanson, 2005).

Knowles contrasted how children learn (pedagogy) in the formal education system with how adults learn (andragogy). The forces that impinge on educating young children have more to do with achieving than with learning. He cited passing tests, scoring high on the Scholastic Aptitude Test, and getting into college or graduate school as the goals of much formal education (Knowles, 1990). He noted that many of the assumptions that underlie the teaching methods used for adults were derived from pedagogy and are inappropriate for adults. He observed that adults learn best in informal, comfortable, flexible, and nonthreatening settings and consequently popularized a different set of assumptions, also called core principles, which apply to all adult learning situations. The assumptions that form the foundation of Knowles theory are: (1) the need to know, (2) the learners' self-concept, (3) the role of the learners' experiences, (4) readiness to learn, (5) orientation to learning, and (6) motivation to learn. These assumptions are discussed in the following section (Knowles et al., 2005; Russell, 2006) along with healthcare examples.

The Need to Know

Adults want to understand why they should learn something new before they are willing to learn it. Adults who initiate new learning projects on their own spend considerable time and effort weighing the cost/benefit ratio before they expend large amounts of time and energy on new projects.

Application to Health Education

In your introductory remarks with adult clients in any individual or group teaching and learning situation, explain the importance of the instructional content and identify the benefits of learning it. Persuade them about the importance of learning the material by making it attractive and interesting. If you are working with a group, each individual has joined it for a different reason, so another approach would be to ask the clients what motivates them to be present and have them share their thoughts with the group. As an educator, this gives you some sense of what motivates each individual and why they are present. Do this by asking questions such as:

- "What do you hope to get from this lesson?"
- "What do you expect from our time together?"
- "What is the best outcome you hope for?"
- "Why have you come out on this beautiful/awful day?"

Another approach is to set up situations in which clients discover for themselves the likely benefits of their efforts. For example, a new first-time mother may have a multitude of questions about the care of her baby. As you work with the mother, ask her questions such as:

- "What are your plans for caring for your baby at home?"
- "Have you thought about the equipment you will need at home to care for your baby?"
- "Will you have any help at home in caring for your baby?"
- "What are your concerns about the care of your new baby?"
- "Is there anything that worries you about the care of your baby?"

The Learners' Self-Concept

As individuals grow into adulthood, they increasingly see themselves as responsible beings in charge of their own lives and capable of making their own decisions. Having achieved maturity, adults wish to be respected and treated as being capable of self-direction. Any attempt to treat them as uninformed children in need of direction in the teaching and learning situation is considered demeaning. It is important to avoid talking down to clients.

Application to Health Education

This need for self-direction often presents a problem for you and clients because the situation may necessitate some client dependency. In the hospital you have information about the acutely ill client's physiologic status and you will be in a better position to decide what information is helpful for them to know. During certain stages of illness the client may relinquish some control and trust your judgment and expert care. You can gently guide them in appropriate learning at this time.

Some clients who become dependent may respond with fear, bitterness, and sarcasm to relinquishing their independence. For example, an older man was rude to the nurses who cared for him while he was suffering from incontinence. He was accustomed to being the boss and his strong self-concept was being challenged by the reality of his new dependency. The nurses were matter-of-fact and unperturbed while changing his soiled linen. As the nurses worked, they taught him that his incontinence was temporary and control would return with time and healing. They understood this response and treated him with respect and courtesy even though he was angry and rude.

Health problems may evoke feelings of unmet dependency needs in the client and complementary issues in you, such as the need to control. An example is a nurse who experiences a dependency problem when dealing with burn clients. The nurse thinks, "If only they would do what I say, they will learn that they will feel and look better in the long run. They do not understand that not moving will effect burn healing. It is up to me to teach them about the consequences of immobility before it is too late. They need to listen to me." This nurse wanted the clients to trust her advice and depend on her. In addition, the nurse is adamant about the nurse's role and her expected behavior of clients. In this case the nurse as educator needs to reflect upon her need to control and take a more empathetic approach to the clients.

The Role of the Learners' Experiences

As people mature, they accumulate an expanding reservoir of experiences, both in quantity and quality. Based on these experiences, adults are able to handle more complex issues and make more thoughtful decisions that take into consideration a number of variables. Experience is something that happens to children, but for adults experience is what defines them. A way to check out this assumption is to ask people of various ages, "Tell me about yourself." You will hear differences in the way children and adults answer.

Application to Health Education

Adults bring a wide range of health experiences that nurses as educators can draw on as a group discusses common issues. Nurses guide the discussion by being a facilitator of learning and provide new information as appropriate. This is in contrast to lecturing to the group with little or no time for discussion. Some members of a group may have more experience with a particular issue than the nurse, and that person can become a resource for the group. For example, a small group of diabetic clients met weekly to discuss their experiences in dealing with this disease. The nurse shared information about the physicians' medical regimen. Several clients in the group who had grappled with diabetes for more than 10 years explained the difficulties of balancing insulin intake, exercise, and nutritional requirements. By encouraging clients to share their experiences, the nurse tapped into a rich reservoir of experience to take advantage of the expertise of group members.

Adult clients learn better when strategies are employed that respect a broad base of knowledge and experience and that make use of it in the teaching and learning situation. Strategies such as discussion, laboratory, simulation, field experience, team projects, and other action-learning approaches are more conducive to the way adults learn and have strong experiential and integrating components. A good place to start is to ask adults what experiences they have had on the topic and then listen to how they interpret that experience and what it meant to them. For example, in teaching team members about a new urinary catheterization procedure, the nurse asked what their past experience has been. Have they done a similar procedure before? Were they familiar with the new equipment? What was their reaction to the new procedure? The nurse listened carefully to what was said and prepared the teaching plan accordingly.

Sometimes having extensive experience is a hindrance to learning according to Knowles (1990). Habits, biases, and presuppositions become a hindrance when the person is not open to looking at health issues in new and different ways. The nurses' role in these situations is to help clients examine troublesome and unresolved health issues and then guide them in looking for alternative ways of doing things. Nurses can encourage clients to examine health habits that are not working for them and find creative ways to make changes.

In summary, it is important to recognize adult learners' experiences and contributions. If their experiences are ignored or devalued, they will likely reject efforts to learn in new ways. We believe this phenomenon is behind the resentment that some adults express when they return to school after years of earning a living and are not respected for what they have accomplished.

Readiness to Learn

It is assumed that children are ready to learn according to their biologic development and academic progress. Developmental readiness is also necessary for adults' learning. The needs of adults, however, are related less to their biologic maturation and more to the developing roles in life that they have chosen or have had thrust upon them. A nurse's first pregnancy is an example. "I was a good student and did well in my OB/GYN experiences and state board examinations. Some years later, when I was pregnant, I went to child birth education classes and was amazed at what I did not know. I listened with keener attention and made many associations that had not occurred to me when I was learning how to attend to women in labor and delivery. My increased interest was caused by a change in role. Now I was the one who was entering the role of pregnant woman and expectant parent."

Readiness to learn in the adult is associated with the ability to meet the developmental tasks associated with each stage in life. Adults face real-life situations and want to learn whatever will help them cope with their present circumstances and evolving social roles. Developing job skills and a professional identity, earning a living, meeting community responsibilities, establishing successful relationships, raising a family, and aging gracefully are some examples of these tasks.

Application to Health Education

Adults often seek out knowledge and skills based on a current health need at a particular time in their lives. Perhaps clients encounter a problem or situation and recognize that they do not have the knowledge or experience to handle it. Many adults are self-directed and find the information they need in the local library or in a class offering at a local college or community learning center. For example, a class entitled "How to Remember" was offered in a setting that attracted retired citizens who had the time, energy, and resources to attend. The enrollment was high because the topic was on memory. Older people experience difficulty in remembering and find it a blow to their self-concept when they are forgetful. This workshop offered attendees an opportunity to address an important need.

Knowles (1990) noted that it is not always necessary to wait for readiness to learn to develop. You can foster readiness through experiences you create when you expose clients to successful role models. For example, encourage clients to participate in community-sponsored health fairs designed to prevent illness and detect early evidence of disease. When clients attend health education classes, they learn how to live more healthfully and how to prevent illness. By anticipating the future, clients can prepare themselves emotionally and intellectually if problems develop.

Orientation to Learning

Adults want to learn when it helps them perform a task or deal more effectively with current problems. This approach to learning is in contrast with learning that occurs in the formal educational system, in which the teacher decides what is to be learned and how the subject matter is to be organized. Adults want learning that helps them in the here and now, not learning that will be useful some time in the future.

Andragogy assumes that adults learn better when life- or task-centered problems are the organizing factor. Adults are reluctant to expend their resources (time, money, and energy) to learn information, skills, and attitudes that they do not see as directly relevant to their current lives or problems they anticipate having. When you take a continuing education program or enroll in a degree advancing program, you want to know, "How can I use this when I go to work tomorrow?"

Application to Health Education

Adult clients expect nurses as educators to be knowledgeable and experientially familiar with the health issues they face. Clients expect health professionals to be in touch with real-life challenges in current society. They look for nurses who show empathy for their situation and respond to them in a professional manner. For example, one popular diabetic nurse was introduced to a group as "one of those nurses who works with diabetic clients in the clinic and has diabetes herself." Adults find information easier to grasp when it is presented in a practical life context. When clients say, "Give us an example," they want you to present a real-life example to which they can relate. Another valuable approach is to set up a simulation or interactive exercise and offer clients the opportunity to role play appropriate behavior in a safe setting.

Organization of content is important to learning and good teaching. Your challenge is to develop an effective teaching plan. A good place to begin is the development of learning objectives to meet the client's needs. This should be a collaborative effort between you and the client. Once the objectives are developed, the teaching plan is organized. A good principle is to teach from the simple to the complex. Clients appreciate content that is presented from the simple to the complex and within a context to which they can relate. Other principles are to use a logical train of thought and to promote association. There are times when presenting the concept and then following it with more specific applications is the most effective way of teaching. There are other times when experiencing a number of events and then looking for their relationship to one another is more meaningful. The point is worth repeating. Once learning objectives are in place, organization of content is important. The most effective type of organization will vary with the objectives, the client, you, and the situation.

Motivation to Learn

According to Knowles (1990), the most effective motivators for adults are internal pressures and personal reasons; some examples of these are the desire for increased job satisfaction, self-esteem, quality of life, etc. Adults also respond to external motivators; for example, they may strive for a better job, a promotion, or a higher salary. Santrock (2008) calls these intrinsic and extrinsic motivators. Intrinsic motivators are like Knowles' internal pressures and are characteristic of an individual who does something for its own sake; for example, the adult may study literature because it is enjoyable. Extrinsic motivators are like Knowles' external motivators, which occur when an individual does something to obtain a reward or avoid a punishment, as noted.

Adults seek out learning experiences for a variety of reasons. Merriam, Caffarella, and Baumgartner (2007), quoting Boshier (1991), identifies seven factors that motivate adults to continue learning: (1) improvement of verbal and written skills, (2) social interaction with others, (3) remediation of past deficiencies, (4) improvement of career or job status, (5) improvement of family relationships, (6) social stimulation, and (7) following interests, seeking new knowledge. These are broad-based and powerful motivators for adults seeking to continue learning.

Carl Rogers (1961) and Abraham Maslow (1987) demonstrated that adults are motivated toward self-improvement and continued growth. In Maslow's terminology, adults strive for self-actualization. However, barriers such as negative self-concept, inability to access resources, time constraints, and programs that violate adult learning principles all interfere with the growth process. Our own experiences as clinicians and teachers working with clients of different ages and abilities leads us to believe that these principles have broad application.

Application to Health Education

During times of illness and stress, clients are more motivated to make changes and modifications to improve their health status. Often health-altering events cause clients to seek help for themselves or their family members. The nurse as educator asks, What is the nature of the client's problem, and what kind of adaptations will he or she have to make? How life-altering are these adaptations; e.g., are they life style changes or do they involve a lengthy rehabilitation regimen? Is the client temporarily or permanently disabled? Depending on the seriousness of the health problem, clients undergo several stages of adjustment and most become motivated to improve their health status.

Nurses also see clients who are undergoing stressful life situations that compound health problems they are experiencing. For example, consider clients going through role changes and life transitions: changing careers requiring new skills, from childless couple to parents, and from being employed to unemployed. A life transition is the process that individuals undergo when their roles change dramatically, as in the death of a significant other, birth, marriage, divorce, moving from a stable environment, and making a radical work change. A life transition may force clients to make a paradigm shift in their thinking. As an educator, you can capture these moments when clients are amenable and motivated to hear your suggestions and encouragement. These times are what educators call teachable moments. It is a time when you have clients' full attention.

Table 6-3 compares the different assumptions of pedagogy and andragogy as those assumptions affect the approach to learning. This information is important because it influences how you approach clients of different ages. It is the theoretical knowledge that undergirds your teaching plan and your approach to health education. Although Table 6-3 makes a distinction between pedagogy and andragogy, principles of andragogy have been reported to be effective in teaching younger clients (Knowles, Holton, & Swanson, 2005; O'Shea, 2003).

TABLE 6-3   A Comparison of Assumptions of Pedagogic and Andragogic Approaches to Learning

Assumptions About Learning	Pedagogy	Andragogy
Need to know	Teacher driven; accepted by learner	Learner driven
Self-concept	Accepts direction from teacher	Self-directed
Role of experience	Happens to the learner	Integrally involved with self-concept; must be acknowledged
Readiness to learn	Biologic and academic development	Evolving social and life roles
Orientation to learning	Subject centered; selected by the teacher	Life-centered; task and problem centered
Motivation	External approval by the teacher	Internal drives and life goals

Modified from Knowles, 1990; Knowles *et al.*, 2005.

EXPERIENTIAL LEARNING

Learning in adulthood is also viewed from experiential learning theory, an approach that combines experience, perception, cognition, and behavioral learning theories. Personal experiences serve as sources of learning and contribute to adult development. Although experiential learning theory is applicable to individuals in all life stages from childhood to old age (Kolb, 1984), we believe it is especially suitable for working with adult clients who have accumulated a wealth of life experiences.

Recall the discussion about Kolb's (1984) model for experiential learning in Chapter 2. From adults' concrete experiences, they formulate observations and reflect on those experiences. This leads to the formation of abstract concepts and generalizations, theories about effective and ineffectiveness. Following this, adults test the implications of new concepts in new situations. Through personal experiences, they continuously modify their thoughts, concepts, and ideas of the world and their environment (Kolb, 1984). In this model, it is not necessarily the outcome that is important; it is the process of learning that is the focus.

Implications for Health Education

Teaching strategies that combine theory and practice with practical application are most effective for adults. Because learning is grounded in experience, not all experiences have resulted in accurate knowledge. Nurses as educators can implant new ideas and information to revise inaccurate perceptions. It is often helpful to begin teaching by asking learners what they know about the topic. If they express inaccurate beliefs and information, discuss these with the client. Nurses are responsible to modify these beliefs by presenting accurate information, but may encounter client resistance to new information. Clients must then decide if they will integrate, substitute, or reject this new information. Recall Figure 3-2, Assimilation and Accommodation.

WORKING WITH FAMILIES

Illness affects not only the client, but also the client's family and significant others. When clients need assistance from others, nurses must be sensitive to their wishes about the degree to which they want family and significant others participating in their health education. Some clients value their privacy, whereas other clients want family and significant others involved. If clients require procedures and follow-up care that they are unable to do themselves, they may request that others be involved. In all cases, it is important to avoid embarrassing clients by sharing unnecessary information with family or significant others. If clients want family and significant others involved, then reveal only information that is essential for communicating the health message.

WORKING WITH GROUPS AND COMMUNITIES

Many social groups, civic organizations, educational institutions, and industries are interested in health education and are looking for guest speakers. If you have a specialty area, consider making yourself available to these groups. It will build your confidence and you will realize ways to contribute to your community. For example, nursing students were invited to present a program on healthful living to members of a local church. Each took a topic and kept their remarks pertinent, brief, and supplemented them with colorful audiovisual aids. They talked about the benefits of good nutrition, adequate sleep, daily exercise, and mental stimulation through a variety of activities. The audience listened and had questions following the students' presentation. Other nursing students met with women members of another church and taught them about early detection of breast cancer. They taught breast self-examination through a video presentation followed by demonstration of the technique on breast models. Both were successful events supported by the fact that many of the women scheduled mammograms at a nearby hospital.

When presenting health education to a group in the community, be sure to make it lively and interesting by using a variety of teaching strategies and instructional materials. Announce your presentation in advance by publishing it in a local newsletter or community newspaper to attract an audience. Doing so provides time for the audience to work it into their daily schedule. Also, give your presentation an interesting and catchy title, something that creates interest. Perhaps the place where you will make your presentation will help to advertise it. When making the presentation, use teaching strategies that encourage active participation such as providing time for discussion. Also plan time for questions and clarification to ensure your message is understood. Active participation stimulates interest. Your presentation will be remembered longer if those attending actively participate.

WORKING WITH HEALTH TEAM MEMBERS

Some of today's care providers have little formal healthcare training, such as nursing assistants, who usually receive about 6 weeks of training. Consequently, some health education may be directed to team member with whom you work. In planning health education for team members, you must know the provisions of the nurse practice act in your state to know the scope of practice for each team member, such as the nursing assistant, licensed practical nurse, and registered nurse. You must also know the general policies and practice guidelines of your employer. Acute care institutions have in-service education departments that handle continuing education for employees but long-term care facilities may or may not.

If it is your responsibility to provide health education to team members, you should first assess their learning needs through either a formal or informal survey. You can also determine learning needs by observing team members as you work with them. While developing learning objectives, keep in mind the three learning domains, cognitive, affective, and psychomotor, and consider in which domain team members need health education. For example, does a team member lack knowledge about the client's health problem and rationale for treatment (cognitive domain)? Is a team member biased in his or her attitude toward caring for certain patients (affective domain)? Does a team member need to refresh his or her skills in performing nursing care procedures (psychomotor domain)? Once you have determined the learning domain in which health education is needed, write the learning objectives. Your next step is to determine how the content should be taught and whether or not it can be done so informally on the job or formally away from the patient care unit. Once this

---

BOX 6-1   Evidence-Based Nursing Practice

Purpose: This study examined older adults' expectations and experiences with cardiac rehabilitation programs.

Method: A descriptive design was used with a convenience sample of 40 older adults from a large urban teaching hospital who had experienced an acute cardiac event to identify their views of cardiac rehabilitation programs using focus groups and individual interviews.

Results: The participants did not have an accurate understanding of what to expect in cardiac rehabilitation programs; however, their experiences with these programs were generally positive. The participants suggested that cardiac rehabilitation programs could be improved by including more socialization opportunities, offering varied forms of exercise, enhancing teaching about stress management, and adapting teaching strategies. A major finding was the report of adverse events during exercise experienced by individuals who did not go to a cardiac rehabilitation program.

Dolansky, M. A., Moore, S. M., & Viscovsky, C. (2006). Older adults' views of cardiac rehabilitation programs. *Journal of Gerontological Nursing, 32*(2), 37–44.

decision is made, select teaching strategies and instructional materials to meet team members' needs. Following your teaching, you need to assess the effectiveness of your teaching. Detailed information about how to prepare a teaching plan is found in subsequent chapters in this text beginning with Chapter 9.

SUMMARY

As adults deal with changes in their business, personal, and professional lives, they realize that learning is, indeed, a lifelong process. Learning in adulthood is influenced by needs related to biologic characteristics, psychosocial stages, and developmental tasks. Adults continue their learning for a variety of reasons, some to meet goals, others for social reasons, and others for the love of learning. Health-related topics to promote, retain, and restore health are numerous and should be individualized for specific client situations.

The assumptions of andragogy were explored and contrasted to pedagogy. Adults engage in learning activities because they have a need to know, perhaps knowledge related to employment or personal issues. Adults want to be respected as competent, capable of self-direction, and valued for their life experiences. Other assumptions of andragogy include readiness to learn, orientation to learning, and motivation to learn. Health education opportunities occur with individuals, families, and groups/communities, as well as with health team members.

EXERCISES

Exercise I—Contrasting Pedagogy and Andragogy

Purpose: Test Knowles ideas about adult learning.

Directions:

1. Identify children at different ages and ask, "Tell me about yourself." Note the answer. If the child asks you, "What do you mean?" answer, "Oh, anything you want to tell me."
2. Repeat the preceding assignment with adults.
3. Note the differences and similarities between the responses of the children and the adults.
4. Discuss your findings with your colleagues.

Exercise II—Orientation to Learning

Purpose: Develop awareness of your own orientation to learning according to Houle.

Directions: Working in small groups:

1. Categorize your orientation to learning according to Houle's findings.
2. Discuss the implications this has for you as a learner and in your role as an educator.
3. Distinguish between andragogy and pedagogy.
4. Discuss how this information is useful with clients.
5. Discuss your reflections with your peers.

Exercise III—Reflection Questions

Purpose: Become aware of how your orientation to learning affects your motivation, learning strategies, and topics of interest.

Directions:

1. What is your motivation for studying health education in nursing?
2. What strategies help you learn?
3. What aspects of nursing interest you the most?
4. What do you hope to gain from your formal education?

Exercise IV—Teaching Team Members

Purpose: Apply adult learning theory to teaching team members.

Directions: Role play the following teaching and learning situations:

1. A newly certified nurse assistant is assigned to care for a client with a hip replacement. On the first postoperative day, the client requests a bed pan and the nurse assistant asks you what she should do. How would you respond?
2. You observe a dietary aide responding to a client's request for more salt on her dinner tray. The client has congestive heart failure and salt is prohibited. You meet the dietary aide as she is about to enter the client's room to deliver the additional salt. How would you handle this situation?
3. You are supervising a new registered nurse graduate who is administering heparin for the first time to a client with a clotting disorder. She asks you to help her properly administer the subcutaneous injection.

4. Your colleague needs to change a complex dressing on a hospitalized client, which is a new procedure to her. You are familiar with the procedure and she asks you for help.

SUPPLEMENTAL ONLINE RESOURCES

Erikson's Stages of Psychosocial Development:
http://psychology.about.com/od/theoriesofpersonality/a/psychosocial.htm
Principles of Adult Learning:
http://honolulu.hawaii.edu/intranet/committees/FacDevCom/guidebk/teachtip/
    adults-2.htm
Oxford Brooks University, theories of learning:
http://www.brookes.ac.uk/services/ocsd/2_learntch/theories.html
Andragogy and technology, integrating adult learning theory:
http://frank.mtsu.edu/~itconf/proceed00/fidishun.htm
Adult learning, emerging perspectives on learning:
http://projects.coe.uga.edu/epltt/index.php?title=Adult_Learning
Motivation theories:
http://changingminds.org/explanations/theories/a_motivation.htm
Motivation theory:
http://ezinearticles.com/?Motivation-Theory&id=410700
National Council on Patient Information and Education:
http://www.talkaboutrx.org/

REFERENCES

Balakas, K. (2009). Developmental theories. In Potter, P. A., & Perry, A. G. *Fundamentals of nursing* (7th ed., pp. 136–147). St. Louis: Mosby Elsevier.

Boshier, R. (1991). Psychometric properties of the alternative form of the education participation scale. *Adult Education Quarterly*, *41*(3), 150–167.

Derrick, M. G. (2003). Creating environments conducive for lifelong learning. *New directions for adult and continuing education*. Wilmington, DE: Wiley Periodicals.

Erikson, E. (1963). *Childhood and society* (2nd ed.). New York: W.W. Norton.

Houle, C. O. (1961). *The inquiring mind*. Madison: University of Wisconsin Press.

Houle, C. O. (1980). *Continuing learning in the professions*. San Francisco: Jossey-Bass.

Knowles, M. S. (1990). *The adult learner: A neglected species* (4th ed.). Houston: Gulf Publishing Company.

Knowles, M. S., Holton E. F. III, & Swanson, R. A. (2005). *The adult learner* (6th ed.). Burlington, MA: Elsevier.

Kolb, D. A. (1984). *Experiential learning*. Englewood Cliffs, NJ: Prentice-Hall.

Maslow, A. H. (1987). *Motivation and personality* (3rd ed.). New York: Harper & Row.

Merriam, S. B., Caffarella, R. S., & Baumgartner, L. M. (2007). *Learning in adulthood* (3rd ed.). San Francisco: Jossey-Bass.

O'Shea, E. (2003). Self-directed learning in nurse education: A review of the literature. *Journal of Advanced Nursing, 43*(1), 62–70.

Rogers, C. R. (1961). *On becoming a person*. Boston: Houghton-Mifflin.

Ruchala, P. (2009). Young to middle adult. In Potter, P. A., & Perry, A. G. (eds.). *Fundamentals of nursing* (7th ed., pp. 177–190). St. Louis: Mosby Elsevier.

Russell, S. S. (2006). An overview of adult-learning processes. *Urologic Nursing, 26*(5), 349–370.

Santrock, J. W. (2008). *A topical approach to life-span development* (4th ed.). Boston: McGraw-Hill.

CHAPTER 7

The Older Learner

The setting sun is as beautiful as the rising sun.
—Japanese proverb

OBJECTIVES

Upon completion of this chapter you will be able to:
- Discuss ageism and the subjective experience of the older client.
- Describe the psychosocial stages, developmental tasks, and physiologic changes characteristic of late adulthood that affect teaching and learning.
- List health education topics for clients in late adulthood related to psychosocial stages, developmental tasks, and normal physiologic changes.
- Identify common chronic diseases of older adults and their implications for health education.
- Describe the importance of cultural assessment before teaching the ethnic elderly.
- Identify the implications of nutritional status on teaching and learning.
- Identify the teaching and learning implications of working with individuals, families, groups/communities, and health team members.

KEY TERMS

ageism
auditory acuity
cognitive functioning
developmental task
frail elderly
old old adult

physiologic change
presbycusis
presbyopia
psychosocial stage
visual acuity
young old adult

INTRODUCTION

Because people are living longer, you will encounter older clients in virtually every healthcare setting. Older clients, like their younger counterparts, also are lifelong learners and have many lived experiences and much wisdom to share. The focus of this chapter is on providing health education to older clients. We do this by first looking at the concept of ageism that permeates United States culture. We then address the psychosocial stages, developmental tasks, and normal physiologic changes characteristic of late adulthood and the implications of these for teaching and learning. Cognitive functioning, an important consideration for all clients, is discussed as it relates to memory and medications. The chapter concludes with a discussion of the ethnic elderly, aging, and nutrition for older learners.

AGEISM

Ageism is a term used to denote discrimination against the elderly (Lueckenotte, 2009) and can lead to disparities in healthcare delivery (Baker & Heitkemper, 2007). Although fascination with youth in the United States is waning, this country still lacks a culture that values everyone, regardless of age or ethnic background. As a nurse you will be working with older clients, so it is important that you examine your attitudes about aging. How you see older clients wittingly or unwittingly influences how you react and treat them. This, in turn, influences how they see and value themselves. This means confronting the myths and stereotypes about the elderly that research and experience have demonstrated are not true. For example, some people believe that many elderly are confused, lonely, and generally in poor health, none of which is true. Many older adults live alone or with family members, have sufficient financial resources, and are in generally good health (Lueckenotte, 2009).

PSYCHOSOCIAL STAGES, DEVELOPMENTAL TASKS, AND PHYSIOLOGIC CHANGES OF LATE ADULTHOOD

The older population, which begins in the mid-to-late sixties, is increasing rapidly and has the longest time span of development of any age group (Santrock, 2008). According to the US Census Bureau News (2008), in 2030 all of the baby boomers will be 65 and older, accounting for nearly one in five US residents. In total numbers, this age group will increase from 38.7 million in 2008 to 88.5 million in 2050. Residents age 85 and older are expected to more than triple, from 5.4 million in 2008 to 19 million in 2050. Two groups contributing to this increase are the aging baby boom generation, the largest cohort of people who were born between 1946 and 1964, and the increase of individuals who are 85 and older (Lueckenotte, 2009).

Gender differences exist among older adults. For example, white women have a life expectancy of 81 years, compared with 76 years for white men. Black women have a life expectancy of 76.9 years, compared with 70 for black men, according to data from the National Center for Health Statistics (2008). These data suggest that aging is increasingly a woman's issue. Less is known about women's health because women have been underrepresented in research. Women generally have fewer financial resources, which makes it difficult to obtain adequate health care. Even so, women are more likely than men to seek health care, both medical and dental.

Because of this rapidly increasing population of older adults, demographers divide this age group into two time periods, the young old (65 to 84) and the old old adult (85+) (Santrock, 2008). The psychosocial stages, developmental tasks, and physiologic changes for both groups follow.

Psychosocial Stages

We continue viewing the psychosocial stages through the work of Erik Erikson (1963; 1982). His eighth developmental stage is *ego integrity versus despair*. In this stage, individuals engage in a life review. They evaluate the meaning of their lives, their accomplishments and failures, and their satisfactions and disappointments. It is a time of reflection, evaluation, interpretation, and often reinterpretation of their experiences. Many look back with satisfaction, knowing they have done their best in spite of failures (integrity), whereas others look back with regret and see themselves as failures (despair). This stage holds the potential for growth, understanding, and the development of wisdom (Balakas, 2009; Santrock, 2008). Wisdom is the positive growth that comes from life's experiences and results in deeper insights, perceptions, and judgments.

Because the life span for humans continues to lengthen, Erikson and his wife Joan further explored the 80- to 90-year-old age group and added a ninth stage. They reversed the order of each of the previous eight stages and added to the positive aspect (mistrust versus trust: hope, despair versus integrity: wisdom, etc.). Placing the negative before the positive emphasizes how the negative aspects of each stage may potentially affect individuals in this age group. Physiologic aging changes occurring during this time result in daily difficulties and reevaluations. It is the final life cycle stage when individuals must come to terms with declining independence, loss of control, and weakening self-esteem and confidence. Individuals who successfully deal with the negative aspects of this stage move on to *gerotranscendence;* i.e., rising above the negative and celebrating the life that remains (Erikson, 1997).

Maslow's hierarchy, discussed in Chapter 4, provides another framework for viewing the importance of individual needs. It is a theory of motivation that applies to the elderly. At certain times in the older person's life, basic needs, such as nutrition, may be the most important, whereas at other times the same individual may be engaged in self-actualization. It is important to assess each individual to determine present needs.

This is also a time of adjusting to transitions and new social roles. With longer lives, adults experience more losses, transitions, and adjustments to new social roles. Major losses include retirement, financial status, and possibly health. Social roles, relationships, and networks also change. The most difficult losses are usually related to the death of loved ones and friends (Lueckenotte, 2009). Your role as an educator in working with older adults is to help them successfully accept, adapt, and adjust to these psychosocial stages.

Developmental Tasks

Developmental tasks refer to the issues and problems that older adults face in living, including their changing social roles. Knowing these help you understand the life stage clients are in and the common issues they face.

In late adulthood, many clients are adjusting to retirement and may use this time to explore new interests and find new activities. Many clients want to continue employment because it gives meaning to their lives. Others continue employment because of difficult economic times. Financial stress is particularly difficult to deal with when resources are limited or insufficient to meet daily needs. Declining financial resources may require a change in the living situation to which the individual must adjust. If clients are receiving a pension, social security, or welfare, they have to learn about that system and how to navigate it. The same is true with navigating Medicare and Medicaid (Knowles, 1990).

Many retired adults expand their interests and hobbies during this time and find satisfaction in volunteer work. Many want to be useful and associate with like-minded individuals. The death of a spouse or significant other will require an adjustment in living. Roles change in retirement and new ones have to be negotiated with the spouse or significant other, children, and grandchildren (Knowles, 1990; Santrock, 2008).

As the educator, you need to be tuned in to clients' changing social roles. Retirement, for example, is a major life style rearrangement for both men and women. For those who have identified themselves by their work without developing strong interests in other areas, retirement may be particularly difficult. These individuals may experience feelings of dependency, powerlessness, and helplessness. For clients about to retire or having difficulty adjusting to retirement, encourage them to gradually disen-

Many older adults lead active, productive lives.
Source: © Andresr/ShutterStock, Inc.

gage from the work role. Help them identify other areas of interest and activities to pursue. Do not overlook the effect on the spouse when one marriage partner retires. Many wives complain about the adjustments they have to make when their spouse retires and begins following them around the house all day.

Physiologic Changes That Affect Teaching and Learning

Older adults experience an increasing number of physiologic changes during this time; however, there is considerable variability in the rate and nature of these changes. Adults aged 65 to 84 are increasingly healthier when compared with previous generations and lead active, productive lives. They have substantial potential for physical strength and fitness, and retain much of their cognitive capacity. Adults age 85 and older are frailer and show a greater loss in cognitive skills. They also experience a decline in general health and well-being (Santrock, 2008). In evaluating the physiologic changes that occur with aging, it is important to distinguish between normal aging and pathologic processes. There is considerable variability in individual aging affected by factors such as genetics, environmental exposures, life style, stress, and cultural factors (Wallace, 2006).

The impact of biologic aging is evident in every body system as well as the person's general appearance. The health of the older person is dependent in part on genetics; that is, what is inherited from the person's parents, along with luck, good health habits, and preventive measures taken (Lueckenotte, 2009). People are unable to control the first two factors, but do have an impact on the last two. Good health habits, preventive measures, and life style patterns such as rest, exercise, nutrition, and stressors greatly affect the health of every individual. In the older person, the long-term, accumulated effects of these patterns become more obvious. In this section we highlight some physiologic changes and pathophysiologic problems that occur with aging and how they affect teaching and learning.

Appearance

The most obvious signs of aging are seen in the skin. Wrinkling and sagging skin, thinning and graying hair, dryness, and pigmentation changes are common. Many skin changes are caused by exposure to sunlight, a problem about which much health education is focused today (Linton, 2007a). Clients with diabetes or cerebral vascular accidents have decreased sensation and must be taught to prevent burns from heating pads, bathing, and cooking (Wallace, 2006). The appearance of the body changes altering the contours of earlier years. Body mass diminishes from the face and extremities and increases in the trunk, abdomen, and hips.

Musculoskeletal System

In the musculoskeletal system, muscle mass and strength diminishes, bone mass declines, and degenerative joint changes can occur. Almost 30% of muscle mass is lost by the seventies. Older adults who regularly exercise retain more bone, muscle mass, and muscle tone when compared with inactive individuals, providing an excellent opportunity for health education. There is a progressive loss of height, especially among women because of osteoporosis; e.g., demineralization of the bones (Lueckenotte, 2009; Roberts, 2007). Expect your older clients to fatigue more easily than younger ones. Their movements may be slower and more rigid. Taking frequent breaks and allotting sufficient time help compensate for this. Older clients are more comfortable sitting in padded chairs with arms.

Cardiovascular System

Cardiovascular changes occur with aging, as evidenced by a decrease in cardiac output, abnormal increases in systolic and/or diastolic blood pressures, and weak peripheral pulses, particularly in the lower extremities. Hypertension, if present, can lead to serious health problems such as heart failure, stroke, renal failure, coronary heart disease, and peripheral vascular disease (Lueckenotte, 2009). Collagen in the heart muscle increases and elastin decreases, affecting myocardial contractility. The heart valves become thickened and fibrotic from lipid accumulation, degeneration of collagen, with fibrosis of the aortic and mitral valves most frequently affected. Coronary blood flow decreases significantly. The number of pacemaker cells in the SA node, and conduction cells in the AV node, the bundle of His, and bundle branches also decrease, which may result in conduction problems. Atherosclerosis and arteriosclerosis are common in the arterial walls, diminishing elasticity and vasomotor tone. Total peripheral resistance is increased, which results in an increase in blood pressure. These changes result from disease, environmental factors, lifetime health behaviors, and aging, and are not solely caused by aging alone. As a result, the older adult is less able to respond to physical and emotional stress (Disabatino & Bucher, 2007). Factors such as obesity, diet, activity, and habits have been implicated as etiologic factors, all of which have implications for nurses as educators, particularly among younger adults.

Respiratory System

Lung function decreases as respiratory muscle strength and mobility of the ribs declines. Osteoporosis is often present, leading to dorsal kyphosis, a curvature in the thoracic spine. The anteroposterior diameter of the thorax increases, giving the chest a barrel-shape appearance. The number of functional alveoli decreases, resulting in an increase in residual volume (the amount of air remaining after maximum expiration). The alveoli are less elastic and relatively more fibrous, which decreases the older person's ability to engage in physically taxing activities. Dyspnea may be evident on little exertion or stress (Kaufman, 2007). With these respiratory changes, clients may fatigue easily and need learning activities adjusted to their abilities.

Changes in the musculoskeletal, cardiovascular, and respiratory systems affect the older client's energy level, strength, and speed. Endurance certainly may be affected, but another influential variable is the person's usual activity level. Older people who lead very active lives tend to have remarkable endurance. They may be able to do a sustained activity familiar to them better than a younger individual who has less practice. Maintaining the functional ability of older adults; that is, maintaining their ability to live independently and perform the activities of daily living, is enhanced with regular exercise. Exercises also can reverse or slow declines in age-related motor performance (Fahlman, Topp, McNevin, Morgan, & Boardley, 2007). Nurses can encourage older adults to participate in exercises by teaching the benefits of a regular program. Ask older clients if they have noticed a decline in their strength and motor functioning. This focuses their attention on the topic, after which you can explain how exercise limits or reverses a decline, retains their independence, and maximizes their ability to engage in the activities of daily living (Schneider, Eveker, Bronder, Meiner, & Binder, 2003).

Exercise improves strength and endurance of people at all ages, including those who reside in nursing homes. Fahlman et al. (2007) found that a structured exercise program in older adults with limited functional ability increased their strength and endurance. For example, nursing students led older clients at senior centers in an exercise program. It was a lively activity, enjoyed by students and participants. If working with institutionalized clients, take into consideration clients' current rest and exercise routine when deciding on the best time to initiate teaching. Clients learn better when well oxygenated by an invigorated circulatory system and when rested enough to have the extra energy needed to focus on learning. Weinrich, Boyd, and Nussbaum (1989), recommend low-impact exercises for the elderly, during which their feet do not leave the floor. They also recommend slowing the speed of exercise and increasing the warm-up and cool-down time. As educators, focus on helping older clients retain as much physical strength and agility as possible.

Gastrointestinal System

Bowel and bladder problems increase with age. Bowel motility decreases, resulting in constipation. Bladder capacity decreases and can result in urinary incontinence. To address bowel changes, nurses should teach clients the benefits of drinking adequate fluids, eating sufficient roughage, and getting regular exercise. Some medications have an effect on intestinal motility and need further evaluation. To address the bladder changes, nurses should identify the cause of the incontinence, work with clients to establish a regular voiding schedule, and teach pelvic floor or Kegel exercises (Wallace, 2006). Bladder capacity and urinary incontinence are conditions to be aware of when planning learning activities. Providing frequent breaks may be necessary.

Neurologic System

Functional changes in the neurologic system occur with aging. Neuron loss occurs, affecting the function of chemical substances (epinephrine and acetylcholine) that enhance or inhibit nerve impulse transmission. Degenerative changes in myelin can interfere with nerve conduction. Voluntary reflexes are slower and the older person's ability to react quickly to stimuli is slowed (Lueckenotte, 2009). In addition to vision and hearing changes, other aging-related neurologic changes include decrease in memory, taste, smell, vibration and position sense, and muscle strength (Hendrickson, 2007).

Some clients have benign essential tremors that affect their upper extremities, head, and voice, a condition commonly seen in older adults. Tremors also may be associated with pathology such as Parkinson's disease or with side-effects of drugs (Millsap, 2007). The presence of tremors affects the type of learning activities in which these clients can successfully engage. Fine hand movements in manipulating equipment or writing tasks are difficult for these clients, so other learning activities should be selected.

Sensory Changes

Sensory changes have an effect on the life style of older clients. The most important sensory changes affecting teaching and learning are vision and hearing impairments. Diminished functional ability in either or both interferes with the older client's ability to communicate orally and in writing with others. This leads to social isolation as clients avoid the strain of hearing a muted or indistinguishable conversation, personal embarrassment associated with responding inappropriately to comments of others, or diminished mobility associated with loss of vision. All senses may be affected by aging, but vision and hearing are the most important to consider as you plan health education. Because of this, we address the functional declines in vision and hearing in greater depth and how to use this information to adapt health education to the abilities of older clients.

Sensory Changes: Vision

In 2006, vision difficulties affected 17% of the older population, 16% of men and 18% of women. Of those who were 85 and over, 27% reported trouble seeing (2008 Older Americans). The lens loses it ability to accommodate as it becomes less elastic, larger, and denser, resulting in a condition called presbyopia (farsightedness). The increased density plus the accumulation of loosened degenerative cells on the iris, cornea, and lens capsule result in increased scattering of light and sensitivity to glare. The lens becomes progressively yellowed and opaque, resulting not only in visual acuity difficulties, but also in the inability to discriminate blues and greens. This is attributed to the decreased ability of the aging, yellowed lens to filter the shorter wavelengths of light (violet, blue, and green). It is easier for older clients to distinguish among warm colors such as yellow, orange, and red (Linton, 2007b). Use of these colors in teaching materials makes it easier for clients to distinguish them.

When teaching older clients, sit or stand in front of them so they have a full view of you. Clients should be able to see your face and mouth as you talk (Lueckenotte, 2009). If you are using visual aids, consider the impact of colors. For example, a color with a longer wavelength, such as yellow, printed on a white background, would not be easy for older eyes to see because there is insufficient contrast between the two colors. A thick black outline surrounding the yellow material would improve readability. Even more effective is a background color such as light blue that contrasts with deep yellow lettering outlined in black. We now examine functional visual changes (visual acuity, glare, dark and light adaptation, and loss of peripheral vision) that affect the teaching and learning process.

Visual Acuity

Virtually everyone will have visual difficulties related to the aging process regardless of sex, race, ethnicity, or socioeconomic status. Many older adults wear glasses for reading or distance vision because of decreased visual acuity. Watch older clients for signs of difficulty. Note how clients read. How close do they hold a book to read? How much reading do they do? If institutional clients wear glasses, be sure they have them on and the lenses are clean to view your instructional materials. Older clients with presbyopia hold their reading materials at arm's length to focus clearly on the print. Symbols, letters, and objects that are small are more difficult to distinguish from one another. Diminishing ability to discriminate between stimuli is evident to older clients in terms of the size of words and pictures and their intensity and color. Small images, which project shorter light waves into the eye, are harder to distinguish, as are crowded or softly colored images. Larger and more intensely colored print is easier to see. There is enough of the image "getting through" the nerve pathways for clients to "fill in" the missing parts. Allowing space between each of the letters also helps.

This is harder to read for a person with aging eyes because the print is fine and there is a lot of it.

This print is easier to read.

Glare

Glare is a serious problem for older clients. It affects their ability to drive at night by leaving them virtually blind in its presence. Glare may come from a variety of sources, such as reflections off of windows and shiny floors. Linton (2007b) recommends soft, incandescent lighting rather than fluorescent lighting to minimize glare. Sheer curtains or rugs can also help reduce glare. If you become involved with the production of instructional materials, avoid using slick, shiny, white paper, which is more likely to produce glare. If you are arranging lighting for elderly clients, make the light brighter but not glaring.

Dark and Light Adaptation

It takes longer for the eyes of older clients to adapt to dark and light. It takes more time for their eyes to adjust if the room is darkened for a DVD, video tape, or a slide show. Plan for this extra time as you prepare the teaching plan. When you turn the lights back on, clients need extra time to readjust their vision. Because pupils become smaller when the lights are turned on, less light is reaching the retina; thus, extra lighting is required (Linton, 2007b). If you are using a physical model or object in teaching, consider placing high-intensity lighting on it. This increases the visibility of the model or object, which is preferable to increasing the light in the entire room. The level of intensity, however, needs to be balanced to avoid glare to which older eyes are more sensitive.

Loss of Peripheral Vision

With the loss of peripheral vision, older clients are unaware of people and learning activities outside of their line of central vision. This may interfere with how your clients relate to others if you are teaching a group. They may not be aware of others sitting next to them or objects located in their peripheral visual fields. As a result they may appear to lack social interaction skills or appear clumsy if they spill something or knock something over. They may not be able to see an object that you may refer to that is outside of their visual field. Do your best to stay in the clients' line of central vision when teaching to address this condition.

Sensory Changes: Hearing

As with vision, some degree of hearing loss caused by changes in the inner ear or tympanic membrane inevitably accompanies the aging process. In 2006, almost one-half of older men and more than one-third of older women reported trouble hearing. Thirty-two percent of those age 65 to 74 and 62% of those age 85 and over had trouble hearing (2008 Older Americans). Presbycusis is associated with aging and is the most common type of hearing loss. It begins in young adulthood and becomes evident usually after age 50. Initially high-pitched sounds beyond the range of human speech are lost. Because these have little functional significance, the individual is unaware of the loss. As the client ages, the loss eventually involves the sounds in the middle and lower ranges. It becomes problematic for clients when the upper sounds are missed and only the lower sounds are heard. Words sound distorted and conversations are difficult to understand, especially in the presence of background noise (Linton, 2007b).

With high tone hearing loss, it is more difficult for clients to discriminate among consonants, such as *s*, *t*, *f*, *g*, *ch*, *sh*, *z*, and *th*, which have high frequencies. Clients with presbycusis have difficulty distinguishing among phonetically similar words. Words are distorted and sentences make little sense. A sentence such as, "I think he should go to the store," might be interpreted as "I wish we could go to the show." As hearing loss progresses, explosive consonants, such as *b*, *d*, *k*, *p*, and *t*, also become distorted (Miller, 1990).

Clients with presbycusis need more time to process information. Rapid speech is difficult for older clients to understand. If you speak rapidly, remember to slow down when you teach older clients. Lower your pitch and speak more slowly and slightly louder. Face clients when you speak so they can see you. They may lip read to fill in what they do not hear. Reduce any background noise if present or move to a quiet room. If clients wear hearing aids, be sure they are operational, in place, and turned on with sufficient volume (Lueckenotte, 2009).

Older clients in a group setting may not want to participate or answer questions for fear of appearing foolish. Hearing loss affects self-confidence and may lead to social isolation. Uninformed healthcare providers may assume that a hard-of-hearing client is demented. Consider the example of a woman who was attempting to communicate with her elderly mother-in-law. "My mother-in-law does not pay attention to anything I say. Even if I practically shout at her it does no good. But let my husband come in the room and just talk to her in a normal voice, and she hears every word he says." The nursing student responded with sensitivity to what may be symptoms of a family conflict. She explained the facts about sound waves to the woman and explained that a woman's voice is likely to contain higher sound frequencies. If she raises her voice in an effort to be heard, it is likely that she also raises the pitch. Tension also results in a rise in voice pitch. If the relationship already suffers from tension, it is likely that the voice with which the woman begins to speak is already higher than her relaxed voice. These factors make her speech less intelligible to an aging person whose hearing is diminishing. The man who "casually" comes into the room is likely to speak in a lower-pitched voice, which has a longer wave length.

Suspect a hearing loss if older clients give an inappropriate response to questions, are unable to follow oral directions without cues, or frequently ask you to repeat a message. If clients watch you closely, turn their ear toward you, get unusually close to you, do not respond to loud environmental noise, speak too loudly or inarticulately, speak in a monotone, or avoid group settings, suspect hearing impairment (Miller, 1990). Remember, however, that not all older clients are hard of hearing. It is distressing for older persons to be spoken to as if they are deaf when they are not.

Implications of Physiologic Changes That Affect Teaching and Learning

Older adults are experiencing many biologic and psychosocial changes in their lives and need differing levels of help adapting to these changes. They are dealing with faltering health and decreasing strength, and biologic changes that alter or limit their activities. They are adjusting to losses, adapting to changing living circumstances, and changing their self-image. They may be enriching their lives by expanding their knowledge, developing new interests, and learning new skills. This is a time rich with opportunities for nurses to recognize unspoken and unmet needs and to take opportunities to provide health education. We now look at how this information helps you to promote, retain, and restore the health of older clients.

Promote and Retain Health

The focus of promoting health is on prevention, whereas the focus of retaining health is on maintaining one's present health status, assuming it is satisfactory. Clients are never too old to start an exercise program, improve their diet, and change unhealthful habits. Table 7-1 lists suggested topics to promote and retain health appropriate for older learners (Hall, 2009; Lueckenotte, 2009). These suggestions are not all inclusive and must be adapted to the circumstances of the individual client.

Restore Health

Restoration of health for the older adult refers to those who are experiencing an acute or chronic illness or disability. The purpose of health education at this time is designed to help clients understand the nature of their health problem, the treatment regimen, and how to deal with the limitations imposed by health problems, disability, or injury. This involves not only working with the client but also with family members and caretakers. Table 7-2 suggests topics related to the restoration of health (Baker & Heitkemper, 2007; Hall, 2009; Lueckenotte, 2009).

TABLE 7-1   Suggested Topics to Promote and Retain Health

Nursing Assessment	Health Education Topics
Biologic aging	• Knowing normal age-related body changes • Knowing age-related changes to body system of interest
General health habits	• Eating well-balanced, nutritious diet • Maintaining adequate hydration • Practicing oral hygiene and dental care • Knowing benefits of exercise program • Coping effectively with physical and mental stress • Visiting regularly with healthcare providers • Participating in meaningful activities
General living conditions	• Maintaining home cleanliness • Evaluating need for mechanical aids to assist in ADLs • Making life style adjustments • Preventing accidents and falls • Creating safe home environment (slip-resistant rugs, night lights, nonskid adhesive strips in tub, shower, handrails on steps, grab bars in bathrooms, smoke detectors, etc.)
Disease and illness prevention	• Avoiding risk factors (smoking, alcohol, etc.) • Modifying behavior to avoid risk factors • Obtaining immunizations (flu, pneumonia) • Having regular physical examinations • Screening procedures (mammograms, cholesterol, vision, hearing, blood pressure, blood sugar) • Knowing medications • Maintaining medication regimen and medication safety • Recognizing symptoms of depression
Sexual habits	• Preventing sexually transmitted diseases • Knowing mode of disease transmission • Knowing partner's sexual history and practices • Using safe sexual practices • Recognizing symptoms
Community services	• Knowing about community luncheon sites • Knowing community senior center services • Knowing county and state governmental senior services

TABLE 7-2 Suggested Topics to Restore Health	
Nursing Assessment	**Health Education Topics**
Acute illness	• Knowing nature and cause of the health problem or disability • Common conditions: urinary tract infections, fluid and electrolyte imbalance (hyponatremia, dehydration), pneumonia, hip fracture, dysrhythmias • Understanding diagnostic tests • Supporting/explaining treatment regimen • Orienting to hospital/clinic environment and routines • Adapting to life style changes
Chronic illness	• Knowing nature and cause of the health problem or disability • Common conditions: hypertension, cardiovascular, stroke, diabetes mellitus, cancer, arthritis • Understanding diagnostic tests • Supporting/explaining treatment regimen • Using physical, occupational, and speech therapies • Managing exacerbations/remissions • Preventing complications • Adapting to life style changes • Adapting home environment • Identifying/using self-help devices • Supporting continued provider supervision
Disability	• Assessing strengths/limitations of disability • Managing activities of daily living • Building on abilities • Identifying/using self-help devices
Accidents	• Knowing nature of injury sustained and impact on function • Managing activities of daily living • Building on abilities • Assessing rehabilitation issues • Preventing accidents and injury • Maintaining safe home environment (slip-resistant rugs, night lights, nonskid adhesive strips in tub, shower, handrails on steps, grab bars in bathrooms, smoke detectors, etc.)
Community services	• Knowing about community luncheon sites • Knowing community senior center services • Knowing county and state governmental senior services

CHRONIC DISEASE AND IMPLICATIONS FOR TEACHING AND LEARNING

Chronic diseases are not a part of normal aging; however, the prevalence of chronic disease is higher among older adults. The increasing number of older Americans means that more of them need the services of the healthcare system. People 65 and older are less likely to have as many acute conditions as younger people; however, they are more apt to have at least one chronic condition for which they likely require assistance. Many clients have more than one chronic condition. The most common chronic diseases in older clients are heart disease, stroke, cancer, and diabetes. Other common chronic diseases are hypertension, asthma, bronchitis, emphysema, arthritis, depression, vision loss, and hearing impairment (2008 Older Americans; Baker & Heikemper, 2007). Race and ethnic differences are present in these conditions. For example, in 2005 to 2006, the prevalence of hypertension and diabetes was higher in non-Hispanic blacks than non-Hispanic whites. Diabetes was higher in Hispanics than in non-Hispanic whites, but these two groups had similar levels of hypertension. Hispanics had lower levels of arthritis than non-Hispanic whites. Many chronic diseases are preventable or modifiable in individuals who are responsive to health education and willing to make changes in their behavior (2008 Older Americans).

Teaching older clients how to adapt to chronic diseases is a major theme in working with them. The causes of chronic diseases are multiple and frequently related to life style. Chronic diseases develop slowly over time. Older clients may not understand their illness, especially if it is characterized by exacerbations and remissions. Clients with chronic diseases may experience depression, which further compounds their ability to function. The depression may be related to the disease and the disability it inflicts, or the many losses that older adults experience at this time of their lives. Working with older clients with chronic diseases challenges you as the educator. Determine how well they understand their disease and the degree to which they are willing to adhere to the prescribed treatment. Clients need to be educated about how to prevent and manage crises, manage the therapeutic regimen, and control symptoms. They also need to know how to organize their time, prevent social isolation, and have a normal life style and interactions with others despite disease. Refresh your memory of specific chronic diseases as it helps you answer older clients' questions.

Teaching related to general health measures is a fruitful area for health education for older clients. General health measures are instrumental in improving health status and helping clients feel better. Consider teaching the virtues of exercising regularly, improving nutritional intake, controlling weight loss or gain, getting adequate rest, managing stress, and cooperating with the medical regimen.

We have enjoyed teaching these topics, especially the classes on exercises, to older clients during their noon meal at community lunch sites for senior citizens. The exercises taught were suitable to the age of clients and involved simple range-of-motion exercises. The clients perked up, began to smile and interact with each other in a way they had not before. Many said they felt better as a result of the classes.

Alcohol continues to be an underestimated and hidden problem for both older men and women (Wallace, 2006). However, the prevalence rate of alcohol use in older women is increasing and is expected to continue increasing over the next 20 years. Alcohol detoxification and excretion from the older body is less efficient than in younger counterparts. Alcohol abuse leads to accidents, nutritional deficiencies, and damage affecting all body systems. Consequently older women are at higher risk for physical, medical, social, and psychological problems. Factors contributing to the increase in alcohol consumption include psychosocial changes older women experience during this time such as retirement, empty nest syndrome, limited mobility, and illness. Their health problems are compounded when alcohol and prescription drugs are synergistic or incompatible (Epstein, Fisher-Elber, & Al-Otaiba, 2007).

The following experience illustrates how one nursing student made a significant difference in the life of an 87-year-old client, Mrs. Green. She is a widow who was happily married with two children, both of whom have now died. She has two granddaughters who live in different cities and do not visit. When Mrs. Green was younger, she was a supervisor in a large corporation and had an active social life. Through the aging process, she has become isolated. She has arthritis, which limits her activity, and cataracts, which limit her sight. These problems, along with a few other physical ailments, have contributed to her becoming a shut in. At first Mrs. Green was hesitant to let the nursing student come to her home. Previously she had some unfortunate experiences with physicians and had not been seen by anyone for more than 2 years. Her failing vision had contributed to a fear of strangers and arthritis had kept her from going out of the house. With some coaxing, and because she was having abdominal pain that she wanted treated, she let the nursing student come to her home.

When the nursing student arrived, Mrs. Green was pleasant but cautious. The student conducted a health history and physical assessment. Through a telephone consultation with the clinic physician, Mrs. Green was diagnosed as having a flare up of an old ulcer and appropriate medication was prescribed. The student returned weekly and, within a month, Mrs. Green learned to trust the nurse. Each week they discussed Mrs. Green's vision and, if it could be improved, how she would be able to continue taking care of herself. At first Mrs. Green was determined never to see a doctor again, but after a few weeks she made an appointment herself, arranged for a ride, and went to see an eye surgeon. A short time later she had surgery to remove a cataract. The surgery made a big difference. When the nursing student made her next visit, she found Mrs. Green was a different person. Mrs. Green did not talk about any of her health problems; rather, she chatted about current events and other interesting topics. Mrs. Green was joyous about the difference the surgery had made in her sight. She had changed from being a lonely, fearful person to being outgoing and cheerful. She still is a shut in because of her age and arthritis, but she no longer lives in a world of haze. Mrs. Green is less isolated now. She is safer and will be able to live in her own home longer.

Finally, never assume that older men and women are not interested in sex. Many individuals continue to be sexually active beyond the expectations and imagination of their younger counterparts (Bouman, Arcelus, & Benbow, 2006). Health education about sexuality in the later years generates more interest than you anticipate. Consider the example of a 70-year-old female client seen in an outpatient clinic. She came in for her routine checkup and renewal of her prescription for vaginal Premarin (estrogen). She exercised regularly, ate nutritious meals, and maintained a long-standing sexual relationship with a 50-year-old man.

Social support networks are important for older adults. People who maintain relationships with others and remain active and involved with group activities fare better in terms of health and happiness (Wallace, 2006). Self-help and peer support groups are also beneficial when clients are dealing with specific health problems. Your role as an educator is to foster these support networks.

COGNITIVE FUNCTIONING

Although there are age-related changes in brain composition, cells, and synapses, they do not necessarily affect thinking and cognition (Millsap, 2007). Current research from longitudinal studies shows that some cognitive (thinking) functions decline with age, but other cognitive processes function at very high levels well into the later years. The decline that does occur is less than was once thought and individuals can compensate for the decline in ways that are not noticeable (Bjorklund & Bee, 2008). It is a common misperception that older adults become cognitively impaired as they age; that is, they become confused, forgetful, and unable to manage their affairs. This is a myth, as cognitive impairments are not part of normal aging (Lueckenotte, 2009; Wallace, 2006). Keep in mind that most older adults live without cognitive difficulties. Those who do show signs of mild cognitive impairment (MCI) should be evaluated by a physician. MCI is characterized by memory loss, language difficulties, disorientation, inability to perform calculations, and impairments in judgment and reasoning because of pathologic processes (Lueckenotte, 2009; Wallace, 2006).

Older learners may lose some ability to concentrate on more than one task at a time, may be slower to process information, and may need more time to learn and process information (Millsap, 2007). You can help clients concentrate by having them focus on only one task at a time, beginning with the most important. Clients may need more time to process information, so speak slowly and seek feedback that indicates they are tracking with you and understanding the message. Having multiple instructional materials to augment your message, focus clients' attention, and reinforce your message. If the information is new, clients may need additional time to absorb it. Repetition facilitates learning.

Memory

If learning is the process of acquiring new knowledge, then memory is the process of retaining that knowledge over time. When memory falters or is lost completely, it is frustrating, particularly to the elderly. Memory is the "ability to retain or store information and retrieve it when needed" (Bjorklund & Bee, 2008, p. 107). Short-term memory loss is more commonly seen with aging than is long-term memory loss. Short-term memory refers to remembering events in the recent past, whereas long-term memory refers to distant events (Stevens, 2005). There is great variation in cognitive functioning among individuals as they age, as people do not all follow a predictable pattern.

The causes of memory loss are many, and include physiologic causes such as cerebrovascular changes and pathologic causes such as disease or trauma, which cause a loss of neural cells. Psychosocial issues can lead to stress, depression, and social isolation (Stevens, 2005). When older clients become aware of memory slippages, they often conclude incorrectly that something is wrong with their brain or that they are losing their mind. Believing that, they become fearful and anxious, which can in itself interfere with the learning process, leading to a self-fulfilling prophecy. Older clients may need to be reminded about the many memory tasks that they perform daily that are accurate and important (Bjorklund & Bee, 2008).

An important variable in memory and learning is the attitude of both clients and nurses. Your message and the client's internal messages (self-talk) matter. Clients may be aware of short-term memory deficits and be discouraged. It may be true that older clients cannot learn as much or as fast as when they were younger. However, older clients can learn when they set the pace of learning to suit their current ability. It also helps when they develop memory aids themselves. You help older clients learn better when you break up the material to be learned into sensible portions and deliver it at a slower pace with adequate space between units.

The following is a description of the memory problems experienced by a 90-year-old woman who came out of retirement at 75, left her home in Colorado, and went to Alaska to teach children in a completely new, remote, and harsh environment. The woman offers nurses the following description and advice: "I go to get something in a room and when I get there, I have forgotten what I needed to get. I forget lists (in my head), and even three items can be troublesome. I cannot recall names of places, people, and things when I need the information, especially if I am in a mildly stressful situation. I leave out an item in a familiar recipe. I forget to turn off the stove under cooking pots so a timer is a must. Sequential directions are easily confused or omitted. Did I take my medication or not? Give me short, specific instructions. Repeat the instructions. Give me a hands-on demonstration of a procedure."

In addition to the preceding client's advice, we recommend that you encourage clients to use written lists and reinforce memory compensation devices like the timer on the stove. Color-coding medication with colored dots help; i.e., put blue dots on the medicine container that is taken at both breakfast and supper. A calendar is very helpful for remembering important appointments. Poems help, too. A woman complained to the nurse that she became confused when she stepped off the elevator to visit the doctor because elevators on both sides would take her to the correct floor. Once she stepped off the elevator, she would forget which way to turn. She finally solved the problem by noting sunlight streaming in one window. She now tells herself, "Turn to the light and then to the right."

We recommend that you encourage older clients to make a record of important information and keep it in a brightly colored folder: name of doctor, name of insurance, important identification numbers, names of medication, and important people's phone numbers. In this folder older clients should also keep questions that occur between visits to the doctor or to you, the nurse.

Interest is an important variable affecting memory and aging. "I remember what I want to remember" one elderly client said. Help clients find a reason for making the effort to learn. Fear, for example, was the motivator for a 96-year-old gentleman who was learning to walk again after a severe accident. The nurses caring for him remarked on his willpower. He replied: "It is not willpower. If I don't keep trying to walk, you will put me in one of those 'places.'" He wanted to remain in his own assisted-living apartment and not be placed in a nursing home.

Interest is closely related to attention. To assess a client's present level of cognitive competence, ask, "How well do you pay attention? What activities help you pay attention? How well do you concentrate?" A good way to foster attention is to involve several senses. For example, establish eye contact with American or Western European clients. Eye contact indicates that they are probably listening attentively. Some clients have hearing deficits, so ask them to restate a message you have given. If the client is willing to repeat the message back to you, you will learn how the client has understood the message, the modality through which the client learns most easily, and the pace that suits the client. "I see what you mean," may indicate that the client is a visual learner. "I get it," may signify a tactile learning style. "I hear you" may indicate the client is an auditory learner.

Most people learn more easily and remember better from visual presentation, and visual aids are widely available for educational purposes. To be sure that the visual channel would be helpful to an individual client, assess the visual cues to which the client attends. You might take the initiative to point out characteristics that are apparent; for example, "Notice that this little pill is red and round, whereas that one is long and green." If the client is an auditory learner, search for auditory cues to enhance learning, such as "Let me spell it for you." or "The name of the pill is Lanoxin, like Lenox china." Clients who are tactile learners can benefit from activities that involve touching or otherwise manipulating the materials. For example, you could give a set of instructions to the client to hold during the teaching session or you could obtain a model (heart) or the actual object (pill) under discussion for the client to manipulate.

Other senses, such as taste and smell, may be incorporated as appropriate. If the medicine is liquid, it may have a distinctive odor. If a wound is being dressed or a discharge needs to be monitored, smell can be an important clue to the progression of healing, as well as a warning sign of necrosis or infection. The involvement of several senses raises the likelihood that learning will occur.

Memory often works through association. To help clients remember a new idea, help them find ways to associate it with ones they already have, and/or help them organize the new information into a gestalt that makes sense for them as individuals. Logical connections are helpful, but imaginative association is usually stronger. The preceding example associating Lanoxin with Lenox china illustrates this.

Memory is enhanced by arousal. We are more apt to remember events to which we have attached emotions. Events associated with pleasant, aggravating, or frightening emotions all seem to have a higher likelihood of being recalled. You may be able to say or do something amusing to clients as a way to help them remember an event or bit of instruction. For example, to help elderly clients living in a high rise facility improve their appearance, a nursing student dressed in mismatched garments with conflicting colors and excessive jewelry. The clients found it very amusing but understood the message.

"Do you understand?" is a tricky question and reveals only whether or not the client acts cooperatively. Not all clients are assertive; many older clients try not to bother the busy nurse. When feeling overloaded, clients may hide their feelings of ignorance, smile politely, and agree when asked this question. This type of response (with a half-hearted "yes" or a smile and a nod) may feel satisfying to a nurse who is very busy, but it is deceptive. When asked for specific feedback, the nurse may discover that the client understood very little. Eliciting this information is done by asking the client, "Tell me what you understand by what I said." Deception is also common whenever there is a perceived difference in status, such as between nurses and clients. Clients may not want to acknowledge they do not understand what the nurse said to avoid disappointing the nurse. Sometimes it may be necessary to check with the client's spouse to see if the client understands and to learn how the client is doing.

Medication and Cognitive Functioning

Medications can interfere with cognitive functioning. Surveys of older adults have found that many take an average of 8 to 10 medications a day (Stevens, 2005). When asked, "What medications are you taking?" clients vary in their reliability as historians. Nurses also vary in their interviewing skills and the amount of thought they give to the clients' answers. It was common for clients seen in a well oldster clinic to list only their prescribed medications. They routinely omitted herbs and over-the-counter medications such as vitamins, laxatives, and pills taken for headache or upset stomach. They also did not mention medications prescribed by other doctors because they did not want to appear to be dissatisfied with the present providers.

When working with confused, elderly clients, be sure to consider the medications they are taking. Clients may be receiving a dose that is too high or multiple medications may be interacting unfavorably. Other considerations are the cumulative effect and side-effects of drugs (Millsap, 2007). The elderly need to be taught how drugs affect them and how to take them safely.

ETHNIC ELDERLY

As the nation moves toward midcentury, the population is expected to become more diverse. By 2050 the minority population is projected to be 235.7 million out of a total US population of 439 million. During the 2008 to 2050 time period, the major growth will be in the Hispanic population, which is projected to nearly triple, from 46.7 to 132.8 million, when nearly one in three US residents will be Hispanic. During this same time period, the black population is projected to increase from 41.1 to 65.7 million, and the Asian population is projected to increase from 15.5 to 40.6 million. The single-race white population will grow only slightly, from 199.8 to 203.3 million (US Census Bureau News, 2008).

Ethnic groups may view old age differently than the dominant white culture. Of the five major cultural groups in the United States, all show greater respect for the elderly when compared with the dominant culture. For example, the elderly in the dominant culture are expected to live apart from their adult children and maintain their independence as long and as much as possible. The elderly in the African-American culture enjoy closer family ties with the extended family than occurs in the dominant culture. The elderly in the Hispanic culture are respected and often live with large, extended families. Elderly Asians enjoy a high level of respect in the family, which increases as they age. The adult children are expected to take care of their aging parents. Elderly in Native-American cultures enjoy a very high level of honor and respect for their accumulated knowledge and wisdom (Schmall, 1996 as cited in Wallace, 2006).

As with any age group, there is great diversity of beliefs and values among the elderly, both across different ethnic groups and within any one particular ethnic group. It is essential that you conduct a thorough cultural assessment to identify the health beliefs and values of the older client, family, or group that you are teaching. To avoid stereotyping, ask if there is a cultural or ethnic group with which they identify and what their beliefs are about health and illness (O'Brien, 2007). Your cultural assessment will identify the health practices of the client and the degree to which the client believes in and adheres to folk practices and Western healthcare practices.

Clients who are immigrants or first-generation residents in the United States may adhere more strongly to the health beliefs and practices of their primary cultural affiliation. These immigrants, who may have come to the United States to join their children, have the unique challenge of relocating to a new culture and language late in life. Other ethnic elderly clients who have lived a lifetime in the United States are more likely to have become assimilated into US culture, to have had some experiences with the nation's healthcare system, and to have better knowledge of its health practices. By assessing health beliefs, values, and practices, you can tailor your health teaching to the individual client.

Language may be a barrier in communicating with the ethnic elderly. The client may speak little or no English. If the latter is the case, find an interpreter to assist you. Family members may serve effectively as interpreters for the elderly because they know the client and are more likely familiar with the client's mode of self-expression. However, this is not always the case. The nurse must be sensitive to family dynamics and use clinical judgment to determine if this is appropriate.

In providing health education, be sure your message is realistic in terms of the client's living situation, support network, educational background, and financial resources. For example, teaching an elderly Hispanic woman about the importance of a daily intake of fresh fruit and vegetables was meaningless because of the client's very limited financial resources. Her situation was compounded because she could not drive and her family lived far away. The client was dependent on neighbors for transportation, which was irregular and unpredictable at best. In another example, an elderly African-American woman had been on medication for hypertension for several years. The clinic nurse noted the client's blood pressure had been elevated during the past 6 months. After a lengthy discussion with the client, the nurse learned that the client had not been taking her medication. Because of her limited financial resources, the client had to make a choice between food and medicine. She had discontinued the medication and waited to see if the nurses and doctors would notice. The nurse reviewed how the medication works in the body, the health problems it helps to prevent, and the importance of taking the medication. She asked the social worker to address the client's financial issues.

If the elderly client is under treatment for a current health problem, inquire about what she or he is doing to treat it. The client may be engaging in a folk practice designed to ameliorate the condition. Listen carefully to the client's self-care practices and determine if these practices are helpful, neutral, or harmful; that is, if they should be preserved, accommodated, or restructured (DeRosa & Kochurka, 2006). Unless the practice is harmful, be supportive of the practice and view it as an adjunct to your nursing and medical interventions. Remember that the mind has a profound influence on health and healing, and we do not yet fully understand the extent of the mind's influence. If clients' practices provide them with meaning and give them a sense of participating in healing, then the practices deserve our respect, not disdain.

NUTRITION

Sufficient food intake and adequate nutrition are important to maintaining health and preventing disease in older adults. Nutritional status is enhanced if sufficient food and adequate nutrition have been a pattern throughout life. Many factors affect nutrition in older adults, including age-related biologic changes, food preferences, financial status, life style, medications, and presence of chronic disease. For healthy eating guidelines, review the Food Guide Pyramid prepared by the US Department of Agriculture at the Web site shown under the Supplemental Online Resources at the end of this chapter. Older adults' food intake should follow those guidelines and be sufficient to meet their energy needs while managing body weight (Biggs, 2007). Proper nutrition is a broad topic that provides many opportunities for nurses to educate clients and their families.

Nutrition affects memory. The body is dependent on many nutrients to manufacture the neurotransmitters that are essential to learning. The B vitamins are essential ingredients in this process. Iron is essential for the transmission of oxygen to the brain, and water is vital to every metabolic process in the body.

Many older adults are dehydrated and do not consume enough liquid daily. This occurs because of physiologic changes, decrease in thirst sensation, and insufficient fluid intake (Biggs, 2007). One of the organs that may shrink with age is the urinary bladder (Wallace, 2006). Some older people tend to drink less in an effort to avoid the inconvenience or embarrassment of needing to empty their bladders more often. This problem of self-imposed dehydration may be exacerbated by a subculture among the older generation that considers bodily functions or attention to them as taboo. If clients are not properly hydrated, their health is endangered and their ability to learn will be impaired.

Although more Americans are valuing fitness, many older adults do not see the connection between exercise, cardiorespiratory functioning, and an oxygenated, nourished brain. Give clients information and choose a time to teach when they are more invigorated, such as when they are sufficiently rested and have the energy to learn and sufficiently stimulated to pay attention.

WORKING WITH FAMILIES

Older clients, as with their younger counterparts, value their privacy and do not wish to be overly dependent on their adult children. Often family members or friends will need to be involved with the older person's care, and it is to them that you direct your health education. When this is necessary, be sensitive to the privacy concerns clients may have. Be respectful and avoid embarrassing elderly clients by sharing unnecessary information about them with others. When you teach family members or friends, reveal only the information that is essential for understanding the health message. If clients live alone and need assistance from family members or friends, identify the care needs and arrange mutually agreeable times for them to visit. If clients live with family, meeting the clients' care needs requires working around the family's employment and other routines.

WORKING WITH GROUPS AND COMMUNITIES

Senior citizen sites, community gathering places such as senior lunch programs, and long-term care facilities provide opportunities for health education. Everyone is invited to participate and many will if for no other reason than to enjoy the social companionship with other like-minded individuals. This is also an opportunity to encourage team members to attend to update their knowledge about your health topic.

When you are presenting health education information to groups of older adults, be sure to make it lively and interesting. Announce your presentation in advance and give it an interesting and catchy title, something that will capture their attention. The institution where you teach can help to advertise your presentation in advance. If possible, use teaching strategies that encourage active participation, such as asking questions and waiting for responses and engaging clients in small group or short dyad learning activities. Your presentation will be more interesting and remembered longer if those attending are active participants. Clients like to be given written materials that they can read in privacy on their own. Brochures and handouts also reinforce your teaching.

WORKING WITH HEALTH TEAM MEMBERS

As the numbers of older adults increase, there is a corresponding need for caregivers to provide health services whether in long-term care facilities or assisted living residences. Providing these services is a growth industry in the United States. Many of today's caregivers have little formal training for their roles and responsibilities, especially in long-term care facilities in which the primary caregiver is a certified nursing assistant. Certified nursing assistants are supervised by a registered nurse; however, the ratio is often unbalanced and the supervisor may be overloaded. Medicare and many states require that nursing assistants and other care providers undergo training. Because of this, there are multiple opportunities for you to provide health education for these valuable team members.

As with teaching adult learners, you must begin by knowing the provisions of the nurse practice act in your state and know the scope of practice for each team member: the nursing assistant, licensed practical nurse, and registered nurse. You must also know the general policies and practice guidelines of your employer. Long-term care institutions may or may not have in-service education departments to provide continuing education for employees. If such a department is available, you can work with the staff to identify the education needs of the team members and plan for appropriate health education.

If no such department is available, it becomes your responsibility to provide health education to your team members. In this case, you should first assess their learning needs. You can identify these as you work with team members and become familiar with their capabilities and deficiencies. While assessing team members, remember the three learning domains—cognitive, affective, and psychomotor—and consider in which domain the team member needs health education. For example, does the team member lack knowledge about the client's medical and nursing diagnoses, and rationale for treatment (cognitive domain)? Does the team member's attitude show a lack of understanding or compassion toward clients (affective domain)? Does the team member know how to safely and accurately perform a needed nursing care procedure (psychomotor domain)? Once you have determined the learning domain in which health education is needed, you can then plan appropriate teaching strategies to address those needs. Your next focus will be to determine whether the content to be taught can be done informally on the job or if the team member needs formal teaching away from the nursing care unit. Following teaching, you need to assess the effectiveness of your teaching. Selecting teaching content, teaching strategies, and instructional materials, and evaluating teaching effectiveness are discussed in subsequent chapters.

SUMMARY

Because of the growing number and ethnic diversity of aging Americans, teaching and learning among this population is increasingly important. Older clients are different from younger and middle-age clients in ways that significantly affect the planning and implementing of health education. Significant variables include psychosocial stages, developmental tasks, and physiologic changes associated with aging. Clients must be assessed individually to identify their particular characteristics and plan health education that meets those needs. Suitable health education topics for assisting clients to promote, retain, and restore health were identified.

Chronic disease is present in many older clients and affects teaching plans. Many clients simply need more information about the nature of their chronic disease and how they can lessen its effect and work cooperatively with the physician to implement the treatment plan. Some clients have nutritional deficiencies that affect learning and are addressed through health education.

Although researchers are not in agreement about the causes and extent of memory changes, many older individuals and their associates are aware of problems with short-term memory. Fortunately, a number of promising and tested remedies are available to the interested older individual. The nurse who is helping older clients learn information, attitude changes, or skills to promote health can make use of research. As the educator, you can adapt learning theories and principles to enhance older clients' chances of success.

EXERCISES

Exercise I—Ageism

Purpose: Develop awareness of your own attitudes toward the elderly.

Directions: Debate the proposition that ageism negatively affects the health care given to the elderly.

1. Divide into two groups, with each group taking opposing sides of the issue. Take 15 minutes to prepare your comments.
2. Reconvene as one group and debate the proposition.

Exercise II

Purpose: Identify suitable health education topics for older adults.

Directions: Divide into three groups and discuss the following client situations, all seen in a well-oldster clinic. Identify what health education topics are important to discuss with each client. Reconvene as a total class and share your findings.

1. A thin 80-year-old woman presents with a chief complaint of multiple subjective symptoms. Her objective findings included low sodium and chloride, elevated calcium, dry eyes and mouth, and other evidence of dehydration. She has a history of COPD, long-standing alcoholism, osteoarthritis, and kyphosis.
2. An obese 65-year-old man has a chief complaint of increased hunger, thirst, and fatigue. He was diagnosed with adult onset diabetes mellitus and appears motivated to learn better self-care and self-management. His blood glucose was 240 MG/DL (65 to 99 is normal). He is employed at local cafeteria where he eats two meals per day.
3. A slightly obese 85-year-old woman presents with a chief complaint of constipation that has been a problem off and on for the past year. Subjectively she complains of periodic abdominal discomfort. Her objective symptom includes a slightly distended abdomen.

Exercise III

Purpose: Analyze the implications of aging physiology on teaching and learning.

Directions: Divide into small groups and discuss how the age-related changes in the following body systems affect teaching and learning. Then list teaching and learning strategies for dealing with each change you identify.

1. Musculoskeletal system
2. Cardiovascular system
3. Respiratory system
4. Neurologic system
5. Sensory changes in vision and hearing

SUPPLEMENTAL ONLINE RESOURCES

Administration on Aging:
http://www.aoa.gov/
AgingStats 2008 Report:
http://www.agingstats.gov/agingstatsdotnet/Main_Site/Data/Data_2008.aspx
ANA Gero Nurse Online:
http://www.geronurseonline.org/
Department of Health and Human Services:
http://www.4woman.gov/
Erikson's Stages of Psychosocial Development
http://psychology.about.com/od/theoriesofpersonality/a/psychosocial.htm
Alzheimer's Association:
http://www.alz.org/index.asp?gclid=CO-9q6qew5gCFRxNagoduVZJ1w
Dementia versus Alzheimer's Disease:
http://www.alzheimerscaregiverresource.com/Dementia-Vs-Alzheimers-Disease-
    Ways-to-Distinguish-the-Two.html
American Heart Association:
http://www.americanheart.org/presenter.jhtml?identifier=1200000
American Lung Association:
http://www.lungusa.org/
Neurological Disorder Resources:
http://faculty.washington.edu/chudler/disorders.html
Geriatrics Resource Center:
http://www.medscape.com/resource/geriatric

National Council on Patient Information and Education:
http://www.talkaboutrx.org/
USDA Food Pyramid:
http://seniorliving.about.com/b/2008/01/22/usda-food-guide-pyramid-updated-
   for-special-needs-of-older-adults.htm
Tufts University Modified MyPyramid for Older Adults:
http://nutrition.tufts.edu/1197972031385/Nutrition-Page-nl2w_1198058402614.
   html

REFERENCES

2008 Older Americans: Key Indicators of Well-being. Retrieved January 15, 2009 from http://www.
   agingstats.gov/agingstatsdotnet/Main_Site/Data/Data_2008.aspx

Balakas, K. (2009). Developmental theories. In Potter, P. A., & Perry, A. G. (eds.). *Fundamentals of
   nursing* (7th ed., pp. 136–147). St. Louis: Mosby Elsevier.

Baker, M. W., & Heitkemper, M. M. (2007). Older adults. In Lewis, S. L., Heitkemper, M. M.,
   Dirksen, S. R., O'Brien, P. G., & Bucher, L. (eds.). *Medical-surgical nursing* (7th ed., pp. 66–84).
   St. Louis: Mosby Elsevier.

Biggs, A. J. (2007). Nutritional considerations. In Linton, A. D., & Lach, H. W. (eds.). *Matteson and
   McConnell's gerontological nursing concepts and practice* (3rd ed., pp. 169–197). St. Louis: Saunders
   Elsevier.

Bjorklund, B. R., & Bee, H. L. (2008). *The journey of adulthood* (6th ed.). Upper Saddle River, NJ:
   Pearson Education.

Bouman, W. P., Arcelus, J., & Benbow, S. M. (2006). Nottingham study of sexuality and ageing
   (NoSSA I). Attitudes regarding sexuality and older people: A review of the literature. *Sexual
   and Relationship Therapy, 21*(2), 149–161.

DeRosa, N., & Kochurka, K. (2006). Implement culturally competent healthcare in your workplace.
   Nursing Management, 37(10), 18–26.

Disabatino, A. J., & Bucher, L. (2007). Nursing assessment cardiovascular system. In Lewis, S. L.,
   Heitkemper, M. M., Dirksen, S. R., O'Brien, P. G., & Bucher, L. (eds.). *Medical-surgical nursing*
   (7th ed., pp. 739–760). St. Louis: Mosby.

Epstein, E. E., Fisher-Elber, K., & Al-Otaiba, A. (2007). Women, aging, and alcohol use disorders.
   Journal of Women and Aging, 19(1–2), 31–48.

Erikson, E. H. (1963). *Childhood and society* (2nd ed.). New York: W.W. Norton.

Erikson, E. H. (1982). *Life cycle completed: A review*. New York: W.W. Norton.

Erikson, E. H., & Erikson, J. M. (1997*). The life cycle completed*. New York: W.W. Norton.

Fahlman, M. M., Topp, R., McNevin, N., Morgan, A. L., & Boardley, D. (2007). Structured exercise in older adults with limited functional ability. *Journal of Gerontological Nursing, 33*(6),
   32–39.

Hall, A. M. (2009). Client education. In Potter, P. A., & Perry, A. G. (eds.). *Fundamentals of nursing*
   (7th ed., pp. 361–383). St. Louis: Mosby Elsevier.

Hendrickson, S. G. (2007). Nursing assessment nervous system. In Lewis, S. L., Heitkemper, M. M., Dirksen, S. R., O'Brien, P. G., & Bucher, L. (eds.). *Medical-surgical nursing* (7th ed., pp. 1441–1466). St. Louis: Mosby.

Kaufman, J. S. (2007). Nursing assessment respiratory system. In Lewis, S. L., Heitkemper, M. M., Dirksen, S. R., O'Brien, P. G., & Bucher, L. (eds.). *Medical-surgical nursing* (7th ed., pp. 509–532). St. Louis: Mosby.

Knowles, M. S. (1990). *The adult learner: A neglected species* (4th ed.). Houston: Gulf Publishing.

Linton, A. D. (2007a). Integument system. In Linton, A. D., & Lach, H. W. (eds.). *Matteson and McConnell's gerontological nursing concepts and practice* (3rd ed., pp. 225–258). St. Louis: Saunders Elsevier.

Linton, A. D. (2007b). Age-related changes in the special senses. In Linton, A. D., & Lach, H. W. (eds.). *Matteson and McConnell's gerontological nursing concepts and practice* (3rd ed., pp. 600–627). St. Louis: Saunders Elsevier.

Lueckenotte, A. (2009). Older Adult. In Potter, P. A., & Perry, A. G. (eds.). *Fundamentals of nursing* (7th ed., pp. 191–214). St. Louis: Mosby Elsevier.

Miller, C. A. (1990). *Nursing care of older adults*. Glenview, IL: Scott, Foresman/Little, Brown Higher Education.

Millsap, P. (2007). Neurological system. In Linton, A. D., & Lach, H. W. (eds.). *Matteson & McConnell's gerontological nursing concepts and practice* (3rd ed., pp. 406–441). St. Louis: Saunders Elsevier.

National Center for Health Statistics. News Release June 11, 2008. Retrieved February 2, 2009 from http://www.cdc.gov/nchs/pressroom/08newsreleases/mortality2006.htm

O'Brien, P. G. (2007). Patient and family teaching. In Lewis, S. L., Heitkemper, M. M., Dirksen, S. R., O'Brien, P. G., & Bucher, L. (eds.). *Medical-surgical nursing* (7th ed., pp. 53–65). St. Louis: Mosby Elsevier.

Roberts, D. (2007). Nursing assessment musculoskeletal system. In Lewis, S. L., Heitkemper, M. M., Dirksen, S. R., O'Brien, P. G., & Bucher, L. (eds.). *Medical-surgical nursing* (7th ed., pp. 1614–1628). St. Louis: Mosby.

Santrock, J. W. (2008). *A topical approach to life-span development* (4th ed.). Boston: McGraw-Hill.

Schmall, V. L. (1996). Family influences. In Lueckenott, A. G. (ed.). *Gerontological nursing* (pp. 136–166). St. Louis: Mosby; as cited in Wallace, M. (2006). Older adult. In Edelman, C. L., & Mandle, C. L. (eds.). *Health promotion throughout the life span* (6th ed., pp. 571–598). St. Louis: Mosby.

Schneider, J. K., Eveker, A., Bronder, D. R., Meiner, S. E., & Binder, E. F. (2003). Exercise training program for older adults. *Journal of Gerontological Nursing, 29*(9), 22–31.

Stevens, G. L. (2005). Geropsychiatric nursing. In Stuart, G., & Sundeen, S. (eds.), *Principles and practice of psychiatric nursing* (8th ed.). St. Louis: Mosby.

US Census Bureau News. Retrieved January 9, 2009 from http://www.census.gov/Press-Release/www/releases/archives/population/012496.html (News Release, August 14, 2008).

Wallace, M. (2006). Older adult. In Edelman, C. L., & Mandle, C. L. (eds.). *Health promotion throughout the life span* (6th ed., pp. 571–598). St. Louis: Mosby.

Weinrich, S. P., Boyd, M., & Nussbaum, J. (1989). Continuing education: Adapting strategies to teach the elderly. *Journal of Gerontological Nursing, 15*(11), 17–21.

CHAPTER 8

The Culturally Diverse Learner

But if everyone is genetically humming the same notes, why do people from different cultures and nations sing different melodies?
—Margaret M. Andrews, 2002, p. xvi

OBJECTIVES

Upon completion of this chapter you will be able to:
- Define the terms *culture, ethnicity, acculturation,* and *culturally competent care.*
- Describe the six culturally based health education outcomes.
- Select a cultural assessment tool to assess a culturally diverse client.
- Describe the culturally related norms, beliefs about health and illness, family influences, and implications for health education for African-American, Asian, Hispanic, and Native-American clients.
- Describe verbal and nonverbal communication relevant to African-American, Asian, Hispanic, and Native-American clients.
- Identify five culturally based actions you can take to provide culturally congruent client education.
- Describe the supporting rationale for culturally based actions in providing culturally congruent client education.

KEY TERMS

acculturation	culture
Blessingway ceremony	curanderismo
confianza	enculturated
cultural competence	ethnicity
cultural factors	evil eye
culturally competent care	familismo
culturally congruent client education	personalismo

INTRODUCTION

This chapter examines the role of culture in the process of client education. *Culture* is defined as "the totality of socially transmitted behavioral patterns, arts, beliefs, values, customs, lifeways, and all other products of human work and thought characteristic of a population of people that guide their world view and decision-making" (Purnell, 2003a, p. 5). *Cultural factors* include beliefs, values, moral principles, habits, dress, language, rules for behavior, economics, politics, dietary practices, and health care (Burchum, 2002). Not only do cultural factors relate to race and ethnicity, but also to behaviors and beliefs characteristic of particular social, ethnic, disabled, age, and gender groups. *Ethnicity* is identity with or membership in a particular racial, national, or cultural group and observance of that group's customs, beliefs, and language.

Knowledge of culture is a critical element in the process of delivering health education. All cultural and ethnic groups hold concepts related to health and illness and associated practices for maintaining well-being or providing treatment when it is indicated. The perception of health and illness is *enculturated* into members of a cultural group. In addition, the individual's socioeconomic, educational, geographic, religious, and other factors shape their cultural and ethnic health beliefs. Over time *acculturation* may occur, which means that members of a group modify or give up traits from the culture of origin as a result of contact with another culture. Demographic changes anticipated over the next decade magnify the importance of addressing racial/ethnic disparities in health care.

CHARACTERISTICS OF CULTURALLY DIVERSE LEARNERS

Shifting Demographics

The US Census Bureau reports that the population of the United States is more racially and ethnically diverse than ever before. The majority population of English-speaking Whites is giving way to a new influx of immigrants from other countries with many different cultures and ethnic backgrounds. In 2006, the number of diverse people in the United States topped 100 million for the first time, which is about one third of the US population. By 2050, half of US residents will be culturally diverse according to Census Bureau projections (US Census Bureau, 2008). This change is not just occurring in the United States. Demographics changes are occurring in many countries worldwide (Flowers, 2009). As a result of this multicultural phenomenon, cultural competence of nurses is becoming more critical to ensure positive outcomes for an increasingly diverse client population. Nurses must also realize that addressing cultural diversity goes beyond knowing the values, beliefs, practices and customs of African Americans, Asians, Hispanics/Latinos, and Native Americans/Alaskan Natives. In addition to racial classification and national origin, there are many other facets of cultural diversity. "Religious affiliation, language, physical size, gender, sexual orientation, age, disability (both physical and mental), political orientation, socioeconomic status, occupational status and geographical location are but a few of the faces of diversity" (Campinha-Bacote, 2003, p. 1).

It is important not to stereotype people of different cultures, but to cultivate an appreciation for individual cultural variations. Andrews (2008a) notes that having an understanding of culture, either your own or others, does not necessarily bring about respect and understanding. "Nursing students, nurses, and other health care providers must have positive experiences with members of other cultures and learn to genuinely value the contributions all cultures make to our multicultural society" (Andrews, 2008a, p. 9).

Healthcare Disparities

The health and life expectancy of Americans is improving, but racial and ethnic minorities have not benefited equally from this progress. Complex sociologic, cultural, political, and economic factors account for this. A major concern is that even those diverse clients with equivalent access to the health care system receive lower-quality care than White patients for many medical conditions (Smith et al., 2007). These differences in health disparities were revealed in the 2002 Institute of Medicine report, *Unequal Treatment: Confronting Racial and Ethnic Disparities in Health Care.* As a result the issue of disparities has become one of importance to healthcare providers. Experts have also noted that without new and more effective interventions, health disparities will be difficult to eliminate and may become an even larger problem as racial and ethnic minorities become a greater proportion of the US population (Smith et al., 2007). To meet the needs of culturally diverse groups, nurse educators must engage in the process of becoming culturally competent.

CULTURAL COMPETENCE

Definition

Campinha-Bacote (1998) defines *cultural competence* as "the process by which the health care professional continuously strives to achieve the ability and availability to effectively work within the cultural context of a client (individual, family, community)" (p. 6). This process requires nurses to see themselves as *becoming* culturally competent, rather than *being* culturally competent. Cross, Bazron, Dennis, and Isaacs (1989) further describes cultural competence as a developmental process that evolves over an extended period of time that includes both individuals and organizations at various levels of awareness, knowledge, and skills along the cultural competence continuum. Practicing cultural competence brings about the practice of *culturally competent care* that is considered to be "the knowledge, skills, and attitudes required to provide quality clinical care to patients from different cultural, ethnic, and racial backgrounds" (Harvard Medical School, 2009). The American Nurses Association (2001) recognizes the need to provide culturally competent care. It states in the association's code that nurses should "practice with compassion and respect for the inherent dignity, worth and uniqueness of every individual."

Campinha-Bacote Cultural Competence Model

Campinha-Bacote's model, *The Process of Cultural Competence in the Delivery of Healthcare Services*, includes the components of cultural desire, cultural awareness, cultural knowledge, cultural skill (conducting culturally sensitive assessments), and cultural encounters (Campinha-Bacote, 2002). Because cultural competence is an important attribute of the nurse as an educator, the five key concepts of the model are described further.

Cultural desire is the most critical concept of cultural competence because it is the nurse's desire that brings about the entire process of cultural competence. This desire must come from the nurse wanting to engage in becoming culturally competent, and not from having to participate in the process. The nurse takes a humble approach to client differences, and as educator, examines her or his personal motivation to work with clients of different cultures. In this important first step the nurse as educator asks, "How will I develop the willingness and patience to work with clients who are different from me?"

Cultural awareness is the self-examination and in-depth exploration of one's own cultural background. This process involves the recognition of the nurse's biases, prejudices, and assumptions about individuals who are different. This means examining past experiences and considering how to handle biases and assumptions. The nurse asks the question, "How will I develop the skill to be objective and open to cultural differences?"

Cultural knowledge is the process of seeking and obtaining a sound educational foundation about diverse cultural and ethnic groups. Obtaining cultural knowledge about the client's health-related beliefs and values involves understanding how clients' interpret their illness and how their view of the world guides their thinking, doing, and being. It is in this part of the model that stereotyping is addressed. Campinha-Bacote (2003) states that "No individual is a stereotype of one's culture of origin, but rather a unique blend of the diversity found within each culture, a unique accumulation of life experiences, and the process of acculturation to other cultures" (p. 7). The nurse as an educator makes a commitment to learning about other cultures, and to grow and evolve in that knowledge.

Cultural encounter is the process that encourages the nurse to directly engage in face-to-face interactions with clients from culturally diverse backgrounds. Interacting with clients from diverse cultural groups has the potential to refine or modify nurses' beliefs about cultural groups and aids in preventing stereotyping. It is important to note that interacting with only three or four members from a specific ethnic group does not make one an "expert" on the cultural group, but these encounters give the nurse as educator valuable experiences to draw from. As the nurse approaches the role of educator it is advisable to look for opportunities to expand knowledge of other cultures either locally or even internationally.

A final component of Campinha-Bacote's model, *cultural skill*, is the ability to collect relevant cultural data regarding the client's presenting problem as well as accurately performing a culturally based, physical assessment. Cultural assessment is defined as "a systematic, comprehensive examination of individuals, families, groups, and communities regarding their health-related cultural beliefs, values and practices" (Campinha-Bacote, 2002, p. 34). Chapter 4 introduces an initial concise cultural assessment designed for the busy nurse (see Box 4-2). As part of achieving cultural skill a variety of more in-depth cultural assessment tools are presented here. These tools should be selected and used to meet the specific needs of the learning situation. The nurse as educator should be aware that the way these tools are implemented through the nurse/client interaction is important. Cultural skill brings all the knowledge from the components of the model together to create culturally competent client interaction.

Cultural Assessment Tools

Andrews' Transcultural Nursing Assessment Guide for Individuals and Families

Andrews (2008b) offers an extensive in-depth assessment tool entitled the *Transcultural Nursing Assessment Guide for Individuals and Families*. The major categories in this guide include: cultural affiliations, values orientation, communication, health-related beliefs and practices, nutrition, socioeconomic considerations, organizations providing cultural support, education, religion, cultural aspects of disease incidence, bicultural variations, and developmental considerations across the life span. This tool focuses on cultural aspects of the health history and the physical examination.

Leininger's Sunrise Model

The Sunrise Model is part of Leininger's *Theory of Cultural Care Diversity and Universality* and includes seven assessments of culturally congruent nursing care. These include a holistic approach that looks at: cultural values and lifeways; religious, philosophical, and spiritual beliefs; economic factors; educational factors; technological factors; kinship and social ties; and political and legal factors (Leininger, 1991).

Purnell's Model for Cultural Competence

Purnell's *Model for Cultural Competence* includes domains of culture for assessing ethnocultural attributes of individuals, families, or groups (Purnell, 2003b). The twelve domains discussed are: inhabited localities and topography, communication, family roles and organizations, workforce issues, bicultural ecology, high-risk behaviors, nutrition, pregnancy and childbearing practices, death rituals, spirituality, healthcare practices, and healthcare practitioners. The strength of this model includes the domain of *bicultural ecology* that identifies specific physical, biological, and physiologic variations in ethnic and racial origins. This is a source of information on cultural variations in physical assessment for nurses as educators.

Giger and Davidhizar's Transcultural Assessment Model

Giger and Davidhizar's Transcultural Assessment Model consists of six cultural phenomena that go across all cultures affecting nursing care. These include communication, space, social organization, time, environmental control, and biological variations (Giger & Davidhizar, 2008). The model applies these concepts to 23 specific cultural groups found in the United States.

Assessing Cultural Competence

The nurse should take time to self-evaluate her or his progress in becoming culturally competent. The following two tools take slightly different approaches to examining cultural competence, but both help the nurse as educator reflect upon the role of culture in client care. Campinha-Bacote and Narayan (2000) state that "*Cultural*

TABLE 8-1	Culhane-Pera *et al.* Levels of Cultural Competence
Level 1	No insight about the influence of culture on health care
Level 2	Minimal emphasis on culture in healthcare setting
Level 3	Acceptance of the role of cultural beliefs, values, and behaviors on health disease, and treatment
Level 4	Incorporation of cultural awareness into daily healthcare practice
Level 5	Integration of attention to culture into all areas of professional life

Adapted from Blue, A. (2009). The Provision of Culturally Competent Health Care. Medical University of South Carolina: Department of Family Medicine. Retrieved on May 17, 2009 at http://www.musc.edu/fm_ruralclerkship/culture.html

awareness is "a continual self-examination of one's own prejudices and biases toward other cultures" (p. 213). Campinha-Bacote (2002) provides the "ASKED" mnemonic to help nurses assess their cultural awareness. The "A" is for awareness, the "S" is for skill, the "K" is for knowledge, the "E" is for encounters, and the "D" is for desire. Nurses as educators ask themselves if they have "A"wareness of biases and prejudices; do they have the "S"kill to conduct a cultural assessment; do they have cultural "K"nowledge; do they have experiences "E"ncountering people of different cultures, and do they have the "D"esire to be culturally competent? This self-assessment assists the nurse when working with diverse clients.

Culhane-Pera, Reif, Egli, Bake, and Kassekert (1997) describe five levels of cultural competence with respect to health care. With this tool nurses can track progress in becoming culturally competent as they advance through the levels (Table 8-1).

CULTURALLY CONGRUENT CLIENT EDUCATION

The definition of culturally congruent client education is drawn from the concept of culturally congruent care initially conceptualized by Leininger (1991). She defines culturally congruent care as, "Those cognitively based assistive, supportive, facilitative, or enabling acts or decisions that are tailor made to fit with individual, group, or institutional cultural values, beliefs, and lifeways in order to provide or support meaningful, beneficial, and satisfying health care to well-being services" (1991, p. 49). Schim, Doorenbos, Benkert, and Miller (2007) further explain Leininger's definition by saying "culturally congruent care is a holistic construct, heavily influenced by negotiated experiences, meanings, mutual understandings, and respect" (p. 105). We use this as a foundation to define culturally congruent client education. *Culturally congruent client education* involves providing meaningful and useful education for clients by incorporating diverse ways of knowing from the viewpoint of various cultural groups. It is a harmonious approach in working with clients that shows sensitivity and respect for individual cultural differences and a willingness to collaborate with them to meet health education needs. Culturally competent nurses who are educators welcome client collaboration and cooperation. They have a foundation of knowledge about client cultures and reflect on their own personal cultural values and beliefs. This self-examination helps them understand how their beliefs influence the way they teach.

The need for culturally congruent client education is based on the fact that diverse clients respond culturally to health and illness. Healthcare disparities are a leading cause of morbidity and mortality in the United States among minorities and those of lower socioeconomic status. Because of this, it is important that nurses incorporate cultural perspectives into all facets of delivery of health education (Anderson, Scrimshaw, Fullilove, Fielding, & Normand, 2003). This approach addresses the need to promote equal access to quality health care and treatment of clients.

Later in this chapter we introduce the Culturally Congruent Health Education Model that brings together culturally based actions, rationale, and culturally based health education outcomes. We do this after we introduce information about the four major cultural groups.

Culturally Specific Client Assessments and Concerns

Cultural factors affect client education interactions. It is important for the nurse as an educator to have an understanding of the cultural factors that shape learners from different cultural groups. Stressors and adaptive behaviors may present considerable barriers to effective client education unless nurses are sensitive to their origins and meanings and are willing to take them into account when working with clients (Falvo, 2004). By taking time to investigate a client's past experiences and cultural perceptions, the nurse takes steps to build rapport with clients, which is a basic component of effective nurse/client relationships.

Clients accept or reject the information given by a nurse based on whether they *perceive* the information as truthful, in their best interest, and congruent with their beliefs. To gain a better understanding of factors related to teaching and learning with cultural groups, we have chosen to present information on the four major ethnic minority groups: African American, Asian, Hispanic, and Native American. They are the major ethnic minorities in the United States as traced by the US Census Bureau.

Four aspects of each group's culture that impact health education are examined: *cultural norms* (aspects of the culture that impact the teaching and learning process), *family influence* (impact and involvement of family in the teaching and learning process), *beliefs about health and illness* (including religious influences and folk medicine that influence perception of heath care), and *implications for health education*. Knowledge of these aspects provide insight for the nurses as educators in planning and implementing teaching plans, but caution is needed to avoid stereotyping. Never assume that all clients from one ethnic group hold the same beliefs.

Black/African American

Cultural Norms

The US Census Bureau (2008) reported that there are approximately 41.1 million Black/African Americans living in the United States, which is about 14% of the total population. This number is expected to grow to 65.7 million, or 15% in 2050.

In preparing to work with African-American clients, the nurse should be aware that the initial client approach and the initial impression that you give is very important. Because interpersonal relationships are highly valued among African Americans, it is important to focus on developing a sound, trusting, and respectful relationship. This begins with consideration of the way that clients are greeted and referred to. Be aware of intracultural variations within the cultural group; for example, different generational groups may have a particular way by which they wish to be identified. Younger clients may want to be called African American; elderly may prefer the terms Negro or colored, and middle-age clients may refer to themselves as Black or Black American (Campinha-Bacote, 2008). Most African Americans prefer to be greeted formally using "Mr." "Mrs." or "Miss" along with their surname because the family name is respected and indicates pride in family heritage. Unless invited, it is best to use the last name and appropriate title instead of first names. It may be necessary to clarify preferences with clients.

The attitude of healthcare professionals is one of the most significant barriers when working with African Americans. Research shows that African-American clients feel they are often treated unfairly or disrespectfully because of their race (Kaiser Family Foundation, 2001). Because of this, African Americans may be suspicious of healthcare professionals and may seek out a physician or nurse only when absolutely necessary. Treating clients with respect is the foundation of the nurse/client relationship. Respect for persons has been broadly defined as the recognition that all persons have dignity and inherent worth. Expressions of respect include treatment with dignity and respect for autonomy and involvement in healthcare decisions. These expressions are associated with client satisfaction with care and increased adherence to treatment regimens. Beach et al. (2005) suggests that clients are able to determine when clinicians demonstrate a valuing attitude. These perceptions correlate with whether the client was treated kindly or rudely. Respectful treatment of African-American clients includes acknowledging clients appropriately as described previously, shaking hands, using eye contact, listening intently, and giving physical and mental comfort.

Family Influence

Understanding the African-American family is an important aspect of teaching clients. Traditional family structure of husband and wife is often found, but many African-American families have a matriarchal system with a single mother, aunt, or grandmother heading the household. The role of the grandmother is one of the most central roles in the African-American family and is afforded great respect (Campinha-

Source: © Patricia Marks/ShutterStock, Inc.

Bacote, 2008). A growing number of grandparents are functioning in the primary parental role. African-American women are expected to assist family members in maintaining good health and determining treatment if a family member is ill. It is important for the nurse to recognize the importance of African-American women in disseminating information and in assisting family members in making decisions (Cherry & Giger, 2008). If present, the African-American man should also be included in the decision-making process. Some African-American families have large supportive extended family networks. It is important to include involved, extended family members in planning and implementing teaching plans where appropriate, because they could unknowingly sabotage the clients' progress if uninformed.

Health Beliefs

Spiritual and religious orientation is important in some African-American families with the majority participating in Protestant denominations. Belief in God and the use of prayer and participation in formal religious service may be part of religious practices. The church community is viewed as a viable support system in developing health-promoting behaviors, and the nurse may consider a partnership with faith-based communities to support client learning.

There is evidence that African-American folk medicine is practiced in all areas of the United States, but the extent of its use is not known. African-American folk medicine is an offshoot of African cultural heritage in the rural South. It can involve treatment by folk practitioners who use witchcraft, voodoo, and magic. Folk medicine may be used for a variety of reasons: lack of access to traditional healthcare services, inability to afford the cost of health care, or humiliating experiences when encountering the mainstream healthcare system (Cherry & Giger, 2008).

Folk medicine perceives illness as either a natural or an unnatural occurrence. Natural illness occurs because a person is affected by natural forces without adequate protection. Unnatural illnesses are perceived as either a punishment from God or the work of the devil, which are more difficult for the nurse to address. Death is viewed as a natural part of living and is handled through strong religious beliefs (Campinha-Bacote, 2008). It is important for the nurse to assess if folk remedies are being used, and if so to assist the client in sorting out what is helpful, neutral, or harmful. This is part of the assessment information necessary to prepare the teaching plan.

Implications for Health Education

When setting up teaching sessions with African-American clients, keep in mind that they may prefer a closer personal space, and that extended family may accompany them. When teaching how to perform psychomotor skills, structure the learning activities in ranked order to produce maximum learning results. If timing is involved with an activity, it is important to be clear about when timing is flexible and when it is not, such as with the giving of medication. Keep in mind that a teaching plan that is congruent with the client's beliefs has a better chance of being successful. The most common health concerns for African Americans requiring health education are listed in Table 8-2.

Asian American

Cultural Norms

The US Census Bureau identified the Asian population as 15.5 million in 2008. It is expected to climb to 40.6 million by 2050. This is an increase from 5.1% to 9.2% of the total US population. Asians Americans emigrate from more than 20 countries and speak more than 100 different languages. The Asian-American population is diverse and represents people from a variety of countries and cultures. The largest subpopulations are persons of Chinese, Filipino, Japanese, Asian Indian, Korean, and Southeast Asian ancestry. Recent Asian immigrants represent the highest foreign born percentage among all racial and ethnic groups in the United States.

Establishing rapport with Asian clients begins with establishing trust. It is important to remember as you approach Asian clients to be aware that their values include hard work, acceptance of what life brings, respect for nature, self-control, respect for

TABLE 8-2   Most Common Disorders Requiring Health Education: African Americans

Ethnic/Racial Group	Most Common Disorders Requiring Health Education
African American	• Heart disease • Hypertension • Stroke • Cancer • Asthma • Influenza/pneumonia • HIV/AIDS • Homicide • Obesity • Sickle cell anemia

elders, and loyalty to family. Cultural values stress politeness in verbal discourse, and if mistrust develops you may find the client reluctant to discuss life style issues and behaviors. Many Asian Americans view relationships in heath care as hierarchical and therefore expect the health professional to take charge (Management Sciences for Health, 2005). Clients may not want to participate in making decisions about their treatment and may appear passive in the process. Nurses as educators should acknowledge their role and use it to their advantage when working with clients. This can be particularly effective in encouraging patients to adopt healthy behaviors and adhere to teaching plans. It is important, however, that the client not feel intimidated by the nurse. Feelings of intimidation may prevent the client from telling you the truth about customs, beliefs, or behaviors that may impact the success of the teaching plan. You should also be aware that some clients may silently decide not to adhere to recommended treatments (MSH, 2005).

Asian clients view health from a variety of perspectives and often combine Eastern and Western perspectives of health. They use acupuncture, acupressure, and the use of herbs in combination with dietary therapy, Western medicine, and supernatural healing to achieve maximum results. When beliefs contradict each other, however, some Asians will *not* adhere to Western medicine. It is also important to be aware that clients do not always disclose the use of Complementary and Alternative Medicine (CAM), which can increase the chances of adverse interaction with conventional Western treatments. Clients may be reluctant to share their use of these methods, fearing disapproval from the nurse and worrying that they might appear disrespectful of Western traditions. To determine use of CAM, you should ask clients directly and clearly what remedies they use. Nurses need to educate themselves about traditional Asian approaches to healing and encourage their clients and their healers to collaborate together for the client's good. A common belief of Asian clients is that Western medicine is very potent and that it can cure illness rapidly (MSH, 2005). This belief may manifest itself by the client reducing dosages. Clients also may stop medication as soon as symptoms are relieved. These are all areas that require attention when preparing teaching plans.

When meeting Asian elders it is a sign of disrespect to look them straight in the eyes. A limp handshake from Asian clients is a way of showing humility and respect. For many, physical contact such as a handshake or hug between a man and a woman is interpreted as a sexual advance. For some Asian subcultures it may be appropriate for you to first address the oldest male in a group or family before greeting other members (MSH, 2005). Be aware that a lack of facial expression or a low level of verbal communication may not indicate a lack of emotion or opinion. Neither does it indicate agreement with the diagnosis or recommended treatment. Try to determine your clients' true feelings or opinions before accepting their apparent acquiescence of the treatment plan. Asian clients tend to be more comfortable with a health professional who shares their language and culture, perhaps because they believe that a person of their own culture will not dismiss their traditional Asian practices and "home remedies" (MSH, 2005).

Family Influence

Traditionally, the Asian family unit is strong, stable, and cohesive for all its members. The family plays a critical role in the ongoing development and support of children through adulthood. The importance of the extended family, emphasized in Asian culture, often results in the extended family being highly involved in the client's care and medical decision making (MSH, 2005). Family members can provide valuable information regarding the client's diet, health behavior, daily activities, and types of alternative medications used. Their involvement in a treatment plan may be vital to the client's ability to adhere to the recommended teaching plan. Families may decide what the client will eat, when to take medication, whether to exercise, and when to

Source: © Monkey Business Images/ShutterStock, Inc.

seek medical attention. The family also exerts influence on youth to prevent antisocial and self-defeating behaviors.

Many Asian immigrants experienced stressful and painful episodes in their native countries that affect their health and influence their perception of the US healthcare system. The effects of war, migration, detention camps or torture, and experiences associated with adjustment to the US culture are all major factors that might result in mistrust, fear, or helplessness keeping the client from taking an active role in their health care.

Nurses as educators need to be sensitive to the diversity and generational differences within the Asian population and decide on an individual basis, whether it is culturally appropriate to involve family members. The culturally competent educator will discuss with the client the patterns of decision making in the family. Understanding and respecting complex and often delicate interactions among family members enables nurses to use the client's family as a valuable resource rather than an intrusion into the nurse/client relationship (MSH, 2005).

Health Beliefs

Asian medical tradition centers on a belief in the interconnectedness of the mind, body, and spirit and the need for balance and a holistic approach to the treatment of illness. Buddhism and other Eastern philosophies teach that art and science coexist and that healing is spiritual as well as scientific (Yee, Mokuau, & Kim, 1999). A common belief held by many Asians is that of Taoism. Originating in China, Tao or "the way," is based on the idea of balancing the natural processes and forces of *yin* and *yang*. *Yin* is negative female energy associated with cold and water, and *Yang* is positive male energy associated with heat and fire. These forces remain in balance through a combination of practices of holistic medicine, acupuncture, herbalism, and meditation. Beliefs about health and illness strongly influence clients' behavior. They may avoid the wind, be reluctant to go out after surgery, or refuse to have blood drawn (MSH, 2005). Many Asians perceive life in fatalistic terms and may feel less able to do something about their illness. Beliefs in supernatural spirits may result in reliance on religion or spiritual healing rituals in addition to Western medicine. All of these factors influence your approach to teaching Asian clients.

Implications for Health Education

As an educator, you need to be a strong encourager as Asian clients need assurance that the recommended treatment plan is the right thing to do. This may mean urging family members to encourage the client. Being an advocate also means helping to

TABLE 8-3   Most Common Disorders Requiring Health Education: Asians

Ethnic/Racial Group	Most Common Disorders Requiring Health Education
Asian	• Cancer • Heart disease • Stroke • Accidents • Diabetes • Tuberculosis • Liver disease

locate other supportive healthcare providers. In some communities, Asian-American organizations (temples, churches, benevolent association, cultural associations, etc.) serve as focal points for social and other activities. Developing contacts with and working through these community-based organizations can be a useful way for you to develop an understanding of the health and social needs of clients (MSH, 2005). Be aware that Asian clients usually expect something concrete such as prescriptions for medications at the conclusion of a teaching session for the meeting to live up to their expectations. Without this, they might be reluctant to return for routine teaching visits or preventive care. Also be aware that Asian women may prefer to work with an educator who is a woman. The most common health concerns for Asians requiring health education are listed in Table 8-3.

Hispanic

Cultural Norms

The US Census Bureau (2008) lists the Hispanic population as 46.7 million and projects it to increase to 132.8 million by 2050. This will be an increase from 15% to 30% of the total US population, making Hispanics the largest ethnic minority group in the US. Hispanics are classified as one ethnic group, but they are actually multiple, culturally similar ethnic subgroups. The subgroups that make up the Hispanic population in the United States are: Mexicans, Puerto Ricans, Cubans, Central Americans, South Americans, Dominicans, and other Hispanics and Latinos.

When working with Hispanic clients it is important to be aware of the different terms used to refer to Hispanics. The US Census Bureau (2001) used the term *Hispanic* to describe any person, regardless of race, creed, or color, whose origins are

Mexican, Puerto Rican, Cuban, Central or South American, or of some other Hispanic origin. *Latino* or Latina refers to a person of Latin-American or Spanish-speaking descent living in the United States. The terms *Hispanic* or *Latino* may be used interchangeably (Zoucha & Zamarripa, 2003). It is not recommended to use the terms *Chicano, Mexicanos,* or *Xicans* unless the client refers to themselves in these ways as these terms may be considered derogatory. The term *Tejano* is used to describe a Texan of Hispanic decent. It is important to ask clients how they would like to be referred to.

Several cultural characteristics impact the way that Hispanic clients perceive interactions with healthcare professionals. The concepts of *respecto* (respect), *personalismo* (personal relationships), and *confianza* (trust) are important concepts for the nurse to be aware of when interacting with Hispanic clients (Gonzalez, Owen, & Esperat, 2008). *Respecto* is a behavior that shows differential attention toward others based on age, sex, social position, economic status, and authority. It is important for you to show respect by addressing Hispanic clients by their surname and title in English or Spanish, such as Mrs. Rodriquez or Senora Rodriquez and by avoiding a condescending attitude. Hispanic clients may avoid eye contact with authority figures. To be respectful, personal or private questions should be approached in an indirect way to avoid client embarrassment. *Personalismo* is about the nurse conveying to the client that they want a personal relationship. This is demonstrated by being friendly and taking interest in the client's life. This is shown by engaging in a greeting that inquires about how they are doing and puts the client at ease. Personal contact and touch are acceptable parts of the relationship and are considered to be important aspects of the nurse/client relationship. Hispanic clients prefer to be close and are comfortable with the nurse giving a handshake, sitting closer, leaning forward, and giving a comforting pat on the shoulder or other gestures that indicates interest in the client. Hispanic clients demonstrate stronger attachment to the healthcare provider than to the healthcare institution and will follow the provider if they move (MSH, 2005). This emphasizes how strongly they value personal relationships. *Confianza*, or trust, develops over time in relation with Hispanic clients. When trust is established between the nurse and the client, it becomes more likely that the client will value the time spent with the nurse and that they will be more likely to adhere with teaching plans.

It can be frightening for clients that cannot speak English to enter the US healthcare system. Studies show that Hispanic clients view nurses who attempted to speak some Spanish as caring and respectful (Gonzalez et al., 2008). It is common for Hispanic clients to appear agreeable on the surface and to be courteous, but if they disagree they may not carry out suggested treatment. It is uncommon for Hispanic clients to be aggressive when interacting with health professionals, but their response may be silence and/or not adhering to the teaching plan. Joking by the nurse is considered rude, insulting, and offensive and may cause stress and result in a negative response (Gonzalez et al., 2008). When under stress Hispanic clients may revert back to using their native language. Hispanic clients also may prefer educators matching their gender.

Family Influence

Family is a highly valued part of Hispanic life and family involvement is often critical in providing health care to the client. Family matters take precedence over work and all other aspects of life. Hispanic families are large, and respect for parental authority is emphasized. Typical Hispanic families are patriarchal with the male family members having the dominant role as head of the household. They are the decision makers. Hispanic men typically have a strong sense of *machismo*. This is an attitude that the man is wiser, smarter, stronger, and more knowledgeable (Zoucha & Zamarripa, 2003). Hispanic women defer to men and have subdued qualities. Mothers may influ-

Source: © Feverpitch/ShutterStock, Inc.

ence family decisions but do not play a dominant role. Any dishonor or shame that may occur for an individual family member is considered a reflection on the entire family. Elderly Hispanics are respected and may live with married children if they are not self-sufficient. Changes in these patterns are seen in the more educated clients and families with higher socioeconomic status. Overall change to a more egalitarian family structure is slow to happen.

Many clients live in multifamily arrangements that include extended family who offer social and economic support. The term *familismo* describes the Hispanic belief in family interdependence that curtails exposure to outside influences, and that may be a major cause of resistance to change (Gonzalez et al., 2008). An important aspect of Hispanic families is that they are the main source of assistance before seeking out any assistance from the community. By including family members, nurses as educators can build greater trust and confidence and in turn increase adherence to teaching plans.

Health Beliefs

Hispanics believe in an external *locus of control*, which is the belief that outside forces control their lives. For some Hispanics, health is viewed as being the result of good luck or a reward from God. Some also believe in the theory of hot and cold imbalances. The basis of this belief is that illness is caused by prolonged exposure to hot or cold. Many of the illnesses are digestive in nature. To ensure good health both hot and cold foods must be taken into the body. It is important for the nurse to be aware that the use of self-medication with alternative therapies is prevalent in Hispanic culture, and this information is seldom reported to health professionals. The nurse should understand that Hispanics will have more respect for the nurse who accepts the spiritual and folk basis of their health beliefs (Gonzalez et al., 2008). If the teaching plan is incongruent with folk beliefs, the nurse as educator should attempt to find compromises or solutions to resolve the incongruence and allow clients to maintain their belief system while following the plan. Folk healers are part of *curanderismo*, which views illness from a religious and social perspective rather the Western scientific perspective. *Curanderas, santera,* and *espiritistas* are folk healers who are sought out to treat illness and are preferred over the medical community because they are personal, less dehumanizing, know the family, and are an integral part of the Hispanic community (Gonzalez et al., 2008).

Implications for Health Education

Begin with an assessment of the Hispanic client's ability to communicate and understand English. Establishing rapport is an essential part of building a trusting relation-

TABLE 8-4 Most Common Disorders Requiring Health Education: Hispanic	
Ethnic/Racial Group	**Most Common Disorders Requiring Health Education**
Hispanic	• Heart disease • Cancer • Accidents • Stroke • Diabetes • Hypertension • Obesity • HIV/AIDS

ship. There should be continuous evaluation of learning by questioning and return demonstration; problem solving should be encouraged. You need to understand the perceived causes for folk-related diseases and show respect for cultural differences, such as amulets that the client might wear to protect from the evil eye or evil spirits. Also be aware that some Hispanics feel that medication is always necessary and many may not believe that their illness is being treated adequately unless medication is ordered (MSH, 2005). Your long-term goal working in the Hispanic community should be to gain understanding of folk medicine beliefs and try to establish a relationship with the healers in the hope of eliciting acceptance and understanding of the rationale for the teaching plan. You need be aware of the client's cultural health beliefs to have an effect on the client's behavior and recovery. The most common health concerns for Hispanics requiring health education are listed in Table 8-4.

Native American

Cultural Norms

The number of American Indians and Alaska natives in the United States is approximately 4.9 million, but that number is projected to increase to 8.6 million by 2050 (US Census, 2008). This will be an increase from 1.6% to 2% of the total US population. The Bureau of Indian Affairs recognizes over 500 different Indian tribes with the largest number being Cherokee and Navajo (Hanley, 2008). Alaska natives are divided into five cultural and linguistic groups: Interior Indians, Aleuts, Southeast Coastal Indians, Northern Eskimos, and Southern Eskimos (Davidhizar & DeLapp, 2008). For the purposes of this discussion, American Indians and Alaska natives are referred to as Native Americans.

The first meeting with Native American clients is considered a time for building rapport and not for carrying out essential work. Native Americans may introduce themselves by stating the clan and the location of their home. They often initially appear silent and reserved; quiet voice tones are usually used when speaking. On greeting they may extend a hand and touch the hand of the other person lightly out of respect, but touch is generally reserved for those people that the client knows well. Eye contact is to be avoided, and pointing at another person should not be done as this is considered rude.

Family Influence

Family is very important to Native American clients and includes all members of the extended family. The primary goal of the family is the development of children and

Source: © ZanyZeus/ShutterStock, Inc.

adolescents. They follow the concept of clanship, in which the nuclear family and extended family are in close relationship (Hanley, 2008). Usually a male member of the family is looked upon as the leader; however, all members of the family may be involved in healthcare decisions. A family member may travel long distances to be with an ill family member. Although men are seen as important, grandmothers and mothers are often at the center of many Native American traditions (Zoucha & Zamarripa, 2003). Elders are a source of cultural information and can provide advice and support to the nurse. The time orientation for many Native Americans is focused on the present, which affects how they perceive future events. This may result in difficulties knowing when to take medications and the importance of being on time for appointments. Many Native Americans believe that the shared space of the *hogan*, or round open room, provides spiritual security and a sense of trust (Hanley, 2008). Some clients may not feel comfortable outside their normal surroundings.

Health Beliefs

Native Americans believe that wellness is a state of harmony with ones' surroundings and with their families. Illness results from something that the client has done to cause disharmony. When they are ill they may seek out the services of a medicine man to find out what is causing disharmony. The different types of medicine men and women include diagnosticians, singers, and herbalists. The use of the healing ceremony is used to return to a harmonious state. The *Blessingway* ceremony attempts to remove ill health by means of stories, songs, rituals, prayers, symbols, and sand paintings (Hanley, 2008). They have *jish*, or medicine bundles, containing symbolic and sacred items such as corn pollen, feathers, stones, arrowheads, and other instruments used for healing and blessing (Hanley, 2008). Pain is considered to be something to be endured, and clients may not ask for pain medication. An important cultural belief is that Native Americans should not touch a dead or dying person, as they believe that the spirit of the deceased may contaminate them. They also may avoid discussing the topics of death and dying. They blend traditional beliefs with Western health practices.

Implications for Health Education

It is important to remember that Native American beliefs depend on clients' personal experiences and the degree of acculturation into US society. If the client uses folk medicine it is important for you to determine which cultural health practices are beneficial, neutral, or harmful to provide culturally congruent care. When teaching Native Americans, you should be aware that they are comfortable with extended periods of silence, so allow them adequate time for information processing. You should use

TABLE 8-5 Most Common Disorders Requiring Health Education: Native Americans	
Ethnic/Racial Group	**Most Common Disorders Requiring Health Education**
Native American	• Heart disease • Cancer • Accidents • Diabetes • Stroke • Alcohol abuse • Hepatitis • Obesity • Sudden infant death syndrome (SIDS)

straightforward and easily understood language, and clarify misconceptions in a direct manner. The most common health concerns for Native Americans requiring health education are listed in Table 8-5.

Cross-Cultural Communication

Cross-cultural communication factors must be considered when nurses interact with clients and their family members from cultural backgrounds that differ from their own (Andrews, 2008c). To be culturally competent, the nurse as educator needs to examine ways in which people from diversified cultural backgrounds communicate. Research has shown that communication between healthcare professionals and clients is linked to client satisfaction, adherence to medical instructions, and health outcomes (Stewart et al., 1999). This discussion on cross-cultural communication focuses on verbal and nonverbal communication, focused communication tools, and the use of interpreters. These factors are reviewed for the four major cultural groups: African American, Asian, Hispanic, and Native American.

Verbal Communication

Some African-American clients speak in what is called African-American English. This dialect, a mixture of English, Creole, and West African languages, is sometimes misinterpreted as uneducated, but is actually a way to share unique cultural ideas and symbolize racial pride and identity (Campinha-Bacote, 2003). You may have to seek clarification if words are not understood. The volume of African-American voices is sometimes louder that those of other cultures, but this should not be interpreted as anger or aggression.

A hallmark of Asian communication is to think before speaking and to be polite. When working with Asian clients you may find that they respond "yes" to a question as a way of being polite or avoiding conflict, even when they do not understand the question being asked (Hoang & Erickson, 1985). Also some Asian clients may feel uncomfortable about giving and receiving compliments or saying "thank you." Their communication style is based on a cultural tradition that emphasizes self-humility in social situations. An interpreter may be needed to communicate with Asian clients.

For Hispanics in the United States, inability to speak and understand English can be a serious complication to receiving health care. Most Hispanics speak some English but many continue to speak Spanish at home with family. Communication may be complicated by the fact that Hispanics often learn a mixture of English and Spanish, which makes it difficult for you to understand. An interpreter may be required to facilitate communication. Hispanic clients expect that nurses will give direct eye contact when interacting with them, but they do not reciprocate with direct eye contact. When looking at or admiring a Hispanic child, it is important to touch the child to avoid giving the child the "evil eye" (Gonzalez et al., 2008).

Communication with Native American clients may require you to use interpreters because many still speak native tribal languages. Another complicating factor when developing teaching plans is that many of the native languages do not have equivalent single words in the English language, which makes understanding difficult. Native Americans consider silence essential to understanding and may pause after questions to carefully consider the answer.

Nonverbal Communication

African-American clients are generally more comfortable with touch and a close personal space. You will see more demonstrative facial expression and use of animated gestures when talking. Using humor is acceptable with African Americans and can be a way to release feelings and reduce stress. Asian clients often will be serene and stoic, suppressing negative emotion. Asians consider the head sacred, and so it is not polite to pat the head (Giger & Davidhizar, 2008). Be aware that the lack of facial expression of Asian clients or a low level of verbal communication may not indicate a lack of emotion or opinion. It is important to determine Asian clients' true feelings or opinions before deciding what they think. Hispanic clients are often tactile in their relationships and show affection for each other. They may appear agreeable on the surface to avoid confrontation especially during health education. Dramatic body language is used when Hispanic clients describe emotional problems (Gonzalez et al., 2008). If a disagreement develops, Hispanic clients may become silent and not adhere to the teaching plan. Native-American clients prefer listening to speaking and rarely practice small talk except among close acquaintances. In social situations when they are angry or uncomfortable, Native Americans may remain silent. Often they will avoid eye contact and may look at the floor while you are talking as a way of showing they are listening intently.

Focused Cultural Assessment Tools

A thorough cultural assessment helps you as the educator to develop a teaching plan and, if possible, should be done in advance of the teaching session. Specific assessment tools for an in-depth cultural assessment were described earlier in the chapter and can be selected based on client needs. Often, however, a client presents with a specific problem that needs immediate attention. In this situation it is important to first assess how the client views their health problems and what he or she believes is the care needed to resolve it. Kleinman (1980) developed the following list of questions that you can use to better gain insight into the client's perception of his or her illness.

1. What do you call your problem (sickness)? What name does it have?
2. What do you think caused your sickness?
3. Why do you think it started when it did?
4. What does your sickness do to you? How does it work?
5. How severe is it? Do you think it will last a short or long time?
6. What do you fear most about your sickness?
7. What are the chief problems that your sickness has caused for you?
8. What kind of treatment do you think you should receive? What are the most important results you hope to receive from the treatment?

Once you have an understanding of the client's perception of the health problem, there may be a need to negotiate the plan of care. The LEARN model is a framework for creating new health patterns through effective listening, education, and negotiation (Berlin & Fowkes, 1983). When using this framework for health education, you should first attempt to understand, then to be understood, and finally to negotiate a teaching plan that fits the client's cultural framework. Negotiation includes a preserve-accommodate-restructure approach (DeRosa & Kochurka, 2006). You should preserve cultural practices that help the client achieve health goals, and accommodate neutral cultural practices that neither help nor hinder the client. Negotiation is called for in restructuring harmful cultural practices that might risk or impair the client's health into healthful ones. This approach of honoring cultural values and practices helps the client feel respected and comfortable, and makes it more likely that they will adhere to the treatment plan.

L: *Listen* with sympathy and understanding to the patient's perception of the problem.
E: *Explain* your perceptions of the problem.
A: *Acknowledge* and discuss the differences and similarities.
R: *Recommend* treatment.
N: *Negotiate* agreement.

Use of Interpreters

Interviewing non-English speaking clients requires a bilingual interpreter for full communication. Even a person who has basic English skills may need the services of an interpreter when placed in teaching situations that require give and take. Whenever possible, use a bilingual team member or trained medical interpreter. The interpreter should possess a high level of fluency and a strong sense of ethics. Family members, children, or friends are not a good choice for interpreting. Using them violates confidentiality, plus they are not trained to understand medical terminology. A professional interpreter has the special skills needed to fully understand what the nurse and client want to say, and to make their messages clear in two languages. In addition, a qualified interpreter knows the role, limitations, and responsibilities that an interpreter needs.

If possible the interpreter should meet the client ahead of time to build rapport. Arrangements should be made in advance because the teaching session will take more time. Prepare ahead of time and focus on the major teaching points and prioritize information. During the session the nurse, client, and interpreter sit so that they form the points of a triangle. When speaking to the client, the nurse looks at the client. Two different interpretive styles are possible in the teaching session: line-by-line and summarization. Using the line-by-line approach ensures accuracy but takes more time. Information needs to be presented on a concrete level because abstract conceptualizations do not readily translate and may confuse the client (Putch, 1985). The nurse chooses words carefully and uses gestures sparingly. A normal tone of voice is used, not too fast or too loud. The nurse and client speak only a sentence or two and then the interpreter is given time to interpret. Simple language is used without medical jargon. Summary translation is faster and works well when teaching simple procedures with which the translator is already familiar. The interpreter summarizes the points that the nurse wants to teach. The interpreter and the nurse observe the non-verbal messages throughout the teaching session. At the end it is important to ask the client to confirm their understanding of what was taught.

The use of on-site medical interpreters or translators is only one way that language access services may be available to nurses. There are also telephone interpreter services, video medical interpreting services, translation software for written materials, bilingual clinical staff, and language classes for staff.

Linguistically and Culturally Appropriate Teaching Strategies and Instructional Materials

Linguistic competence is the capacity of an organization and its personnel to communicate effectively, and convey information in a manner that is easily understood by diverse audiences including persons of limited English proficiency, those who are not literate or have low health literacy skills, and individuals with disabilities (Goode & Jones, 2006). To address cultural linguistic competence, The National Standards on Culturally and Linguistically Appropriate Services Standards (CLAS) were developed by the US Department of Health and Human Services Office of Minority Health (2001) to ensure that all people entering the healthcare system receive equitable and effective treatment in a culturally and linguistically appropriate manner. The standards are intended to be inclusive of all cultures and not limited to any particular population group. They are designed to address the needs of racial, ethnic, and linguistic population groups that experience unequal access to health services. These standards serve as guidelines for nurses and can be accessed online through the Office of Minority Health.

Healthy People 2010 (2009) defines health literacy as "the degree to which individuals have the capacity to obtain, process, and understand basic health information and services needed to make appropriate health decisions." Research shows that health literacy is the single best predictor of client health status (Campinha-Bacote, 2008). Low health literacy affects older people, immigrants, the impoverished, and minorities. It is often brought about by inadequate communication between clients and nurses. Clients frequently attempt to hide their inability to read, and the nurse cannot judge literacy level solely by clients' years of education. Clients with low reading ability and comprehension skills may not able to express what is not understood and therefore may choose to conceal their low literacy skills (Maurer & Smith, 2004). Ways to reduce low health literacy include limiting the amount of medical jargon, using pictures or models to explain important health concepts, assuring understanding with "show me" techniques, and encouraging clients to ask questions. Additional information about health literacy can be found in Chapter 11. Sockalingam (2007) identifies six principles to create culturally competent health materials that should be considered when choosing, adapting, or creating health promoting instructional materials:

1. Acknowledge the unique issues of biculturalism and bilingual status of both healthcare providers and the service populations.
2. Incorporate client preferences in choosing instructional materials. Health messages should demonstrate respect for client uniqueness and cultural difference.
3. Involve members of the target population in the creation of instructional materials.
4. Use the family as the focal point of intervention when developing health messages.
5. Base health education and promotion on cultural aspects of epidemiology (concepts of causation and cure).
6. Education and promotion should exist in concert with natural and informal health care and support systems within the community (Sockalingam, 2007).

Culturally appropriate teaching strategies and instructional materials are necessary when the client's particular culture dictates how a problem should be addressed. These teaching strategies and instructional materials include the following:

- Use a variety of teaching strategies and instructional materials that are culturally and language specific. This includes use of written materials (posters, brochures, etc.), short films, and computer-assisted instruction, group teaching, and Web sites.
- Consider clients' cultures and language skills when developing learning objectives, teaching strategies, and instructional materials.
- Facilitate comparable learning opportunities for clients with differing characteristics and learning styles. For example, consider learning opportunities for clients who differ in race, sex, disability, ethnicity, religion, socioeconomic status, and ability.
- Incorporate learning objectives for personal development based on cultural beliefs.
- Clearly communicate learning objectives.
- Use concrete terms, choose words that do not have multiple meanings, and avoid medical jargon and slang.

BOX 8-1   Six-Step Approach to Delivering Culturally Congruent Care

1. Cultivate attitudes associated with culturally competent care and health education.

2. Recognize the impact of culture on the beliefs, values, and practices of clients and team members.

3. Obtain background information about the client's culture.

4. Perform a cultural assessment.

5. Plan culturally sensitive health education using a "preserve-accommodate-restructure" framework.

6. Avoid defensiveness and recover from cultural mistakes.

- Give clients an overview of the teaching plan and tell them about the learning objectives. Relate the plan to previous learning and summarize the main points.
- Provide frequent review of the content learned.
- Facilitate independence in thinking and action by helping clients to find answers themselves.
- Promote on-task behavior by keeping clients actively involved.
- Check with clients during the teaching session to see if they have any questions about what they are doing and if they understand the content.
- Provide frequent feedback and reinforcement.

DeRosa and Kochurka (2006) developed a six-step approach to providing culturally competent care, which we have adapted to apply to nurses providing culturally congruent health education. These steps are found in Box 8-1.

CULTURALLY CONGRUENT CLIENT EDUCATION MODEL

The increasingly multicultural profile of the US population requires that nurses provide culturally congruent care. Providing culturally congruent client education has the potential to improve health outcomes, increase the efficiency of healthcare professionals, and result in greater client satisfaction with services (Brach & Fraser, 2000). The Culturally Congruent Client Education Model brings together the concepts presented in this chapter to summarize the essential framework of what it means

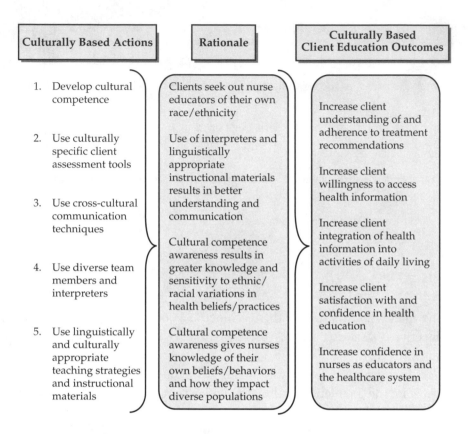

FIGURE 8-1   The Culturally Based Congruent Client Education Model.

to provide culturally congruent client education. The three major components of the model are: culturally based actions, rationale, and culturally based health education outcomes (Figure 8-1).

Culturally Based Actions

The culturally based actions in this model begin with the first action, which is to *develop cultural competence*. This chapter provides Caminha-Bacote's cultural competence model that identified the steps in the process of becoming culturally competent: cultural desire, cultural awareness, cultural knowledge, cultural skill, and cultural encounters.

The second culturally based action is using *culturally specific client assessment tools* to develop individualized teaching plans. This chapter presented in-depth assessment tools by a variety of authors as well as a focused assessment option to gather client information. The nurse chooses the cultural assessment tool that is appropriate for the situation.

The third culturally based action is using knowledge of *cross-cultural communication techniques* to interact with clients in developing teaching plans. A preserve-accommodate-restructure approach (DeRosa & Kochurka, 2006) is taken in working with clients so that cultural practices are preserved except for those that hinder the client's health. The LEARN technique of L: listen, E: explain, A: acknowledge, R: recommend, and N: negotiate is an example of using cross-cultural communication (Berlin & Fowkes, 1983). It is a negotiation framework that supports a cross-cultural approach to client communication.

The fourth culturally based action is to use *diverse team members and interpreters* that reflect the client's culture. Diverse clients are more likely to access and use health care services when they encounter health professionals of their own race and ethnicity (Purnell, 2003a). The correct use of interpreters or bilingual team members is an important culturally based action that allows for cultural congruency. Lack of interpreter services is a significant factor associated with client dissatisfaction and poor comprehension.

The fifth culturally based action is using *linguistically and culturally appropriate teaching strategies and instructional materials* to enhance and support learning. This action involves providing culturally appropriate oral and written language services to clients with limited proficiency. This action increases client adherence to treatment and improving the quality of health education.

Rationale

Nurses as educators gain knowledge through developing cultural competence, which includes becoming aware of their own beliefs and behaviors as well as those of clients. The use of assessment tools facilitates gathering clients' cultural data that can be used to build individualized teaching plans. When possible, nurses of the clients' race or ethnicity should be involved in teaching clients. A goal for the future is to increase the number of culturally diverse nurses to meet this need. The use of interpreters and linguistically appropriate instructional materials are actions that result in better understanding, adherence to treatment plans, and improved cross-cultural communication.

Culturally Based Client Education Outcomes

Culturally based actions result in meeting the needs of diverse populations. The desired culturally based client education outcomes are to meet the needs of diverse populations by increasing client understanding of treatment and adherence to treatment recommendations. When nurses take the recommended culturally based actions, clients are more willing to access health information. This increases their satisfaction with health education and increases their confidence in nurses as educators. These outcomes result in clients who are better able to integrate health teaching into their activities of daily living.

BOX 8-2   Evidence-Based Nursing Practice

Collins, C.A., Decker, S.J. & Esquibel, K.A. (2006) Definitions of health: comparison of Hispanic and African-American elders. *The Journal of Multicultural Nursing & Health 12*(1), 14–19.

Purpose: This study described the definitions of health in Hispanic and African American elders.

Method: The study used a qualitative framework in a doctoral-level multicultural nursing course. Quasi-statistics and a semi-structured interview format were used to tabulate the frequency of themes. A convenience sample of Hispanic and African American clients at senior citizen centers was used. Data were gathered throughout the class and was shared with the class which was a study limitation.

Results: The participants shared some differences but more similarities in their definitions. Eight reoccurring themes were identified: spirituality, without pain/feeling good, positive attitude with good mentality, high priority, independent/active, health promotion/maintenance, socialization, and helping others. The findings of the study were consistent with the literature and emphasized the importance of avoiding stereotyping individuals from any cultural background.

SUMMARY

This chapter looked at the importance of cultural competence for nurses who provide health education. Changing demographics and disparities in health care are powerful reasons that necessitate that nurses become culturally competent. Becoming culturally competent is a developmental process and involves self-awareness and insight into the workings of other cultures. To provide meaningful health education it is important for nurses to adapt the Culturally Congruent Client Education Model that looks at culturally based actions, their rationale, and outcomes.

EXERCISES

Exercise I—Health Beliefs and Home Remedies

Purpose: Examine the health beliefs of various cultural/ethnic/racial groups.

Directions:

1. Divide into small groups composed of individuals who are most culturally/ethnically/racially *alike*.
2. Discuss how your parents and grandparents (a) defined good health and poor health (b) list the home remedies they used to treat individuals in poor health.
3. Share your findings with the entire class. How were your findings similar? Dissimilar?
4. What did you learn about individuals who are supposedly "alike?"

Exercise II—Health Beliefs and Home Remedies

Purpose: Examine the health beliefs of various cultural/ethnic/racial groups.

Directions:

1. Divide into small groups composed of individuals who are most culturally/ethnically/racially *unlike* each other.
2. Compare and contrast the findings discovered in Exercise I. How were the beliefs about good health and poor health alike? Different?
3. Compare and contrast the various home remedies identified in Exercise I. How were the home remedies across the cultural/ethnic/racial groups alike? Different?
4. Share your findings with the entire class.

Exercise III—Cultural Reflection

Purpose: Reflect on the health education needs of various cultural/ethnic/racial groups.

Directions:

1. As an individual, reflect on the new knowledge you gained from participating in Exercises I and II. What are the implications for health education? How will this impact you in your role as an educator? Take about 15 minutes for reflection.

2. As a group, share your thoughts and conclusions with others in your class. Did others have similar thoughts and conclusions?

3. Using the Campinha-Bacote's mnemonic "ASKED" questions found in this chapter, discuss how this exercise made you more culturally competent.

Exercise IV—Application of the Culturally Congruent Client Education Model

Purpose: Apply the Culturally Congruent Client Education Model.

Directions: Identify a culturally diverse client for whom you want to provide culturally congruent care. Go through the culturally based actions identified in the model to develop a plan that meets the needs of the client. Ask yourself these questions:

1. Are you culturally competent?
2. How will you expand your knowledge of the culture?
3. What culturally specific client assessment tools will you use?
4. What cross-cultural communication techniques will you use?
5. Are there diverse team members or interpreters whose skill you can tap?
6. What linguistically and culturally appropriate teaching strategies and instructional materials will you use?

SUPPLEMENTAL ONLINE RESOURCES

Office of Minority Health
http://www.omhrc.gov/templates/browse.aspx?lvl=2&lvlID=11
National Center for Cultural Competence
http://www11.georgetown.edu/research/gucchd/nccc/
Resources for cross-cultural health care:
http://www.diversityrx.org/HTML/DIVRX.htm
Ethnomed:
http://healthlinks.washington.edu/clinical?ethnomed/htopics.html
Ethnomed: Patient Education All Languages:
http://www.ethnomed.org/ethnomed/patient_ed/
Learn More about Best Practices for Improving Linguistic Competency *A Patient-Centered Guide to Implementing Language Access Services in Healthcare Organizations:*
www.thinkculturalhealth.org/LanguageAccessServices.asp

One Size Does Not Fit All: Meeting the Health Care Needs of Diverse Populations:
www.jointcommission.org/PatientSafety/HLC/one_size_meeting_need_of_
diverse_populations.htm

Toolkit to Reduce Racial and Ethnic Disparities in Health Care – Section 3: Language Access:
www.rwjf.org/files/research/nhpctoolkit.pdf

The Exchange—"Talking About Language and Health":
http://www.health-exchange.net/language.html

REFERENCES

American Nurses Association (2001). *Code for nurses.* Washington, DC: ANA Publishing.

Anderson, L. M., Scrimshaw, S. C., Fullilove, M. T., Fielding, J. E., & Normand, J. (2003). Task Force on Community Preventive Services. Culturally competent healthcare systems: A systematic review. *American Journal of Preventive Medicine, 24*(3), Supplement 1, pp. 68–79.

Andrews, M. M. (2002). Forward. In Leininger, M., & McFarland, M. R. (eds.). *Transcultural nursing: Concepts, theories, research and practice* (3rd ed., pp. xvi). New York: McGraw-Hill.

Andrews, M. M. (2008a). Theoretical foundations of transcultural nursing. In Andrews, M. M., & Boyle, J. S. (eds.). *Transcultural concepts in nursing care* (5th ed., pp. 3–14). Philadelphia: Wolters Kluwer/Lippincott Williams & Wilkins.

Andrews, M. M. (2008b). Cultural competence in the health history and physical examination. In Andrews, M. M., & Boyle, J. S. (eds.). *Transcultural concepts in nursing care* (5th ed., pp. 34–65). Philadelphia: Wolters Kluwer/Lippincott Williams & Wilkins.

Andrews, M. M. (2008c). Culturally competent nursing care. In Andrews, M. M., & Boyle, J. S. (eds.). *Transcultural concepts in nursing care* (5th ed., pp. 15–33). Philadelphia: Wolters Kluwer/Lippincott Williams & Wilkins.

Andrews, M. M., & Boyle, J. S. (2008). *Transcultural concepts in nursing care* (5th ed.). Philadelphia: Wolters Kluwer/Lippincott Williams &Wilkins.

Beach, M. T., Sugarman, J., Johnson, R., Arbelaez, J. J., Duggan, P. S., & Cooper, L. A. (2005). Higher satisfaction, adherence, and receipt of preventive care? *Annals of Family Medicine, 3*(4), 331–338.

Berlin, E. A., & Fowkes, W. C. Jr. (1983). A teaching framework for cross-cultural health care. *Western Journal of Medicine, 139*, 934–938.

Blue, A. (2009). *The provision of culturally competent health care.* Medical University of South Carolina; Depart of Family Medicine Retrieved on May 17, 2009 from http://www.musc.edu/fm_ruralclerkship/culture.html

Brach, C., & Fraser, I. (2000). Can cultural competency reduce racial and ethnic disparities? A review and conceptual model. *Medical Care Research and Review, 57*(1), 181–217.

Burchum, J. L. R. (2002). Cultural competence: An evolutionary perspective. *Nursing Forum, 37*(4), 5–15.

Campinha-Bacote, J. (1998). *The process of cultural competence in the delivery of healthcare services: A culturally competent model of care* (3rd ed.). Cincinnati: Transcultural C.A.R.E. Associates.

Campinha-Bacote, J. (2002). The process of cultural competence in the delivery of healthcare services: A model of care. *Journal of Transcultural Nursing, 13*(3), 181–184.

Campinha-Bacote, J. (January 31, 2003). Many faces: Addressing diversity in health care *Online Journal of Issues in Nursing, 8*(1), Manuscript 2.

Campinha-Bacote, J. (2008). People of African American heritage. In Purnell, L. D., & Paulanka, B. J. (eds.). *Transcultural health care* (3rd ed., pp. 56–74). Philadelphia: F.A. Davis.

Campinha-Bacote, J., & Narayan, M. (2000). Culturally competent health care in the home. *Home Care Provider, 5*(6), 213–219.

Cherry, B., & Giger, J. N. (2008). African-Americans. In Giger, J. N., & Davidhizar, R. E. (eds.). *Transcultural nursing: Assessment and intervention* (5th ed., pp. 190–238). St. Louis: Mosby Elsevier.

Cross, T., Bazron, B., Dennis, K., & Isaacs, M. (1989). *Towards a culturally competent system of care: A monograph on effective services for minority children who are severely emotionally disturbed: Volume I.* Washington, DC: Georgetown University Child Development Center.

Culhane-Pera, K. A., Reif, C., Egli, E., Bake, N. J., & Kassekert, R. (1997). A curriculum for multicultural education in family medicine. *Family Medicine, 29*(10), 719–723.

Davidhizar, R. E., & DeLapp, T. D. (2008). American Eskimos: The Yup'ik and Inupiat. In Giger, J. N., & Davidhizar, R. E. (eds.). *Transcultural nursing: Assessment and intervention* (5th ed., pp. 323–356). St. Louis: Mosby Elsevier.

DeRosa, N., & Kochurka, K. (2006). Implement culturally competent healthcare in your workplace. *Nursing Management, 37*(10), 18–26.

Falvo, D. R. (2004). *Effective patient education: A guide to increased compliance.* Sudbury, MA: Jones and Bartlett.

Flowers, D. L. (August, 2009). Culturally competent nursing care a challenge for the 21st Century. *Critical Care Nurse, 24*(4), 48–52.

Giger, J. N., & Davidhizar, R. E. (2008). *Transcultural nursing: Assessment and intervention* (4th ed.). St. Louis: Mosby Elsevier.

Gonzalez, E. W., Owen, D. C., & Esperat, C. R. (2008). Mexican Americans. In Giger, J. N., & Davidhizar, R. E. (eds.). *Transcultural nursing: Assessment and intervention* (5th ed., pp. 239–275). St. Louis: Mosby Elsevier.

Goode, T., & Jones, W. (2006). *Definition of linguistic competence.* Washington, DC: National Center for Cultural Competence. Georgetown University Center for Child and Human Development.

Hanley, C. E. (2008). Navajos. In Giger, J. N., & Davidhizar, R. E. (eds.). *Transcultural nursing: Assessment and intervention* (5th ed., pp. 276–299). St. Louis: Mosby Elsevier.

Harvard Medical School (2009). *Culturally competent care online resource center.* Retrieved on May 16, 2009 from http://medweb.med.harvard.edu/cccec/about/index.htm

Healthy People 2010. (2009). US Department of Health, Education and Welfare, Public Health Service. Washington DC: US Government Retrieved on May 23, 2009 from http://www.healthypeople.gov/LHI/lhiwhat.htm

Healthy People 2010 (2009). *Health communications.* (Definition of health literacy.) Retrieved on June 22, 2009 from http://www.healthypeople.gov/document/html/volume1/11healthcom.htm#_Toc490471359

Healthy People 2010. (2009). US Department of Health, Education and Welfare, Public Health Service. Washington DC: US Government Retrieved on May 23, 2009 from http://www.healthypeople.gov/LHI/lhiwhat.htm

Hoang, G. N., & Erickson, R. V. (1985). Cultural barriers to effective medical care among Indochinese patients. *Annual Review of Medicine, 36*(2), 229–239.

Kaiser Family Foundation (2001, December). *Generation Rx.com: How young people use the Internet for health information.* Retrieved on June 28, 2009 from www.kff.org/entmedia/20011211a-index.cfm

Kleinman, A. (1980). *Patients and healers in the context of culture.* Berkeley, CA: University of California Press.

Leininger, M. (1991). *Culture care diversity and universality: A theory of nursing.* New York: National League for Nursing.

Leininger, M. M., & McFarland, M. R. (2006). *Culture care diversity and universality: A worldwide theory of nursing* (2nd ed.). Sudbury, MA: Jones and Bartlett.

Management Sciences for Health (MSH) and the US Department of Health and Human Services, Health Resources and Administration, Bureau of Primary Health Care. Introduction to Cultural Competence. (2005). *The provider's guide to quality & culture.* Boston: Management Sciences for Health. Retrieved on June 22, 2009 from http://erc.msh.org/aapi/cc1.html

Maurer, F., & Smith, C. (2004). *Community/public health nursing practice: Health for families and populations.* St. Louis: Elsevier Health Sciences.

Purnell, L. D. (2003a). Transcultural diversity and health care. In Purnell, L. D., & Paulanka, B. J. (eds.). *Transcultural health care: A culturally competent approach* (pp. 1–18). Philadelphia: F.A. Davis.

Purnell, L. D. (2003b). The Purnell model for cultural competence. In Purnell, L. D., & Paulanka, B. J. (eds.). *Transcultural health care: A culturally competent approach* (pp. 19–55). Philadelphia: F.A. Davis.

Putch, R. W. (1985). Cross-cultural communication: The special case of interpreters in health care. *Journal of the American Medical Association, 254*(23), 3344–3348.

Schim, S. M., Doorenbos, A., Benkert, R., & Miller, J. (2007). Culturally congruent care: Putting the puzzle together. *Journal of Transcultural Nursing, 18*(2), 103–110.

Smith, W. R., Betancourt, J. R., Wynia, M. K., Bussey-Jones, J., Stone, V. E., Phillips, C. O., et al. (2007). Position paper: Recommendations for teaching about racial and ethnic disparities in health and health care. *Annals of Internal Medicine, 147*(9), 654–650.

Sockalingam, S. (2007). *Developing culturally and linguistically competent health education materials: A guide for the state of New Jersey.* Retrieved on June 8, 2009 from http://www.state.nj.us/health/fhs/asthma/documents/pacnj_guide.pdf

Stewart, M., Brown, J. B., Boon, H., Galajda, J., Meredith, L., & Sangster, M. (1999). Evidence on patient-doctor communication. *Cancer Prevention and Control, 3*(1), 25–30.

US Census Bureau (2001). *Profiles of general demographic characteristics. 2000 Census of population and housing.* Washington, DC: Government Printing Office.

US Census Bureau News. News Release, August 14, 2008. *An older and more diverse nation by mid-century.* Retrieved on January, 9, 2009, from http://www.census.gov/Press Release/www/releases/archives/population/012496.html

US Department of Health and Human Services Office of Minority Health (2001). Retrieved on June 8, 2009 from http://www.omhrc.gov/assets/pdf/checked/executive.pdf

Yee, B., Mokuau, N., & Kim, S. (Eds). (1999). *Developing cultural competence in asian and pacific islander communities: Opportunities in primary health care and substance abuse prevention.* Washington, DC: US Department of Health and Human Services (DHHS Publication No. SMA 98–3193).

Zoucha, R., & Zamarripa, C. A. (2003). People of Mexican heritage. In Purnell, L. D., & Paulanka, B. J. (eds.). *Transcultural health care* (3rd ed., pp. 309–324). Philadelphia: F.A. Davis.

PART IV

Planning and Implementing Health Education

CHAPTER 9

Learning Objectives

. . . if you are not sure where you are going,
you may end up someplace else
—Inspired by Mager, 1997

Upon completion of this chapter you will be able to:
- Identify two purposes for stating learning objectives.
- Discuss five factors to consider before writing learning objectives.
- Describe how selection of content is affected by time and environmental constraints.
- Differentiate among words commonly used in writing objectives that have few interpretations and words that have many interpretations.
- Formulate learning objectives in each of the three learning domains using the ABCD method of writing learning objectives.
- Select the appropriate hierarchical level for each of the three learning domains.
- State the rationale for selection of content for the teaching plan in any teaching and learning situation.
- Describe the four sections of a teaching plan.

KEY TERMS

affective	learning objectives
cognitive	levels of complexity
conditions	performance
content	psychomotor
criteria	taxonomy
goal	

INTRODUCTION

Beginning with this chapter, we illustrate the steps of developing a teaching plan and show its progression in subsequent chapters. Developing a teaching plan helps you see the totality of the approach to client education and keeps you on track in carrying out the plan. The teaching plan has four sections: (1) learning objectives, (2) teaching content, (3) teaching strategies and instructional materials, and (4) evaluation. To optimize learning as you move through the chapter, we suggest you identify a client for whom you wish to provide health education and begin to develop a teaching plan appropriate to that client. In this chapter we address the first step of the teaching plan, which is to write learning objectives.

LEARNING OBJECTIVES DEFINED

Objectives provide direction and indicate the desired end point of an effort or activity (Merriam-Webster, 2007). In health education, objectives for learning are essential to providing a framework around which the nurse as an educator builds the teaching plan. Objectives clarify what you intend to teach and what the client is to learn.

The word *goal* is often used interchangeably with *objective*, but goal has a broader meaning than objective. Goals are statements that refer to the overarching learning outcomes to be achieved over a period of time. They are the general intentions or aims for what is to be learned. Objectives are included under goals and are more focused, yet consistent with the goals. They address specific behaviors to be learned. *Objectives* are precise, measurable, and obtainable statements describing what will be learned and who will do what, when, and how.

Objectives must be met before the goal can be achieved (Bastable & Doody, 2008). An example of a goal for an obese client is to learn weight management, whereas objectives would focus on specific behaviors to bring about that goal. Three examples of learning objectives related to weight management include:

1. The client will explain in writing when and how to weigh him or herself so as to maintain a healthy weight over time.
2. The client will state three ways to eat healthy foods each day.
3. The client will make the association between physical activity and weight control in a personal written reflection at the end of the learning session.

Clearly stated goals and learning objectives give direction to both the learner and the nurse as educator. They keep the teaching and learning process on track to achieve the desired learning outcomes. The main purpose for establishing learning objectives is to focus the instruction and guide the planning, implementation, and evaluation of

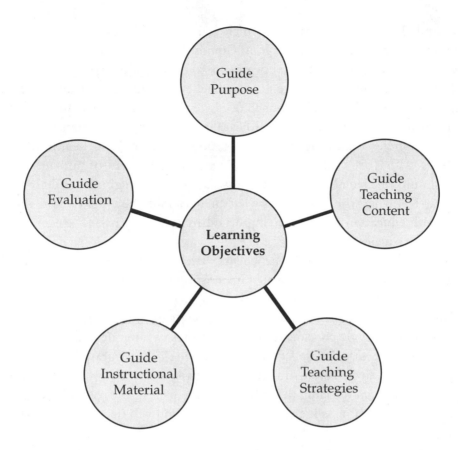

FIGURE 9-1   Learning Objectives as the Basis for the Teaching Plan

the desired learning. Evaluating learning objectives reveals client learning as well as the educator's effectiveness in the teaching and learning process. Figure 9-1 illustrates the critical role of clearly stated learning objectives in developing the teaching plan.

In the education literature objectives are referred to as behavioral objectives, instructional objectives, and learning objectives. We prefer learning objectives and use that term in this chapter to develop the teaching plan.

FACTORS TO CONSIDER BEFORE WRITING LEARNING OBJECTIVES

Before writing learning objectives you need to take into account five factors that affect your approach. The first factor is to consider your educational philosophy, the educational philosophy of the client's healthcare provider, and beliefs about education held by the institution at which you work. Recall that hospitals are required by the accrediting body, the Joint Commission, to provide health education. Clinics may also have educational protocols to follow. Questions to ask include, What does the client's healthcare provider believe about the role and purpose of health education? What and how much does the client's provider want you to teach and the client to know? Does the healthcare institution have a statement of philosophy and policies regarding health education? Does it have health education guidelines? What are your beliefs about the type and extent of information that clients should receive about their diagnoses, treatment regimen, and alternative therapies? Knowing who determines what clients should be taught and the institution's health education policies are important to know to work as a team in meeting the client's needs.

A second factor is to identify what clients want to learn. Ask the client what his or her expectations are and plan to collaborate in writing the learning objectives. Engaging the learner helps the client to be motivated and attentive.

A third factor is to assess what you think clients need to learn. Part of your assessment should include consideration of the client's developmental, emotional, and experiential readiness, as these factors influence one's ability grasp information. An example of using these factors in writing objectives is that clients in denial are less likely to benefit from teaching than those who are willing to face their health challenges. Another example is if a client cannot read, you will need to choose learning objectives that do not depend on reading ability. The objectives should be appropriate to the abilities of the learner. For example, young clients should not be expected to acquire knowledge or perform skills that are beyond their developmental level. A client paralyzed from a cerebral vascular accident (stroke) should not be expected to engage in tasks requiring muscular control that he or she is incapable of performing.

A fourth factor when establishing learning objectives is the time available for teaching and learning. Nurses and clients are busy, so you need to identify the time constraints and make the best use of the time available. This may involve collaborating with colleagues who could teach at other times or after discharge. Some health information takes time to be learned, which may mean establishing priorities, selecting intermediate objectives, and making arrangements to provide for continuity of teaching. This includes communicating clearly to colleagues how far the client has progressed in learning and what remains to be taught and learned.

A fifth and final factor affecting the establishment of learning objectives is the environment in which the learning will take place. This includes the physical environment as well as the psychological atmosphere. Before writing learning objectives the environment needs to be considered. For example:

- What is the physical environment like? Is it conducive to learning?
- Is functional audiovisual equipment available?
- Are instructional materials available?
- Is the learning atmosphere unhurried?
- Is there sufficient space? Is the space comfortable?
- Is there a nonthreatening atmosphere in which clients feel free to learn?

WRITING LEARNING OBJECTIVES

Once you identify what you wish clients to know and be able to do, the next step is drafting the text that clearly and specifically tells them what they can expect to learn. Learning objectives are composed of four parts adapted from Mager (1997), who is credited with first focusing the educational community on learning objectives. The parts are distinguished as the ABCD approach to writing learning objectives and include the following:

- *Audience* (who the learner is)
- *Behavior* (what the learner is to do)
- *Conditions* (the conditions under which the learner is to perform)
- *Degree* (how well the learner is to perform)

A summary of the parts of the ABCD approach to writing learning objectives is shown in Table 9-1. The writing **in bold** describes the addition of each part of the learning objective writing process.

We introduce you to writing learning objectives by reviewing each of the four parts, but before doing this, there are two general guidelines to be aware of according to Mager (1997):

- Objectives should be written from the perspective of the learner, not the teacher.
  Correct: Describe how a pacemaker affects the heart rate.
  Incorrect: Teach how a pacemaker affects the heart rate.
- Objectives should focus on a learning outcome, not the process for achieving the outcome.
  Correct: Count the pulse rate for 1 minute.
  Incorrect: Learn how to obtain the pulse rate for 1 minute.

TABLE 9-1 The ABCD Approach to Writing Learning Objectives		
Objective Part	**Description**	**Example**
Audience	To whom is the objective applied	**The client will**
Behavior	What will the client do? What is the action verb? What is the learning domain addressed?	The client will **create a time line of the main events that occur with hypoglycemia.**
Conditions	How will the action be accomplished? What specifics about the situation must be met?	The client will create a time line of the main events that occur with hypoglycemia, **by drawing a diagram of the process using a list of items provided by the teacher.**
Degree	What is the degree of accuracy to be observed? How will the client be considered proficient?	The client will create a time line of the main events that occur with hypoglycemia, by drawing a diagram of the process using a list of items provided by the teacher **in the order that the events normally occur.**

Audience

The first step in the ABCD approach to writing learning objectives is to identify the *Audience* or the person to whom the objective is directed. This part of the learning objective describes who the learner is. For example, the audience may be a student, a learner, or a diabetic patient. In our case, the learner is the client, so the objective begins with: The client will. . . .

Behavior

The second step in writing learning objectives is to clearly state the *Behavior* that the client will do and how he or she will demonstrate the knowledge, attitude, or skill you are attempting to teach. Behavior is about the activity in which the client is to engage. The activity can be visible, such as writing or doing, or invisible, such as adding or solving; however, the results are visible or audible.

Behavior is best described through action verbs that have few interpretations. Avoid using ambiguous verbs such as "learn" or "know," and verbs that express the nurse's view, such as "inform" or "teach." Appropriate verbs are action verbs written from the learner's perspective that states precisely what the client will do following instruction. Examples of poorly and clearly stated verbs are shown in Table 9-2.

Table 9-3 provides a sample list of verbs with few interpretations and vague verbs that have many interpretations that are useful when writing objectives (Gronlund & Brookhart, 2009; Slavin, 2009).

Domains of Learning

Verbs are categorized by the domains of learning and hierarchies within the domains. Bloom, Englehart, Furst, Hill, and Krathwohl (1956) were pioneers in categorizing the domains and levels. They classified various academic achievements according to educational outcomes and called the classification system the Taxonomy of Learning Objectives (Anderson et al., 2001). The domains of learning help make clear what is expected of different levels of intellectual behavior. By writing learning objectives, nurses as educators take an active role in health education. As health education becomes an increasingly large part of health and illness care, nurses must be knowledgeable about how to structure, write, and evaluate learning objectives. Learning objectives should be written in all three domains. The three domains of learning are the:

- *Cognitive domain* that emphasizes thinking
- *Affective domain* that emphasizes attitudes and feelings
- *Psychomotor domain* that emphasizes doing and performing skills

TABLE 9-2   Poorly and Clearly Stated Objectives

Poorly Stated Objectives	Clearly Stated Objectives
The client will **know** the symptoms of diabetes.	The client will **be able to verbally state** the signs and symptoms of hyperglycemia and state why they occur.
The client will **understand** the distinction between hypoglycemia and hyperglycemia.	The client will **be able to identify the signs and symptoms** of hypoglycemia and hyperglycemia from a list on a written exam.
The client will **know how** to test his or her blood sugar.	The client will **demonstrate the proper use of** the glucometer to test his or her blood sugar.

TABLE 9-3 Verbs with Few and Many Interpretations	
Verbs with Few Interpretations	**Verbs with Many Interpretations**
To apply	To appreciate
To compare	To be familiar with
To contrast	To be interested in
To construct	To believe
To define	To enjoy
To describe	To feel
To demonstrate	To grasp the significance of
To explain	To have faith in
To identify	To internalize
To list	To know
To order	To learn
To recall	To think
To recite	To understand
To recognize	To *really* understand
To select	
To solve	
To state	
To verbalize	
To write	

It is important to choose the correct verb to illustrate the domain for which you are writing objectives. In writing learning objectives, you will soon realize that many behaviors do not fall exclusively in one of the three domains. Learners learn "as an integrated whole" (Harrow, 1972); however, you must isolate the particular behavior that is your concern. For example, irrigating a colostomy is not only a psychomotor activity, it also requires cognition and an affective response. Thus, learning objectives may involve more than one domain.

Cognitive Domain

We now examine the domains of learning by looking first at the cognitive domain. The cognitive domain is concerned with knowledge, beliefs, and reasoning. Bloom initially divided the cognitive domain into six levels or hierarchies. The initial six levels were: knowledge, comprehension, application, analysis, synthesis, and evaluation. During the 1990s the taxonomy was updated. The changes included renaming the six categories, changing the categories from noun to verb form, and rearranging the categories. This new taxonomy reflects a more active form of thinking evident in Twenty-first century learning. The new cognitive levels are: remembering, understanding, applying, analyzing, evaluating, and creating (Anderson et al., 2001) (Figure 9-2).

The six categories are examined in further detail in Table 9-4, which gives the category description, verbs, and sample objectives. Table 9-5 includes a detailed list of verbs that can be used to write cognitive objectives.

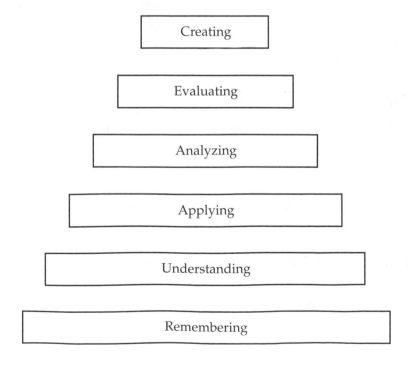

FIGURE 9-2 Hierarchy of the Cognitive Domain.

TABLE 9-4	Cognitive Categories with Sample Objectives		
Cognitive Categories	**Description**	**Verb**	**Sample Objective**
Remembering	Client recalls information.	define	The client will define the terms hypoglycemia and hyperglycemia.
Understanding	Client explains ideas and concepts.	describe	The client will describe the signs and symptoms of insulin shock.
Applying	Client grasps ideas and concepts.	interpret	The client will interpret his or her blood sugar level to determine if more insulin is needed.
Analyzing	Client distinguishes between different parts.	compare, contrast	The client will compare and contrast the signs and symptoms of hypoglycemia and hyperglycemia.
Evaluating	Client justifies a stand or takes a position.	support	The client will support the need to keep blood sugar within normal limits.
Creating	Client creates a new product or point of view.	design	The client will design a calendar to keep track of daily blood sugar levels.

Affective Domain

The next classification of objectives is the affective domain, which is related to the client's attitudes, interests, attention, awareness, and values. The cognitive domain was previously listed in increasing order of complexity, but the affective domain is listed in increasing order of depth into the client's emotions and value system. Affective objectives are more difficult to isolate and express accurately and consequently difficult to evaluate through measurement. The levels of the affective domain are receiving, responding, valuing, organization, and characterizion by value (Krathwohl, Bloom, & Masia, 1964). Table 9-6 illustrates the description, verbs, and sample objectives of the five levels of the affective domain. Table 9-7 reviews verbs in depth used for affective objectives.

Psychomotor Domain

In contrast to affective learning, psychomotor skills are concerned with physical movement and coordination, which is easier to identify and to measure because they

TABLE 9-5   Sample Verbs for Cognitive Objectives

Remembering	Defines	Lists	Recalls	Reproduces	Tells
	Identifies	Matches	Records	Selects	Underlines
	Indicates	Names	Repeats	Shows	
	Labels	Points	Reports	States	
Understanding	Describes	Explains	Identifies	Paraphrases	Rewrites
	Discusses	Expresses	Increases	Reiterates	Summarizes
	Draws	Generalizes	Locates	Restates	Translates
	Estimates	Gives example	Outlines	Reviews	
Applying	Applies	Draws	Investigates	Predicts	Selects
	Calculates	Eliminates	Manipulates	Prepares	Shops
	Changes	Formulates	Measures	Produces	Shows
	Computes	Illustrates	Modifies	Proposes	Solves
	Demonstrates	Implements	Negotiates	Revises	Uses
	Designs	Infers	Operates	Relates	
	Develops	Interprets	Orders	Schedules	
Analyzing	Appraises	Calculates	Criticizes	Distinguishes	Relates
	Analyzes	Categorizes	Debates	Identifies	Selects
	Arranges	Classifies	Diagrams	Illustrates	Separates
	Assigns	Compares	Differentiates	Infers	Subdivides
	Breaks down	Contrasts	Discriminates	Outlines	Tests
Evaluating	Appraises	Contrasts	Distinguishes	Interprets	Selects
	Assesses	Criticizes	Estimates	Judges	Summarizes
	Calibrates	Debates	Evaluates	Justifies	Supports
	Compares	Defends	Explains	Measures	Values
	Computes	Describes		Relates	
	Concludes	Discriminates		Revises	
Creating	Arranges	Compiles	Devises	Orders	Reorganizes
	Assembles	Composes	Estimates	Organizes	Revises
	Blends	Constructs	Formulates	Paraphrases	Rewrites
	Categorizes	Contrasts	Generates	Plans	Simplifies
	Classifies	Correlates	Integrates	Prepares	Summarizes
	Collects	Creates	Manages	Rearranges	Teaches
	Combines	Defends	Mixes	Reconstructs	Writes
	Compares	Designs	Modifies	Relates	

Adapted from Gronlund and Brookhart, 2009; and Gronlund, 2004.

TABLE 9-6	Affective Categories and Sample Objectives		
Affective Categories	**Description**	**Verbs**	**Sample Objective**
Receiving	Client is aware of or attending to something in the environment.	listen to	The client will listen to a presentation on colostomy care and share the information with family members.
Responding	Client shows new behaviors as a result of experience.	choose	The client will choose to discuss his feelings about caring for his colostomy in a support group.
Valuing	Client shows involvement or commitment.	express	The client will express agreement with the guidelines for maintaining sterile technique in wound care.
Organization	Client integrates a new value ranking it among priorities.	select	The client will select foods that meet the requirements of a diabetic diet.
Characterization by value	Client acts consistently with the new value.	display	The client will display acceptance that he has a chronic illness by taking his medication.

are readily observable. Learning a physical skill, such as walking with crutches, manipulating a syringe, or doing a procedure, usually involves substantial psychomotor learning. More than one level of learning exists in the psychomotor domain. For example, hand washing is less complex than cleaning a wound. In these psychomotor activities, the level of skill is readily observable.

Several systems for defining psychomotor learning are available in the literature (Harrow, 1972; Simpson, 1972). We have chosen to adapt and abbreviate the system developed by Simpson (1972) because it appears to have the most relevance for client education. Table 9-8 reviews the description and gives sample objectives in the psychomotor domain. Table 9-9 reviews in detail verbs for writing objectives in the psychomotor domain.

Conditions

The third step in the ABCD process of writing learning objectives is to define the *Conditions* under which the client will perform the desired task. This includes specify-

TABLE 9-7   Sample Verbs for Affective Objectives

Receiving	Accepts	Focuses	Names
	Admits	Follows	Observes
	Allows	Heeds	Pays attention
	Asks	Identifies	Replies
	Attends	Listens	Stays
	Describes	Looks	Uses
Responding	Agrees	Discusses	Replies
	Answers	Explains	Reports
	Assists	Labels	Selects
	Attempts	Participates	Shows
	Chooses	Performs	States willingness
	Complies	Practices	Tries
	Conforms	Reacts	Verbalizes
Valuing	Asks	Differentiates	Justifies
	Asserts	Disagrees	Proposes
	Assists	Explains	Reports
	Attempts	Follows	Selects
	Chooses	Gives	Volunteers
	Completes	Helps	Works
	Describes	Initiates	
	Defends	Joins	
Organization	Adheres	Completes	Modifies
	Alters	Defends	Orders
	Arranges	Generalizes	Organizes
	Chooses	Explains	Relates
	Combines	Expresses	Resolves
	Compares	Integrates	Synthesizes
Internalizing values (Characterization)	Acts	Describes	Performs
	Adheres	Discriminates	Practices
	Asserts	Displays	Revises
	Assists	Endures	Solves
	Commits	Explains	Uses
	Defends	Influences	

Adapted from Gronlund and Brookhart, 2009; and Gronlund 2004.

TABLE 9-8   Psychomotor Categories and Sample Objectives

Psychomotor Categories	Description	Verb	Sample Objective
Perception	The client attains sensory awareness of clues associated with the task to be performed.	watches	The client watches the nurse perform a colostomy irrigation.
Set	The client exhibits readiness to take action through verbal expressions or body language.	expresses	The client expresses willingness to try to do part of the colostomy irrigation.
Guided response	The client exerts efforts to imitate observed behavior; attempts to comply with directions and coaching.	performs	The client will perform colostomy irrigation with assistance.
Mechanism	The client achieves the ability to perform the skill, which is becoming a habit.	demonstrates	The client will demonstrate how to irrigate a colostomy without assistance.
Complex overt response	The client performs the skill easily and independently in sequence with attention to details.	coordinates	The client coordinates complete colostomy care, and makes adjustments as needed in the process.
Adaption	The client achieves the ability to alter the skill to suit conditions and performs the skill automatically as needed.	adapts	The client adapts skill knowledge and performs colostomy care while on a camping trip.

TABLE 9-9 Sample Verbs for Psychomotor Objectives

Perception	Attends	Contrasts	Distinguishes	Looks	Selects
	Chooses	Describes	Focuses on	Observes	Separates
	Compares	Detects	Identifies	Perceives	
	Concentrates	Differentiates	Isolates	Relates	
Set	Aims	Begins	Gets ready	Reacts	Starts
	Aligns	Copies	Positions	Responds	Tries
	Attempts	Displays	Prepares	Stands up	Volunteers
	Asks	Expresses	Proceeds	Shows	
Guided	Aligns	Combs	Holds	Presses	Solves
response	Applies	Compiles	Inserts	Produces	Splints
	Arises	Constructs	Joins	Pulls	Spreads
	Arranges	Cools	Leans	Pushes	Squeezes
	Assembles	Coordinates	Lifts	Raises	Stands
	Attaches	Counts	Locates	Reassembles	Starts
	Attempts	Connects	Lowers	Reclines	Sticks
Mechanism	Auscultates	Covers	Makes	Removes	Stimulates
	Avoids	Crawls	Manipulates	Repairs	Stops
	Balances	Cuts	Mends	Replaces	Synchronizes
	Bathes	Demonstrates	Molds	Restores	Stoops
	Boils	Disconnects	Navigates	Rubs	Tears
	Breathes	Discriminates	Opens	Runs	Tests
Complex	Brushes	Dissects	Operates	Scrubs	Ties
overt response	Builds	Examines	Palpates	Secures	Turns
	Calibrates	Fastens	Parts	Separates	Transfers
	Catheterizes	Finds	Places	Sews	Hypes
	Changes	Folds	Picks up	Shakes	Ventilates
	Chooses	Grasps	Pinches	Sharpens	Walks
	Cleans	Guides	Pivots	Shortens	Washes
	Cleanses	Heats	Pours	Simulates	Weighs
	Closes	Hops	Practices	Slides	Wipes
Adaptation	Adapts	Creates	Modifies	Reverses	Substitutes
	Alters	Composes	Rearranges	Revises	Swaps
	Changes	Designs	Remodels	Rotates	Switches
	Converts	Diverts	Reorganizes	Shifts	Varies
	Corrects	Exchanges	Replaces	Reformulates	

Adapted from Gronlund and Brookhart, 2009; and Gronlund 2004.

TABLE 9-10	Audience, Behavior, and Condition	
Audience	**Behavior**	**Condition**
The client will	perform a colostomy irrigation	given a syringe and a basin
The client will	verbally tell the pulse rate	when asked by the nurse

ing situations/restraints during which the objective must be met, or describing important conditions under which the performance is expected to occur. The statement of conditions is not always necessary to a clear statement of objectives, but it should be included when pertinent. Conditions might be stated with the following phrases:

Given a list of . . . when provided with . . . without using . . . by the end of this lesson . . . the learner will be denied . . . under special conditions of . . . (Table 9-10).

Degree

Degree refers to the quality or level of performance that is considered acceptable and should be specified or implied when writing objectives. The degree may be based on practice standards of which the nurse should aware. The degree defines what level the client must perform the task at so as to determine if learning is successful. The criteria might include concepts such as *amount*. For instance, clients may be considered successful if they are able to slow their pulse during relaxation training by five beats per minute. *Accuracy* is an important criterion when a client is preparing an insulin injection. The degree might specify *without error*. Other criteria might be *without any verbal guidance* or *from memory*. Table 9-11 summarizes how the parts of the ABCD method of writing learning objectives come together to give a complete picture of client expectations.

TABLE 9-11	Audience, Behavior, Condition, Degree		
Audience	**Behavior**	**Condition**	**Degree**
The client will	perform a colostomy irrigation	given a syringe and a basin	without any verbal guidance from the nurse
The client will	verbally tell the pulse rate	when asked by the nurse	under which she should not take Lanoxin

SELECTION OF CONTENT

The time has come for you to select appropriate content to develop a teaching plan. Based on a client or clients that you have identified, assessment data you have collected, and the learning objectives you have written, you must now select appropriate content for teaching. In Chapters 5 through 8 ample suggestions are given for teaching content appropriate to various age groups and health problems. To clarify and illustrate the process of developing the teaching plan, we created a vignette and will expand on it in the remaining chapters of this text. The format we have chosen is widely applicable and shows the pertinent information that should be included in the teaching plan.

CASE EXAMPLE: MRS. ROSA LOPEZ

Our client is Mrs. Rosa Lopez, a 40-year-old woman of mixed race with African-American and Mexican heritage. She is a single mother supporting two teenage children, a son and daughter, who live at home. She is a teacher's aid at a public school and has stress at work. She is also busy raising her children and volunteering at her church. She was recently diagnosed with hypertension. The doctor prescribed an antihypertensive medication and recommended she limit her sodium intake to 2000 mg per day.

She has a family history of hypertension, but is reluctant to take medication to treat it. She stated that the hypertension is not bothering her and does not understand why it is necessary to take medication for it. Her behavior emphasizes the fact that hypertension is an invisible disease with multiple factors contributing to its etiology and treatment, including medications, nutrition, weight management, and stress reduction. We determined that she has educational needs in the three domains of learning: cognitive, affective, and psychomotor. Although there are many things our client needs to learn about hypertension, for purposes of illustrating a teaching plan, we will provide an example of one learning objective in each of the domains. Recall that the learning domains are not isolated entities; rather, learning in the domains overlap. For example, psychomotor and affective objectives have cognitive components.

Our teaching plan has four columns. The first contains the learning objectives, the second identifies the content in an outline form, the third column lists the teaching strategies and instructional materials, and the fourth column lists the evaluation methods. We have included only four columns because we want the teaching plan to be serviceable, a plan from which you can actually teach. Four columns are all we believe is practical to include on one page.

TABLE 9-12   Sample Teaching Plan for Mrs. Rosa Lopez

Learning Objectives	Content Outline	Strategies and Materials	Evaluation
By the end of this lesson, the client will be able to:	Greeting and introductions	This column is completed in Chapters 10 and 11	Examples are provided in Chapters 12 and 13

1. Explain the relationship between excessive sodium intake and hypertension. (cognitive)	Hypertension
	  Definition
	  Fluid retention
	Excess sodium intake
	  Role in fluid retention
	  Sodium and salt relationship
	  Sodium is 40% of table salt(sodium chloride)
	Fluid retention and C-V system
			Verbal questions
			
			Paper and pencil test

2. Choose to limit the intake of sodium to 2000 mg/day by working with the nurse to prepare a dietary plan. (affective)	Four components of dietary plan: 1. Remove salt shaker from table. 2. Use no salt in cooking. 3. Avoid canned or processed foods that are high in sodium. 4. Use low-sodium seasonings such as herbs and spices.		Short term: attitude scale Long term: implementation of dietary changes
3. Demonstrate accurately obtaining self-blood pressure reading using home digital equipment without any verbal guidance. (psychomotor)	Techniques for obtaining blood pressure: 1. Read equipment directions. 2. Locate brachial artery. 3. Place arm in cuff. 4. Inflate cuff. 5. Release air in cuff. 6. Record findings.		Checklist to obtain blood pressure Record of blood pressure readings

SUMMARY

This chapter defined learning objectives as precise, measurable, and attainable statements that describe what will be learned and who will do what, when, and how. Five factors were discussed that should be considered before writing learning objectives. A four-part process for writing objectives was presented: Audience, Behavior, Conditions, and Degree. The process emphasized writing clear and specific learning objectives. Examples of objectives were given of using the ABCD method in each of the learning domains: cognitive, affective, and psychomotor. The correct choice of verbs for each domain was emphasized. Next we looked at the selection of content for the teaching plan. The chapter concluded with the introduction of the case example of Mrs. Rosa Lopez and a format for the teaching plan that will be developed in the subsequent chapters of this book.

EXERCISES

Exercise I—Writing Objectives in Each Learning Domain

Purpose:

- Differentiate among cognitive, affective, and psychomotor learning domains.
- Write clear statements to describe client learning outcomes in each domain.

Directions:

1. The following statements are incorrectly written learning objectives.
2. State the learning domain(s) and level of complexity inferred by each objective.
3. Correct the objectives using the ABCD method of Audience, Behavior, Conditions, and Degree.
4. You may rewrite more than one correct objective for each incorrect objective.
5. Use verbs with few meanings listed in this chapter.

Incorrectly written learning objectives:

1. Client will be integrating the mastery and competency of passive exercises to support attitudes of adequacy and self-esteem.
2. Client will be able to perform at some level a return demonstration of the presented passive exercises despite his physical limitations.
3. To teach the client to cough and deep breathe preoperatively.

4. To demonstrate to the client the use of the circle bed traction and abduction splint preoperatively.

5. Client will understand the importance of food groups that comprise a healthy diet.

Exercise II—Writing Learning Objectives for Clients

Purpose: Write learning objectives using the ABCD method of Audience, Behavior, Conditions, and Degree.

Directions: Divide into small working groups and (1) identify appropriate teaching content, (2) state the rationale for the content you have selected, and (3) write at least one learning objective using the ABCD method in each of the three domains appropriate to each client situation.

1. John Martinez is a 50-year-old farm worker who was admitted to the coronary care unit 4 days ago. This is his first myocardial infarction and states that he has never been ill a day in his life. He lives with his wife and their four teenaged children. He speaks very little English.

2. Suzie Scofield is a blind 6-year-old African-American girl who has been admitted to the pediatric unit in preparation for a tonsillectomy tomorrow. Suzie lives with her mother, one older brother, and one younger sister. Her mother is a licensed practical nurse at the hospital.

3. Delores Johnson is a 30-year-old woman with a stormy 10-year history of ulcerative colitis. She has been hospitalized again for medical treatment. The doctors are trying to persuade Ms. Johnson to accept surgery, an ileostomy. She is a buyer for a large department store and travels in her work. She is married and has no children, but would like to become pregnant some time in the near future.

Exercise III—Writing Learning Objectives for Health Team Members

Purpose:

- Apply theory to teaching health team members.
- Write learning objectives using the ABCD method of Audience, Behavior, Conditions, and Degree.

Directions:

1. Develop a teaching plan for teaching health team members.
2. Think about possible learning deficits and potentials among the team members you plan to teach.
3. Write one learning objective in each learning domain: cognitive, affective, and psychomotor.
4. After you are satisfied with each objective, refer back to the information in this chapter. Determine the level of depth or complexity at which you have written the objective and consider if it is too high or too low and rework as necessary.
5. After you are satisfied that the objective is at the level you believe is appropriate, write the level beside that objective.
6. Work in small groups and consult with each other.

Exercise IV—Sample Nursing Diagnosis and Related Health Education

Purpose: Illustrate a sample nursing diagnosis and related health education.

Direction: Discuss the following situation and the implications for health education.

Situation: Acute Care/Home Care for Todd Smith.

Todd is a 10-year-old white boy who has been diagnosed with osteomyelitis. He is in the hospital to receive aggressive, intravenous, antibiotic treatment. Your job is to prepare him and his mother for self-care of a central venous catheter at home, administration of antibiotics, maintenance of a clean insertion site, clamping off the catheter, administration of medications by learning to remove air before injection, and maintenance of a patent catheter.

Nursing Diagnosis:

- High risk for skin integrity impairment related to central venous catheter placement as evidenced by possible redness and swelling at the site
- Todd and mother's fear and anxiety related to insufficient knowledge of catheter care as evidenced by their questions

Expected Outcomes/Learning Objectives:

1. Client describes to the nurse the correct route of the catheter in the body.

2. Client expresses confidence in his ability to assist his mother with catheter care within 1 week of insertion.
3. Client assists mother with catheter care without contamination while following the established protocol.
4. Client assists mother with established protocol for IV antibiotic administration twice daily without contamination.
5. Client keeps catheter securely bandaged between IV treatments according to the protocol.
6. Client keeps catheter clean and dry during bathing according to the protocol.
7. Client verbalizes to the nurse signs and symptoms of incipient infection, side-effects of antibiotics, and allergic reactions immediately upon observing them.

Health Education Interventions:

1. Assess client's previous experiences with changing dressings, administering medication by syringe, and incision care.
2. Explain the anatomy and physiology components of the procedure.
3. Demonstrate full protocols for catheter care, IV antibiotic administration, and incision care.
4. Invite and reinforce step-by-step participation by the mother and client in the procedures.
5. Explain the signs and symptoms of incipient infection, side-effects of antibiotics, and allergic reactions.

Discussion:

This situation is a good example of the value of audiovisual aids, objects and models, reinforcement, and demonstration/return demonstration. Using the real equipment as well as pictures and charts will facilitate teaching the mother and client the necessary skills. You should watch facial expressions for signs of comprehension, overload, or both. Choose activities that are likely to promote immediate success. Encourage the mother and client to participate at their own pace. Build gradually by giving mother and client things to hold before giving them things to do. For example, have them handle the bandage and then apply it. Assure them that they do not have to do the entire procedure until they are ready.

Explain your collaborative relationship with the home health nurse who will pick up where you have left off. Assure them that the home health nurse will be with them the first time any of the protocols are performed at home. Send home a videotape of the procedure that they have already watched in the hospital.

SUPPLEMENTAL ONLINE RESOURCES

Bloom's learning domains:
http://coe.sdsu.edu/eet/Articles/BloomsLD/start.htm
Bloom's taxonomy:
http://coe.sdsu.edu/eet/Articles/BloomsT/start.htm
Learning domains or Bloom's taxonomy:
http://www.nwlink.com/~donclark/hrd/bloom.html
Bloom's revised taxonomy:
http://coe.sdsu.edu/eet/Articles/bloomrev/start.htm

REFERENCES

Anderson, L. W., Krathwohl, D. R., Airasian, P. W., Cruikshank, K. A., Mayer, R. E., Pintrich, P. R., Raths, J., & Wittrock, M. C. (eds.). (2001). *A taxonomy for learning, teaching, and assessing: A revision of Bloom's taxonomy of educational objectives*. New York: Longman.

Bastable, S. B., & Doody, J. A. (2008). Behavioral objectives. In Bestable, S. B. *Nurse as educator: Principles of teaching and learning for nursing practice* (3rd ed., pp. 383–427). Sudbury, MA: Jones and Bartlett.

Bloom, B. S., Englehart, M. D., Furst, E. J., Hill, W. H., & Krathwohl, D. R. (1956). *Taxonomy of educational objectives: The classification of educational goals. Handbook I: Cognitive domain*. New York: David McKay.

Gronlund, N. E. (2004). *Writing instructional objectives for teaching and assessment* (7th ed.). Upper Saddle River, NJ: Pearson Education.

Gronlund, N. E., & Brookhart, S. M. (2009). *Gronlund's writing instructional objectives* (8th ed.). Upper Saddle River, NJ: Pearson Education.

Harrow, A. J. (1972). *A taxonomy of the psychomotor domain: A guide for developing behavioral objectives*. New York : David McKay.

Krathwohl, D. R., Bloom, B. S., & Masia, B. B. (1964). *Taxonomy of educational objectives: The classification of educational goals. Handbook II: Affective domain*. New York: David McKay.

Mager, R. F. (1997). Preparing *instructional objectives* (3rd ed.). Atlanta: CEP Press.

Merriam-Webster's Dictionary and Thesaurus. (2007). Springfield, MA: Merriam-Webster Inc.

Simpson, E. J. (1972). *The psychomotor domain* (vol. 3). Washington, DC: Gryphon House.

Slavin, R. E. (2009). *Educational psychology: Theory and practice* (9th ed.). Upper Saddle River, NJ: Pearson Education.

CHAPTER 10

Teaching Strategies

The mediocre teacher tells.
The good teacher explains.
The superior teacher demonstrates.
The great teacher inspires.
—William Arthur Ward (1918 to 1994)

OBJECTIVES

Upon completion of this chapter you will be able to:
- Define the term *teaching strategy*.
- Compare and contrast teacher-directed, teacher-facilitated, and learner-directed teaching strategies according to their advantages and disadvantages.
- Describe the "teachable moment."
- Contrast formal and informal teaching.
- State at least two examples of teaching strategies for achieving learning objectives in each of the following domains: cognitive, affective, and psychomotor.
- Identify three factors that affect the choice of teaching strategies.
- Demonstrate selected teaching strategies when implementing a teaching plan.

KEY TERMS

computer-assisted learning
demonstration
games
group activities/teaching
guest lecture
learner-directed strategy
lecture
lecture with discussion
levels of prevention
one-to-one instruction

peer counseling
programmed instruction
return demonstration
role play
simulation
teacher-directed strategy
teacher-facilitated strategy
teaching strategy
team teaching

INTRODUCTION

Teaching is the active process by which information is shared with others in order to provide them with the information needed to make behavioral changes. *Learning* is the process of assimilating information with a resultant change in behavior. The purposes of client teaching are to promote, retain, and restore health. Learning needs related to health education include three levels of prevention: primary prevention (health maintenance), secondary prevention (diagnosis and treatment), and tertiary prevention (follow-up). Health teaching in these areas is used to prevent disease and provide nurses with starting points in making effective, positive changes in the health status of clients. The challenge for nurses as educators is to choose teaching strategies that nurture health-promoting habits, values, and attitudes.

This chapter looks at the use of teaching strategies when preparing teaching plans for health education. A *teaching strategy* is defined as an instructional method that presents content in a way that is designed to bring about specific changes in learners. Teaching strategies include activities that are done by learners as well as teachers. They are a part of the teaching and learning process, which is a planned interaction that promotes a behavioral change. An important distinction in the current nurse's role as an educator includes facilitating learning rather than being a source of all knowledge. The nurse helps learners construct their own knowledge rather than telling them things they are expected to memorize. The client as learner is the center of all teaching and as a result no one single teaching strategy is effective all the time for all learners (Killen, 2000).

TYPES OF TEACHING STRATEGIES

Different teaching strategies are simply different ways of helping clients achieve the learning objectives. The choices range from a totally teacher-dominated approach in which clients are passive recipients of information, to totally independent learning in which the teacher plays no active role. In between these extremes there are several major strategies and numerous variations of each strategy. No single teaching strategy is better than another in all circumstances. Your choice of teaching strategy is influenced by the outcome you want for the client. Different types of learning can be facilitated by different strategies. There is an array of teaching strategies from which to choose. This chapter discusses different teaching strategies and factors to consider in selecting them. We discuss teaching strategies under three broad headings: teacher-directed strategies, teacher-facilitated strategies, and learner-directed strategies.

TEACHER-DIRECTED STRATEGIES

Teacher-directed strategies are those in which the teacher presents information in a highly structured format, directing the activities of learners. These strategies include one-to-one individualized instruction, lecture format, lecture with discussion/question and answer, demonstration/return demonstration, and team teaching. These strategies are described, the necessary preparation identified, and the advantages and disadvantages discussed.

One-to-One Individual Instruction

One-to-one individualized instruction is either formal or informal and includes clients alone or clients and family members as appropriate. *Formal* one-to-one individual instruction occurs when nurses meet individually with clients at a planned time for the purpose of providing health education. A common clinical example is pre-op teaching. The nurse selects the meeting location, time, and the content to be covered based on the client's schedule for surgery. Meeting face to face allows the nurse to give clients personalized attention. This is a good format to use initially to provide basic knowledge in an atmosphere that gives the client the opportunity to ask questions and get immediate feedback. Individual teaching allows clients to share confidential information and problems. This format is adaptable to the needs of clients with low health literacy skills, physical impairments, or emotional difficulties (Rankin, Stallings, & London, 2005).

Plan formal one-to-one individual instruction ahead of time. Planning involves creating an outline of the content that sequences learning and choosing supplemental materials specific to the client's background and experiences. When sequencing information, teach basic concepts first and then variations and adjustments. Clients are more interested in learning what is meaningful to them, so it is helpful to begin with what clients have identified as a need or concern.

The most frequent type of teaching is *informal* one-to-one individual instruction that occurs at the bedside while interacting with clients for other reasons. These interactions turn into *teachable moments*, those unplanned moments when nurses recognize a client's readiness to learn and capture the opportunity to facilitate learning. Romano (2009) states that "The reality of the complex environment we practice in requires us to do much of our teaching on the fly, which can be effective if done right and done often" (p. 141). Be alert to your interactions with clients that characterize teachable moments and use clinical judgment to determine when teaching is appropriate. Opportune times to teach are before procedures, after a doctor's visit, transporting a client, or awaiting test results. Other opportune times to teach include when:

- The client asks questions and shows facial expression of curiosity or puzzlement.
- The client voices concern about specific issues.
- The client makes innocent comments that indicate misunderstanding.
- The client shows nonverbal signs of confusion/frustration/discouragement.
- The family voices concerns.

When in teachable moments, constantly assess the clients' knowledge by listening and developing what Lowenstein and Reeder (2009) identify as "meta-cognitive empathy." In other words, be aware of what the learner does and does not understand by evaluating his or her responses to pointed questions. Ask what he or she knows about the illness, what he or she considers to be positive life style behaviors, and what life style changes are needed to improve health. Avoid starting your conversation by telling clients what you think they need to know. Listen carefully to identify thoughts that may need strengthening or reinforcing. This also includes correcting misunderstandings, adding knowledge that may need supplementing, or referral to appropriate resources (Lowenstein & Reeder, 2009). Information that you glean from informal conversations helps you to construct a mini-teaching plan with appropriate teaching strategies on the spot to address client concerns. Although informal client education takes place spontaneously, you still need to present information in a clear, organized manner based on the client's level of need (Falvo, 2004). Present information to clients when they are ready to receive it and in amounts they are able to comprehend.

Another form of one-to-one individual instruction is telehealth, which is the use of electronic and telecommunications technologies to support long distance clinical health care. This strategy is used for client care and health-related education. It uses video conferencing to connect the nurse and client. Some of the technologies used in telehealth include videoconferencing, Internet access, streaming media, and wireless communications. There are significant barriers in making this a part of daily healthcare practices. This is a technology that is currently being used and will likely become more popular in the future. It has great potential for health education in the future, especially for home-bound clients and clients in remote areas.

Advantages of one-to-one individual instruction are the personal approach to the client, the active learner role in a give-and-take relationship with the nurse, and the flexible format in an informal atmosphere. Individualized teaching also is done through phone calls, e-mail, and telehealth. Disadvantages include lack of sharing with and support from other clients and their families. This strategy exacts a high cost in terms of staff time for instruction (Rankin, Stallings, & London, 2005).

Lecture

A lecture is an oral presentation of a given subject delivered before an audience or class for the purpose of instruction. Lectures are given in person, televised, audio taped or podcasting. The nurse presents information on a topic that is divided into three major segments: the introduction (5 minutes), body, and conclusion (5 minutes) (Woodring & Woodring, 2007). Usually in health education the lecture is short, lasting from 15 to 20 minutes. The introduction is your opportunity to gain the attention of the audience and state what clients should gain from the lecture. The body of the lecture should explain the main concepts and convey the critical information clients need to know. The conclusion summarizes the information that was presented and makes a link between what was taught and what the clients will be able to practically use. The lecture format is an efficient, versatile, and economical teaching strategy than can be used when the amount of time is limited or when a group of clients and family members can benefit from core factual information (Lewis, Heitkemper, Dirksen, O'Brien, & Bucher, 2007).

Preparation for giving a lecture requires planning ahead of time and includes knowing the learners, clarifying learning objectives, knowing the topic, and organizing and sequencing the content. Visual reinforcement such as a PowerPoint presentation or handouts are used to emphasize the key points. Keep in mind that an individual's optimal attention span is approximately 1 minute per year of age up to the age of 45. For example, a 5 year old has a 5-minute attention span, whereas a 21 year old has a 21-minute attention span (Woodring & Woodring, 2007). This illustrates the importance of varying the presentation pace and including other supplemental strategies to add interest. The effectiveness of the lecture strategy is dependent on the skill of the speaker. Table 10-1 offers suggestions for how to successfully prepare to give a lecture and avoid pitfalls.

The advantage of the lecture strategy is that you can address a large numbers of clients in one setting. It is also useful for poor readers, permits auditory learners to receive succinct information quickly, and enables the speaker to make facts more interesting and understandable by clarifying confusing points. Disadvantages of the lecture strategy are that clients are in a passive learner role. It provides little feedback opportunity for clients. Eighty percent of lecture information is forgotten within 1 day (Woodring & Woodring, 2007). A modification of the lecture strategy that addresses disadvantages is the interactive lecture, in which the nurse gives clients

TABLE 10-1 Suggestions for the Lecturer		
Stage of Lecture Preparation	**Suggestions**	**Avoid**
Preparation stage (weeks in advance)	• Specify the date, time, and location of the lecture. • Visit the venue the lecture will be held at if possible. • Clarify the purpose and objectives of the lecture. • Cover only three to five main points. • Gather evidence-based research on the topic. • Analyze the audience: consider age, culture, socioeconomic factors, and language. • Make sure tone and examples are appropriate to the audience. • Prepare an outline and notes for the presentation. • Practice giving the lecture. • Choose appropriate attire. • Check to be sure technology is working and accessible. • Prepare handouts in advance. • Prepare in advance for questions.	• Procrastinating • Lack of preparation • Trying to "wing it" at the last minute
Giving the presentation (introduction)	• Introduce yourself. • State the purpose and objectives of the lecture. • Get the attention of the audience. • Remain calm and cope with anxiety. • Place a glass of water on the podium for dry throat. • Gain learner attention by showing enthusiasm and self-confidence. • Smile and look at the audience frequently. • Speak clearly, strongly, and loudly; use a microphone if needed. • Use a conversational pace when speaking. • Use natural gestures. • Use language and expressions appropriate to the audience. • Provide handouts with an outline of the presentation if appropriate.	• Distracting mannerisms or gestures such as pacing, clearing the throat • Saying you are nervous • Apologizing • Looking down at your notes

(continues)

Stage of Lecture Preparation	Suggestions	Avoid
Giving the presentation (body of the lecture)	• Define the main concepts and principles. • Provide smooth transitions between topics. • Do not try to provide every detail pertaining to your topic. • Talk from notes, do not read from notes. • Use humor, stories, analogies, or metaphors to make a point. • If appropriate, move from behind the podium to engage the audience. • Use appropriate audiovisuals. • Provide a change of pace in longer presentations—combine strategies. • Provide 15-minute breaks if the lecture is longer than 20 minutes.	• Repeating phrases or expressions such as "umm" or "you know" • Turning your back on the audience • Reading from notes • Talking "down" to the audience
Giving the presentation (conclusion)	• Stay within the time allotted. • Review the key points and emphasize practical learning aspects. • Provide the opportunity for learners to ask questions if time allows. • Admit when you do not know an answer. • Thank the audience for their attention.	• Do not abruptly stop speaking and leave the podium • Speaking longer than the specified time

TABLE 10-1 Suggestions for the Lecturer *(continued)*

something to do during the lecture. This strategy includes segments of lecture combined with segments in which clients are interacting with each other and the teacher. An example is lecture followed by clients answering questions using clickers or clients interacting in pairs or small groups to answer questions.

Guest Lecture

Guest lecturers are a good choice for teacher-directed learning, as it provides role models with whom clients can identify. An example of an appropriate guest speaker is to invite a person who has quit smoking to talk with a group of clients trying to stop smoking. The testimony of a guest lecturer can have a powerful effect on clients and be a source of motivation. Some important aspects of the guest lecturer strategy are the following:

- The guest lecturer should be chosen carefully and be fully informed of the learning objectives he or she is expected to cover.
- If possible, attend a presentation or talk with someone who has attended a presentation by the guest lecturer in order to determine if the presentation is appropriate.
- Provide the guest lecturer with exact information about time, place, and location. Plan to have someone meet and orient him or her to the venue.
- Check with the guest lecturer to identify the equipment or special tools that will be needed ahead of time.

Lecture with Discussion/Question and Answer

Lecture is most effective when used with discussion that involves clients. Discussion is a two-way verbal interaction that involves talking, listening, asking questions, and answering questions. The use of discussion or exchange of points of view assists clients to become active participants in the learning process. This strategy is a good choice when clients have previous experience with a subject and have information to share. It promotes understanding and application of knowledge. It also fosters the development of desirable attitudes (Rankin, Stallings, & London, 2005).

There are several different types of discussions. *Open discussions* occur when clients determine the topic and the role of the nurse is to ask questions that lead learners to consider various ideas. With this type, the nurse needs to define terms and encourage differing points of view. *Planned discussion* occurs when the nurse determines the content of the discussion, plans questions in advance, and guides clients toward a predetermined goal or conclusion. *Formal debate* is a type of formal discussion in which clients present opposing viewpoints, usually in a structured format.

Nurses play a big part in the discussion strategy by choosing the type of discussion and forming focus questions that guide clients toward the learning outcomes that are the focus of the lesson. Questions serve many purposes in the teaching and learning process. Questions help to assess what clients already know, stimulate interest in a new topic, discern whether or not clients grasped the main points, explore ideas, and promote higher levels of thinking. It is important to prepare questions ahead of time and then to modify them as needed.

As the teacher, you shape the discussion by the manner in which contributions are treated. If clients feel that their contributions are valued and used, they experience freedom to express themselves. Do not dominate the discussion, but use the time to identify and correct inaccurate information and guide the discussion. Encourage participation by all clients; do not let the conversation be dominated by a few group members. It is important to maintain a nonthreatening environment that encourages informal sharing. A disadvantage is that this strategy takes more time depending on the topic and the number of participants.

An important skill is the ability to manage the discussion and facilitate learning. This requires thought and preparation. The first task in leading a discussion is to get the discussion started. It is often helpful to begin by reviewing the objectives of the session with the group. Another approach is to summarize past information and then ask group members their opinions. Sometimes a skilled teacher will make a controversial statement to stimulate the group's participation. Once the discussion is in progress, there are several ways to keep it on track by focusing, refocusing, changing the focus, and recapping what has been said (deTornyay & Thompson, 1982).

Focusing is keeping the group discussion centered on the learning objectives. One way to focus the group is to ask questions that specifically direct the group's attention to the point(s) you wish to make. This can be done by asking open-ended or questions such as, "What do you find is the most interesting part of . . . ?"

Refocusing is getting the group discussion back on the topic when it has strayed from the original topic. Sometimes groups bring interesting but irrelevant information into the discussion. You refocus the group by saying something such as, "Let's get back to our topic." There may be times the group has deviated from the topic and you must choose whether or not to refocus the discussion. This is a judgment call because the new topic may be important to discuss. The group may need to deal with the new topic before they can focus on anything else. When a group has discussed a topic sufficiently and no new information or ideas are forthcoming, then it is time to *change the focus* of the discussion. You might say, "Now that we've discussed the . . . let us examine another aspect of . . . " *Recapping* is summarizing the discussion to help clients to see relationships and draw conclusions.

Using Questions as a Teaching Strategy

Questioning is a useful teaching strategy to stimulate thinking. Types of questions that are useful in client education are: remembering/factual, understanding/describing, clarifying, and higher-order questions. *Remembering/factual questions* begin with words such as: who, what, where, or when. For example, "What is the normal range for blood pressure?" *Understanding/describing questions* require clients to organize thoughts in a logical relationship and respond with a longer answer. For example, "Describe the signs and symptoms of insulin shock." *Clarifying questions* help clients clarify an idea that is based on their own statements and go beyond a superficial response. For example, "I don't quite understand what you mean; please tell me more."

Higher-order questions help clients think critically and require considerable thought. Higher-order questions have a place in health education in group discussions and when working one-to-one with clients who are confronted with complex health decisions. Higher-order questions help clients compare/contrast (find similarities and differences), analyze (examine the parts/elements), and evaluate (determine the value of) information. Examples of these questions are found in Table 10-2.

Questions also prompt clients to examine their assumptions (unstated beliefs taken for granted) and make inferences (drawing conclusions/deducing) (Merriam-Webster, 2007). A sample question to identify assumptions is, "Why must a surgery consent form be signed before your operation?" A sample question to make inferences is, "After reading this pamphlet about the risk of heart attacks in people with high cholesterol, what would you infer about the foods you usually eat?"

Clients often find themselves in situations in which there are few right and wrong answers. They simply must make the best decision in difficult circumstances. There is a danger of not thinking critically about the consequences of these decisions (Browne & Keeley, 2007). Clients often hear contradictory opinions when they are under the care of specialists, and sorting through this information requires thought. As educators, encourage clients and their families to think through all aspects of a situation. For example, "Your family doctor and the surgeon told you different opinions about treatment. What are the pros and cons of each? What are the long-range results of having open-heart surgery or taking medication and changing your life-style?" Table 10-2 helps you in using questioning as a teaching strategy. The examples complement the cognitive categories hierarchy found in Chapter 9.

Problems with the Discussion Strategy

A disadvantage of the discussion strategy is that it requires additional time, depending on the topic and the number of participants. When using this strategy, you give up some control because you allow clients to share some of the leadership. At times, this means that clients diverge on a topic that is very different from what you had in mind and you need to decide whether or not to refocus the group.

Another problem with the discussion strategy occurs if the participants lose interest. This is evident when they start side conversations, yawn, become restless, and

TABLE 10-2   Examples of Types of Questions

Sample Question	Type of Question
What is your . . . ?	Remembering/factual
Who is your . . . ?	Remembering/factual
Describe the signs of . . .	Understanding/describing
Describe how you do this at home . . .	Understanding/describing
Tell me what you mean when . . .	Clarifying
Describe how you . . .	Clarifying
How does . . . compare with . . . ?	Comparing/contrasting
How are . . . and . . . alike and different?	Comparing/contrasting
Give me an example of . . .	Applying
How will you manage . . . at home?	Applying
How would . . . work for you?	Analyzing
What can you infer from . . . ?	Analyzing
How does . . . relate to . . . ?	Synthesizing
How has your past experience . . . ?	Synthesizing
Which . . . will work best for you and why?	Evaluating
What are the pros and cons of . . . ?	Evaluating
How will you design . . . ?	Creating
How would you create . . . ?	Creating

look glassy eyed. At this point you should consider changing your strategy. For instance, you could conduct a group activity and have the participants move their chairs into a new arrangement that is more appropriate for the activity. Or you could have everyone stand up and stretch or perhaps call for a 15-minute break. Another option is to change the topic of the discussion.

Other problems with the discussion strategy are the nonparticipant, the overparticipant, and the rude participant. Once the participants know each other and are comfortable being together, most clients will participate. If you have a very quiet, nonparticipant in the group, you can encourage that person to speak up. For example, after some participants have commented, you can say, "What do some of the rest of you think about this?" It rarely helps to call on a specific participant unless the learning objective is to learn to be verbally assertive. Keep the environment welcoming and usually the quiet ones eventually share their thoughts.

Handling the overly talkative participant can be a challenge. This is a client who is outgoing, has lots of ideas, and likes to talk. There are several ways to handle this situation. For example, you can say to the over-participant, "That is a great idea. Now, what do some of the rest of you think?" or "Do you all agree with . . . ?" or "Does . . . speak for all of you?" It helps when you look away from the over-participant and look at other members of the group. If the over-participant continues to talk, you can say, "Now I'd like to hear from some others in the group." If the person is simply impossible, you may need to have a private conversation with the person away from the group. This is also true for the rude participant.

Demonstration/Return Demonstration

Demonstration is performing a practical activity in order to teach skills. This strategy requires that clients have an adequate sense of sight and manual dexterity. Demonstration is useful for cognitive and psychomotor learning (Rankin, Stallings, & London, 2005). An example of the demonstration strategy is teaching child care skills to parents of an ill child. Demonstration can be done in person or by video. It involves a single client or small or large groups.

Begin by informing the clients about the learning objectives and the purpose of the demonstration. It is important for you to understand the procedure before attempting to perform for others. Gather the essential equipment at the beginning of the demonstration to avoid fumbling and false starts when your clients are present. Be sure that all clients are positioned so they can see the demonstration and hear your comments. Provide a running commentary throughout the demonstration to focus the attention of clients on the relevant components. If possible, hold the demonstration in the actual place where clients will carry out the procedure. Clarify and repeat your demonstration as needed and then have each client return the demonstration. Be sure to define unfamiliar terms and have a discussion period after the demonstration to answer questions. The entire process should last no more than 15 to 20 minutes (Lewis et al., 2007). If clients are learning motor skills, provide time for clients to practice as soon as possible after the demonstration. Table 10-3 reviews the steps to follow when performing a demonstration.

TABLE 10-3 Demonstration Guidelines	
Phase	**Guidelines**
Predemonstration phase	• Assess client needs. • Identify learning objectives. • Become familiar with the procedure. • Choose the location. • Gather essential equipment and supplies.
Demonstration phase	• Inform client(s) of objectives and purpose. • Define unfamiliar terms. • Be sure clients can see and hear. • Give commentary about the procedure. • Clarify and repeat as needed.
Postdemonstration	• Provide time for discussion and questions. • Limit time to 20 minutes. • Provide time for practice as soon as possible.

Team Teaching

Team teaching occurs when two or more teachers with different preparation, abilities, and skills cooperate and share with one another the responsibilities for planning, teaching, and evaluating client learning. In team teaching, teachers combine their strengths to make the presentation stronger. Refer to the guidelines for effective team teaching found in Box 10-1.

BOX 10-1   Guidelines for Effective Team Teaching
1. All team members participate in formulation of the objectives.
2. All team members contribute to the specific planning of each member's presentation.
3. All team members should be conversant with the specific plans of the other team members.
4. All team members should carry on teaching functions in the presence of others whose roles might be to assist, observe client reactions, and offer constructive criticism in subsequent discussion.
5. All team members participate in periodic evaluation of the class.
6. Conflicts should be viewed as opportunities for growth. They should be addressed before the team encounters the clients.
Babcock, D.E. and Miller, M. A. (1994). *Client education: Theory & practice*. St. Louis: Mosby.

TEACHER-FACILITATED STRATEGIES

Teacher-facilitated strategies are viewed as a bridge between teacher-directed strategies and learner-directed strategies. The teacher takes the role of facilitator of learning rather than directing the process. The strategies in this group include group activities/teaching, role play, and simulation.

Group Activities/Teaching

Teaching in groups occurs when two or more clients work together on an activity. All approaches to group work have the distinguishing feature that clients are working together without direct intervention by the teacher for at least some of the time (Killen, 2000). The principal reason to use this teaching strategy is to offer greater active learning opportunities. Cognitive and affective learning objectives are addressed through group activities. Some examples of situations in which group work might be an appropriate teaching strategy are (Killen, 2000):

- When you want to increase clients' depth of understanding of course content by having them explore it and discuss their understating with other learners
- When you want clients to exchange ideas and learn from one another by exploring issues from many perspectives
- When you want to enhance clients' motivation and increase their active participation in learning

You facilitate the group process by making the learning objectives clear and explaining the directions for the group activities. You should also develop guidelines to help clients participate productively in the group process. Some disadvantages of group activities/teaching are that clients who are accustomed to teacher-directed strategies may have difficulty changing their expectations. Some clients may find the activities a waste of time. Also, you may find it difficult to assess individual clients fairly when they have worked within a group. Group work requires preparation and an adequate room arrangement to accommodate the planned activities. High-ability learners may lose their incentive to learn when placed in mixed-ability groups (Curry, 1997).

Role Play

In role play clients act out their own situation or that of another person. Role playing requires maturity, confidence, and flexibility on the part of clients (Lewis et al., 2007).

This strategy is effective in meeting cognitive, affective, and psychomotor learning objectives. The strategy is most often used when clients need to examine their attitudes and behaviors, when they need to understand the viewpoints and attitudes of others, and when they need to practice carrying out ideas or decisions (Lewis et al., 2007).

Assertiveness training is an example of a situation in which role-playing works well. Your role is as a facilitator, which is to give instructions and provide time for feedback and evaluation. It is important to remember that this strategy takes extra time and some clients may feel uncomfortable and inhibited with this method.

Simulation

Patient simulation is a unique teaching strategy that allows clients to refine and apply their skills in realistic healthcare situations and participate in learning experiences tailored to their educational needs. A patient simulator is a highly sophisticated, technologically advanced mannequin in adult, child, or infant size. These mannequins fully integrate with computer software that supports the development of preplanned scenarios that mimic a wide variety of clinical situations (Beyea & Kibokovich, 2004). Most patient simulators produce lung, heart, and bowel sounds; have anatomically correct pulses; and respond to medical and pharmacologic interventions with the expected physiologic responses. Patient simulators can be programmed to speak and interact like actual patients. A benefit of using simulation is that learning can occur without fear of harming a real patient (Beyea & Kibokovich, 2004). An important part of the simulation experience requires the teacher to create the simulation scenario and be familiar with the technology. The teacher also must be knowledgeable about conducting the simulation and have a debriefing session afterward to integrate learning.

Educators have just begun to explore the usefulness of patient simulation in health care. It is being used to develop, maintain, and evaluate nursing competencies so it is useful for teaching team members. Patient simulation provides a way to help healthcare team members make transitions to actual patient care. This strategy enhances client safety while helping team members to develop clinical skills that reduce the potential for errors (Beyea & Kibokovich, 2004). It is likely that this technology will eventually be used in client education to address specific learning needs of clients. Your role as teacher is to create the learning scenario, facilitate the learning experience, and conduct the debriefing. Disadvantages of this strategy are the cost of the mannequins, software, and support technology.

Simulated experiences do not always require high-fidelity equipment to be effective. It is possible to create lifelike environments to help clients learn to maneuver safely and use trial-and-error to learn how to handle real life situations. An example is rehabilitation programs that use mock city streets to help disabled clients learn to be independent (Steward-Gelinas & Romano, 2009).

LEARNER-DIRECTED STRATEGIES

Learner-directed strategies focus on clients as the initiators and designers of the learning process. These strategies include the use of games, self-directed instruction (computer-assisted strategies and program instruction), and peer counseling groups.

Games

A game is an organized, active competition or contest engaged in by players who act individually or collectively as a team. The objective of a game is winning. Rules define the method of play and the criteria for winning. Instructional games use a body of knowledge or set of skills that must be drawn on as resources. Games provide a pleasurable structure for providing information, testing the level and application of skills and knowledge, and offering practice in simulated situations. They are often used with pediatric patients for preoperative teaching that introduces them to hospital procedures, environment, and staff before surgery (Rankin, Stallings, & London, 2005). During a game, clients take a course of action and view the consequences in a nonthreatening way. Problem solving can be incorporated into the game. Clients should succeed yet be challenged in the exercise. Games may use flash cards, pictures, or computer programs. They may be modifications of popular games such as Bingo, Scrabble, or crossword puzzles. A benefit is that most games are relatively inexpensive to purchase or make. Before introducing a game, evaluate its appropriateness for each specific client. An important aspect of games it that they should be fun, as there is a clear relationship between learning and fun (Baranich & Currie, 2004).

Self-Directed Learning (Computer-Assisted Strategies and Programmed Instruction)

Self-directed learning is the process of clients engaging in learning activities that they define rather than the teacher (Schmidt, 2000). Clients who use this strategy identify their learning needs, formulate goals, identify resources, select and implement learning strategies, and evaluate learning outcomes. Clients demonstrate the initiative and consciously accept responsibility for their own learning. This involves searching out information and resources. Clients' focus on information-gathering, and when used effectively this strategy has many advantages over teaching-directed strategies. Some of the advantages of this strategy are (Killen, 2000):

- It encourages clients to ask questions and investigate, discover, and create answers for themselves, rather than waiting for someone to provide the answers for them.
- It enables clients to develop a deeper level of understanding of the subject than would be possible if teaching strategies such as lecture were used.
- It shows clients that their existing knowledge is valuable and can form the basis for future learning.

Clients use this strategy when they access the Internet and resource centers in libraries and hospitals to find information about health and illness. Personal computer competency is a necessary skill for clients who want to search online. They need to be taught how to identify reliable and accurate information. Encourage them to use Web sites from the government, universities, or reputable medical or health-related associations (Lewis et al., 2007).

Programmed instruction is another self-directed learning strategy that comes prepackaged from a book or computer software company. All of the steps necessary to systematically learn the information are presented sequentially. The information is broken into small steps called frames. Clients are required to make frequent responses as they work through the information. Immediate feedback is given about the correctness or accuracy of responses. Programmed instruction is particularly useful for clients who are independent learners and who learn better when they have no time constraints.

Peer Counseling

Peer counseling is a self-help activity that is learner directed. The members of a peer counseling group provide support for one another by giving information, sharing experiences, and accepting and understanding each other. Peer counseling also provides useful suggestions about a problem or concern. Support groups help clients improve their coping skills, provide motivation to get further help, or take a more active role in their treatment. Participation gives clients hope and the knowledge that they are not alone. Peer counseling groups exist for clients with virtually all health-related problems such as cancer, diabetes, and disabilities. You can refer clients or family members to a peer counseling group to help with follow-up care after initial treatment. Research indicates attending support groups is beneficial. Studies indicate that clients who participate in support groups, in addition to their medical treatments report less anxiety and depression and actually live longer than those who did not attend (Campbell, Phaneuf, & Deane, 2004). It is speculated that having the social support of others in the group boosts the immune system by reducing anxiety and psychological stress. Support groups take place in person, on the Internet, or by phone. Peer counseling helps clients connect with others who share the same problem. It helps to improve coping skills, motivate to get further help, or take a more active role in treatment. Support groups give hope.

SELECTING THE RIGHT TEACHING STRATEGY

We now review important factors to take into consideration when selecting teaching strategies to implement the teaching plan. There are many factors to consider, but the most important is to choose a strategy based on what you want clients to be able to do as a result of your teaching. To select appropriate teaching strategies the following factors are briefly reviewed: the learners' educational needs and learning objectives, characteristics of the client and the teacher, the learning context, and the content to be taught. Figure 10-1 illustrates these factors.

The first factor to consider in selecting teaching strategies is to determine the clients' *educational needs and learning objectives*. Carefully listen to what clients want to know and determine what they need to know. Determine their current health knowledge and if they have misinformation or a history of health problems. Consider their readiness to learn, ability to learn, motivation to learn, and barriers to learning. Each of these impacts how you state the learning objectives and your choice of teaching strategies. Most teaching plans have learning objectives in each of the three domains: cognitive, affective, and psychomotor. When you are clear about the clients' expected learning objectives, appropriate teaching strategies can be considered. When choosing teaching strategies it is important to consider whether the client has the necessary ability, including the intellectual, emotional, and physical ability to learn the skill (Onega & Devers, 2007). Keep in mind that the client's age, developmental stage, sensory impairments, educational background, nature of the illness, and culture should be taken into consideration. Teaching strategies should match the client' strengths and needs and help them reach the level of mastery you set for them. For example, a client with hearing problems does not respond well to a lecture format. A client with poor vision does not learn through the use of demonstration. Also consider the time frame available for teaching. Choose a strategy that allows you to achieve the objectives within the available time frame. If you need to present information as quickly as possible to a group, the lecture method is the best choice.

The second factor to consider in selecting teaching strategies is the *characteristics of the learner and teacher*. Knowing clients' learning styles is particularly important

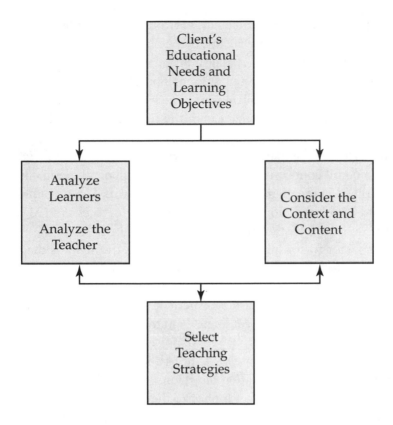

FIGURE 10-1   Selecting Teaching Strategies.

when selecting teaching strategies. Learning styles are characteristic ways that learn-ers perceive, interact with, and respond to their environment. They are the learners' preferred mode of gaining knowledge. Styles are auditory (through hearing), visual (through seeing), kinesthetic (through the whole body), or a combination of these. As the teacher, you should also be aware of your preferred teaching and learning styles. Your clients will achieve learning objectives more quickly if your teaching style is compatible with their learning style. Based on this information about styles, choose among the teacher-directed, teacher-facilitated, or learner-directed approaches. Se-lecting among these approaches is more complex than just choosing one. A variety of teaching strategies helps to maintain learners' attention and increases achievement. For example, supplement the lecture with a group activity (Kindsvatter, Wilen, & Ishler, 1988).

The third factor to consider in selecting teaching strategies is the *learning context*. Learning context refers to the circumstances surrounding teaching and learning and includes both the physical and psychological environment. The physical environment may be the hospital, long-term care facility, private home, school, worksite, and community. Consider the need for privacy and sufficient space. Ensuring privacy and minimizing extraneous noises and interruptions are important.

If you are teaching a group of clients using the lecture strategy, assess the physical environment. Arrive at the location ahead of the time to confirm that the environment is adequate, seating is sufficient, comfortable, and arranged to support learning. Environmental factors are important and affect client learning (Dunn, 1983).

The psychological context is important and must support the teaching strategies. Be actively involved in creating the psychological context. The psychological environment should be relaxed, nonthreatening, and inviting to clients. Maintain a respectful, warm, and enthusiastic attitude.

The fourth factor to consider in selecting teaching strategies is the *content to be learned.* Content is the basic information you want to teach. You should choose teaching strategies to facilitate the efficient and successful accomplishment of learning objectives. Your task is to structure learning experiences that encourage clients to think in particular ways about the things you want them to learn (Killen, 2000). Choose the simplest, clearest, and most succinct manner of presentation (Onega & Devers, 2008). Focus first on must-know content and save nice-to-know information if time allows. Be aware of and take into consideration the clients' current knowledge and previous experiences related to the content. Emphasize the relevance of the content to the client's age and life style. You will find that certain content lends itself to specific strategies. For example, children will respond well to teaching strategies that permit them to participate actively. Would a lecture be an appropriate strategy to teach hand-washing to a class of 6 year olds? Probably not. A hands-on demonstration better meets the needs of this group.

Schedule and pace learning according to the clients' needs and abilities. When giving information, use simple but accurate words. Avoid using medical jargon and periodically check for understanding and interpretation of the information. Avoid information overload; repetition helps to emphasize important points. Using more than one teaching strategy enhances learning. Written materials clarify information and give clients something to refer to at home. Verbal and written communication should complement each other (Falvo, 2004). Finally, remember that interactive teaching strategies are more effective than those that are not (Killen, 2000).

In Table 10-4 we summarize the various teaching strategies, learning domains, and a description of the strategy.

Table 10-5 summarizes this information to help you choose strategies that fit the learning needs and objectives.

TABLE 10-4 Teaching Strategy, Learning Domain, and Description

Teaching Strategy	Learning Domain	Description
Teacher-Directed		
Lecture	Cognitive	• Teacher-directed content and pace • Feedback determined by teacher • Use with individuals or groups • Encourages retention of facts
One-on-one discussion	Affective Cognitive	• Teacher-directed content and pace • Encourages participation by clients • Permits reinforcement and repetition at client's level • Supports introduction of sensitive subjects
Guest lecturer	Cognitive Affective	• Teacher-directed content and pace • Modeling by an expert
Team teaching	Cognitive	• Teacher-directed content and pace • Use with groups • Encourages retention of facts • Offers varied viewpoints • Members present based on their teaching strengths
Lecture with discussion/ question and answer	Cognitive Affective	• Teacher controls most content and pace • Teacher must know the content and be prepared to answer questions • Use with individuals and groups • Teacher confirms understanding by asking questions
Demonstration	Cognitive Psychomotor	• Teacher-directed content and pace • Modeling of skills and behaviors by teacher • Gives commentary with demonstration • Use with individuals and groups • Does not include "hands-on" experience
Demonstration/ return demonstration/ practice	Cognitive	• Teacher-facilitated content and pace • Allows repetition and immediate feedback • Includes "hands-on" experience

(continues)

TABLE 10-4 Teaching Strategy, Learning Domain, and Description *(continued)*

Teaching Strategy	Learning Domain	Description
Teacher-facilitated		
Group activities/ discussion	Affective Cognitive	• Teacher-facilitated content and pace • Clients obtain assistance from supportive group • Group members learn from one another
Role playing	Affective Cognitive	• Teacher-facilitated content and pace • Encourages expression of values, attitudes, and emotions • Can assist in the development of communication skills • Involves active participation by client
Simulation	Cognitive Affective Psychomotor	• Teacher-facilitated • Use with individuals and groups • Group members learn from one another • Encourages expression of values, attitudes, and emotions
Learner-directed		
Peer group	Affective Cognitive	• Client-directed • Support and modeling from clients with similar issues • Encourages expression of values, attitudes, and emotions
Games	Cognitive	• Client-directed • Permits reinforcement and repetition at client's level • Offers practice and application of skills • Fun, competitive • Individual or with a partner
Computer-assisted instruction	Cognitive	• Client-directed • Promotes individual initiative and responsibility for learning • Stimulates information gathering and questioning

TABLE 10-5   Teaching Strategies: Advantages and Disadvantages

Teaching Strategy	Advantages	Disadvantages
Lecture	• Easy to organize • Predictable • Efficient • Good for large group • Allows teacher control	• Lacks client feedback • Lacks client participation • Can create information overload
One-on-one individual instruction	• Personalized attention • Provides basic knowledge • Immediate feedback • Clients can share confidential information • Adaptable to clients with low health literacy skills, physical impairments, or emotional difficulties • Flexible and informal	• Lack of sharing with and support from other clients and family • High cost in terms of staff time
Guest lecturer	• Source of motivation • Role modeling	• May not follow learning objectives • May deviate from topic • May exceed the allotted time
Lecture with discussion/ question and answer	• Continual feedback • Attitude development and modification • Picks up confusion and helps resolve difficulties • Vehicle for clients to network with each other • Active learning process • Assess client's knowledge	• Teacher can dominate the discussion • Takes more time • Nonparticipant • Over-participant
Demonstration/ return demonstration	• Activates many senses • Clarifies the "whys" of principles • Correlates theory with practice • Commands interest	• Takes a lot of time • Does not cover all aspects of cognitive learning • Must have adequate sight and manual dexterity • Practice is needed

(continues)

TABLE 10-5   Teaching Strategies: Advantages and Disadvantages *(continued)*

Teaching Strategy	Advantages	Disadvantages
Team teaching	• Enhances teaching by using competencies of more than one teacher • Allows teachers to learn from each other • Accentuates divergent points of view	• Lacks continuity and internal consistency • Requires more planning time • Makes group processing slower • Forces teachers to give up autonomy
Group activities/ teaching	• Increases depth of client understanding • Encourages clients to exchange ideas • Clients learn from one another • Increases active participation and learning	• Clients may find activities a waste of time • Clients may have difficulties changing their expectations • Requires increased preparation time • Adequate room accommodations are needed • Some learners lose interest in mixed-ability groups
Role play	• Helps examine attitudes and behaviors • Helps examine viewpoints of others • A way to practice carrying out ideas or decisions	• Requires maturity, confidence, and flexibility from clients • May embarrass clients • Requires some self-disclosure
Simulation	• Mimics clinical situations • Requires hands-on participation • Learning without fear of harming a real person • Beneficial in evaluating competencies • Promotes the greatest transfer of learning	• The cost of mannequins and support technology • Scenarios have to be developed and carried out • Time consuming • Requires teachers who are familiar with the technology and process
Games	• Fun • Challenging • Competitive • Active learning • Encourages problem solving • Relatively inexpensive • Application of knowledge	• Makes achievement of outcomes difficult to assess • Some clients may not like them • Cost and development of games • Not effective for presenting information

(continues)

TABLE 10-5   Teaching Strategies: Advantages and Disadvantages *(continued)*

Teaching Strategy	Advantages	Disadvantages
Computer-assisted learning and programmed instruction	• Allows clients to go at their own pace • Repeat a section at will • Breaks material down into manageable increments • Saves teacher time	• Depends on motivation of learner • Does not account for unplanned feedback, which can distract clients
Peer counseling	• Clients provide support for each other • Useful suggestions about a problem or concern • Helps clients improve coping skills • Provides motivation • Gives hope	• Challenge is for clients to stay in contact with the group • Information may be incorrect • May not be suitable for all clients

CASE EXAMPLE: MRS. ROSA LOPEZ

In Chapter 9 we started a teaching plan for Mrs. Rosa Lopez. We now expand on the teaching plan to include teaching strategies. Refer to Table 10-5 to see how to include teaching strategies in the teaching plan. The cognitive objective is to increase knowledge, and because our example is an individual client, we would use the strategy of one-to-one discussion to increase her knowledge about the relationship between excessive sodium intake and hypertension. Discussion is a useful strategy for assessing what the client already knows and building on that knowledge. We identify specific questions to ask her during the discussion in addition to answering her questions.

The affective objective seeks to have the client choose to limit the intake of sodium to 2000 mg/day by working with the nurse to prepare a dietary plan. We note that Mrs. Lopez is at the valuing level, so we would have her think through the steps of how she will prepare a dietary plan and put it into effect. This is important because she is not only cooking for herself, but also for her two children. We would have her identify any barriers she sees to preparing a dietary plan and explore how she can work around those barriers.

The psychomotor objective seeks to have the client accurately obtain her own blood pressure reading and record it without any verbal guidance. We would use the strategy of demonstration/return demonstration to achieve this. We would have Mrs. Lopez read the directions as we demonstrate how to take the blood pressure using the

TABLE 10-6　Sample Teaching Plan for Mrs. Rosa Lopez

Learning Objectives	Content Outline	Strategies and Materials	Evaluation
By the end of this lesson, the client will be able to:	Greeting and introductions		Examples are provided in Chapters 12 and 13
1. Explain the relationship between excessive sodium intake and hypertension. (cognitive)	Hypertension Definition Fluid retention Excess sodium intake Role in fluid retention Sodium and salt relationship Sodium is 40% of table salt (sodium chloride) Fluid retention and C-V system	Talking/ discussion Answer questions Discussion question: "What is the relationship between sodium intake and hypertension?"	Verbal questions Paper and pencil test
2. Choose to limit the intake of sodium to 2000 mg/day by working with the nurse to prepare a dietary plan. (affective)	Four components of dietary plan: 1. Remove salt shaker from table. 2. Use no salt in cooking. 3. Avoid canned or processed foods that are high in sodium. 4. Use low-sodium seasonings, such as herbs and spices.	Talking/ discussion Answer questions. Read sample labels for sodium content. Discussion question: "How can you incorporate these changes into your meal planning and usual diet?"	Short term: attitude scale Long term: implementation of dietary changes
3. Demonstrate accurately obtaining self-blood pressure reading using home digital equipment without any verbal guidance. (psychomotor)	Techniques for obtaining blood pressure: 1. Read equipment directions. 2. Locate brachial artery 3. Place arm in cuff 4. Inflate cuff. 5. Release air in cuff 6. Record findings	Talking/ discussion Demonstrate procedure. Have client demonstrate procedure. Answer questions. Develop record-keeping system.	Blood pressure Checklist to Obtain blood Pressure Record of blood pressure readings

client's own digital equipment. Mrs. Lopez would then perform a return demonstration using the equipment and record the findings using the procedural guidelines (Table 10-6).

Before instructing Mrs. Lopez, we would arrange a room to facilitate learning. The room should be quiet and have comfortable seating with a table nearby for the digital blood pressure equipment. The room should have a clearly visible place to hang the chart explaining hypertension and its relationship to excess sodium. The room should have the pamphlets and handouts we give to Mrs. Lopez. It would be desirable to have a computer available with Internet access to demonstrate how to search online for information about low sodium culturally appropriate diets. If a computer is not available and Mrs. Lopez is Internet savvy, we would walk her through the requisite search steps and suggest Web sites for her to investigate at home.

The digital blood pressure equipment would be placed on the table and ready for use. Mrs. Lopez would read the directions as we demonstrate how to use the equipment. Then she would perform a return demonstration using the procedure checklist and record the findings. Mrs. Lopez would be given an opportunity to evaluate her own performance based on the guidelines in the checklist. When the procedure is performed correctly, we would compliment her and reinforce her newly acquired skills.

BOX 10-2   Evidence-Based Nursing Practice

White, S., Park, Y. S., Israel, T., & Cordero, E. (2009). Longitudinal evaluation of peer health education on a college campus: Impact on health behaviors. *Journal of American College Health, 57*(3), 497–505.

Purpose: This study compared the differences in health education outcomes related to alcohol and drug use, eating and nutrition, and sexual health over time between a randomly selected group of students who either did or did not make contact with peer health educators.

Method: A Web-based survey was administered to a cohort of 2000 randomly selected undergraduate students over a 3-year period. The survey contained measures of knowledge, attitudes, and behaviors for the three targeted health topics. Frequency of peer contact by type and year was noted.

Results: Students who had contact with peer health educators were significantly more likely over time to report less alcohol consumption and fewer related negative consequences. No significant differences in sexual health behaviors were found.

SUMMARY

Teaching strategies involve much more than transmitting information. It is the process of collaborating with clients to achieve the learning objectives. This chapter emphasized the importance of engaging clients in the teaching and learning process so they can benefit from their experiences. The desired learning objectives, characteristics of the client, the learning context, and the content must guide the choice of learning strategies. When selecting teaching strategies, there are teacher-directed, teacher-facilitated, and learner-directed strategies from which to choose. Base your choice on the learning objectives and desired outcomes for the teaching content. Once you choose an overall strategy, select instructional materials to complement your teaching strategies. It is important to vary your approach to instruction, keeping in mind that clients have different needs, abilities, and learning preferences. Chapter 11 discusses instructional materials that supplement your teaching strategies.

EXERCISES

Exercise I—Choosing Learning Strategies

Purpose: Distinguish among teacher-directed, teacher-facilitated, and learner-directed teaching strategies

Directions:

1. Make a list of various topics that require client health education.
2. Review the list and describe whether each topic should be addressed through teacher-directed, teacher-facilitated, or learner-directed teaching strategies.
3. Identify the specific type of teacher-directed, teacher-facilitated, or learner-directed teaching strategy that you would use.
4. Discuss how each group member made his or her decisions and why.

Exercise II—Develop and Implement a Teaching Plan

Purpose: Select appropriate strategies to teach a self-selected topic.

Directions:

1. Divide into groups of five or six members.
2. Identify topics about which each member wants to know more.

3. Each member should choose a topic and then independently:
   a. Prepare two learning objectives using the ABCD method of writing objectives.
   b. Prepare a teaching plan that includes an outline of the content.
   c. Select suitable teaching strategies.
4. Each member then makes a 15-minute presentation of his or her teaching plan.
5. Share and reflect on the experience of presenting your teaching plan.

SUPPLEMENTAL ONLINE RESOURCES

Learning Principles, Teaching Strategies, and Learning Activities:
http://faculty.nwacc.edu/sverwey/learning%20principles,%20teaching%20strate
gies,%20&%20learning%20activities.htm#Teaching_Strategies/Learning_
Activities
Teaching Strategies:
http://pedagogy.merlot.org/TeachingStrategies.html
Bloom's Taxonomy:
http://www.learningandteaching.info/learning/bloomtax.htm
Learning Principles:
http://faculty.nwacc.edu/sverwey/learning%20principles,%20teaching%20strate
gies,%20&%20learning%20activities.htm#Teaching_Strategies/Learning_
Activities

REFERENCES

Babcock, D. E. & Miller, M. A. (1994). Client education: Theory & practice. St. Louis: Mosby.

Baranich, K. L., & Currie, C. C. (2004). Using games to teach motivate and engage. *The Games Journal*, September/October, pp. 6–9. Retrieved on July 23, 2009 from http://www.stc.org/intercom/PDFs/2004/20040910_06-09.pdf.

Beyea, S., & Kibikovich, L. (2004). Human patient simulation: A teaching strategy. *AORN Journal*, 8(4), 738–742.

Browne, M. N., & Keeley, S. M. (2007). *Asking the right questions: A guide to critical thinking* (8th ed.). Upper Saddle River, NJ: Pearson Prentice Hall.

Campbell, H. S, Phaneuf, M. R., & Deane, K. (2004). Cancer peer support programs: Do they work? *Patient Education and Counseling*, 55(1), 3–15.

Curry, A. (1997). *Mixed ability groups in mathematical classrooms*. Unpublished independent study, faculty of education, University of Newcastle as cited in Killen, R. (2000). *Effective teaching strategies: Lessons from research and practice* (4th ed.). Lansdowne, So. Africa: Juta & Co.

deTornyay, R., & Thompson, M. A. (1982). *Strategies for teaching nursing*. New York : John Wiley and Sons.

Dunn, R. (1983). Can students identify their own learning styles? *Educational Leadership, 40*(5), 60–62.

Falvo, D. R. (2004). *Effective patient education: A guide to increased compliance.* Sudbury, MA: Jones and Bartlett.

Killen, R. (2000). *Effective teaching strategies: Lessons from research and practice* (4th ed.). Lansdowne, So. Africa: Juta & Co.

Kindsvatter, R., Wilen, W., & Ishler, M. (1988). *Dynamics of effective teaching.* New York: Longman.

Lewis, S. L., Heitkemper, M. M., Dirksen, S. R., O'Brien, P. G., & Bucher, L. (2007). *Medical surgical nursing: Assessment and management of clinical problems.* St. Louis: Mosby Elsevier.

Lowenstein, A., & Reeder, J. A. (2009). Making learning stick. In Lowenstein, A., Foord-May, A. L., & Romano, J. C. *Teaching strategies for health education and health promotion: Working with patients, families, and communities* (pp. 151–177). Sudbury, MA: Jones and Bartlett.

Merriam-Webster's Dictionary and Thesaurus (2007). Springfield, MA: Merriam-Webster Inc.

Onega, L. L., & Devers, E. (2008). Health education and group process. In Stanhope, M., & Lancaster, J. *Public health nursing: population-centered health care in the community* (2nd cd., pp. 290–315). St. Louis: Mosby Elsevier.

Rankin, S. H., Stallings, K. D., & London, F. (2005). *Patient education in health and illness* (5th ed.). Philadelphia: Lippincott Williams & Wilkins.

Romano, J. C. (2009). Teaching on the fly. In Lowenstein, A. F., Foord-May, L., & Romano, J. C. *Teaching strategies for health education and health promotion: Working with patients, families, and communities* (pp. 139–150). Sudbury, MA: Jones and Bartlett.

Schmidt, H. G. (2000). Assumptions underlying self directed learning may be false. *Medical Education, 34*(4), 243–245.

Steward-Gelinas, D., & Romano, J. (2009). Individualized instruction. In Lowenstein, A. Foord-May, A. L., & Romano, J. C. *Teaching strategies for health education and health promotion: working with patients, families, and communities* (pp. 117–128). Sudbury, MA: Jones and Bartlett.

Ward, W. A. (1918–1994). In Llera, A. (2009, January 8). *The truly great teacher inspires.* Retrieved July 8, 2009, from http://ezinearticles.com/?The-Truly-Great-Teacher-Inspires&id=1861319.

Woodring, B. C., & Woodring, R. C. (2007). Lecture is not a four-letter word. In Bradshaw, M. J., & Lowenstein, A. J. *Innovative teaching strategies in nursing and related health professions* (4th ed., pp. 109–130). Sudbury, MA: Jones and Bartlett.

CHAPTER 11

Instructional Materials

Tell me,
I forget.

Show me,
I remember.

Involve me,
I understand.
—Ancient Proverb

OBJECTIVES

Upon completion of this chapter you will be able to:
- State at least two purposes of instructional materials.
- Describe the importance of health literacy in evaluating instructional materials.
- Evaluate the readability and appropriateness of selected health education materials.
- Identify reliable sources for obtaining health-related pamphlets and brochures.
- List five criteria for evaluating the accuracy and reliability of Web sites.
- Critique the advantages and disadvantages of at least 10 types of media.

KEY TERMS

35-mm slides
analogy
appropriateness
audiocassettes
brochures
bulletin boards
computer-assisted instruction
digital camera
DVD-audio
DVD-video
education pathways
e-mail
flip charts
health literacy
instructional handouts
Internet

LCD projector
objects and models
overhead projector
pamphlets
photographs
posters
PowerPoint slides
readability
replica
story board
symbol
transparencies
videotapes
whiteboards/chalkboards
World Wide Web

INTRODUCTION

In the previous chapter we focused on teaching strategies that facilitate client learning. In this chapter we examine a number of instructional materials that help you supplement the teaching strategies to achieve the learning objectives.

Instructional materials are the actual matter or substance physically manipulated with the aim of promoting client learning. These materials are used by the teacher as well as the client. Instructional materials provide ways to use all senses to enhance learning. Some materials allow for the physical contact that kinesthetic learners need, whereas others enhance and reinforce cognitive knowledge. Still other materials invite emotional involvement, which is crucial for changing attitudes.

Instructional materials serve several purposes (Pohl, 1981). These purposes include extending the client's sensory experience, introducing variety into the teaching and learning process, giving meaning to abstractions, and making otherwise complicated explanations understandable. Pohl identified a number of factors to consider when determining which instructional materials to use. These factors include assessment of the topic being presented, the client(s) being addressed, and the materials available.

It is important to emphasize that instructional materials do not take the place of an effective teacher. Instructional materials enrich the learning experience of clients if they are appropriate to the learning objectives. Instructional materials must be carefully examined, evaluated, and selected on the basis of how they supplement the learning objectives to achieve the educational outcomes. The clinical judgment of nurses as educators is essential in this process.

Although instructional materials are available from a number of different sources, they may not be more effective than those materials that you develop yourself. By tapping into your creativity, you can develop materials that are specific to the health concerns of clients served by your employer or healthcare institution.

In this chapter we discuss health literacy and examples of instructional materials such as print media, multimedia, and the Internet and the World Wide Web (Web). There are a variety of instructional materials available and each has advantages and disadvantages for any specific teaching and learning situation. We discuss these advantages and disadvantages of selected materials along with their purposes and helpful hints in using them.

HEALTH LITERACY

Health literacy is an important consideration in selecting instructional materials, especially printed materials given to clients in the form of pamphlets, instructional handouts, and materials downloaded from the Web. To benefit from these materials, clients must be able to read and make sense of the information. For this reason, we begin this chapter by discussing the importance of health literacy.

Health literacy is receiving increasing attention by health professionals and has particular importance for nurses as educators. We introduced the topic of health literacy in Chapter 4 and included a quick and accurate assessment tool, the Newest Vital Sign, to determine a client's ability to read and apply information from a nutrition label. According to the National Assessment of Adult Literacy, in the United States in 2003, approximately 22% (47 million) of the population had basic health literacy skill and 14% (30 million) had below basic skills (NCES, 2003). Combined, these groups represent 36% (77 million) of the population. Individuals in these groups have difficulty processing and understanding basic health information and services and making appropriate health decisions. According to Clancy (2008), those with basic or below basic health literacy skills have now increased to almost 90 million. This latter figure is important and indicates a substantial health literacy problem that affects you in preparing teaching plans. According to Doak, Doak, and Root (1996), the adult population reads at the eighth to ninth grade level.

Health literacy and intelligence are not the same and should not be confused (Doak, Doak, & Root, 1996). Many factors affect health literacy. It is defined as "the wide range of skills and competencies that people develop over their lifetimes to seek out, comprehend, evaluate, and use health information and concepts to make informed choices, reduce health risks, and increase quality of life" (Zarcadoolas, Pleasant, & Greer, 2006, p. 55). This definition goes beyond reading ability, numeracy skills, and the ability to follow verbal directions. It includes the ability to act on health information, access appropriate healthcare services, and navigate the healthcare system.

Health literacy is required to understand how to take medications, follow a treatment regimen, follow directions to prepare for diagnostic examinations, and respond to radio and television public warnings about the recall of unhealthful products, equipment, and drugs. Health literacy is required for communicating with healthcare providers, describing symptoms, and understanding treatment recommendations. It is also required to critically evaluate newspapers and magazine advertisements and determine the credibility of information found on the Internet. It involves being able to fill out complex forms, understand insurance coverage, and navigate the healthcare system. It is fundamental to making informed decisions about promoting, retaining, and restoring health.

Low health literacy is observed across the demographic spectrum. However, it is more often seen in clients age 65 and older, clients with limited English-speaking skills, racial and ethnic minorities, and clients who have not attended or completed high school (NCES, 2003). It is easy to assume that clients who appear middle class, well groomed, and articulate are also health literate, but this is not always the case (Doak, Doak, & Root, 1996). Even clients who are well educated can have difficulty understanding health-related information. Consider the diabetic client who did not understand how to use the food exchanges or the client on a fat-restricted diet who thought that pork was a "white meat" and therefore low in fat.

Low health literacy has a financial impact. Clients with low literacy skills have poorer health outcomes and adhere less to medical recommendations than those with higher literacy skills. They have higher rates of hospitalization and use emergency services more, perhaps attributed to using fewer preventive and treatment services (Levy & Royne, 2009). The ramifications of low health literacy are particularly important in the treatment of clients with chronic illnesses, who must manage their own health and implement life style changes for success (Seligman et al., 2007).

TYPES OF INSTRUCTIONAL MATERIALS

We are fortunate today to have an abundance of instructional materials to facilitate learning that appeal to all learning styles: visual, auditory, and kinesthetic. However, it is important to remember that they cannot substitute for good teaching. Instructional materials enrich and supplement the teaching and learning process. They do not replace the teacher. They help clients understand concepts and retain information when teachers use a variety of materials. Illustrations quickly bring to life concepts that may take many words to describe. A teacher is essential to assess client needs, develop the teaching plan, provide guidance, answer questions, and evaluate teaching effectiveness. Take-home handouts remind clients about your teaching.

In selecting instructional materials you are constrained by what is available where you are employed. Make use of what your employer has available and, if possible, recommend the purchase of new materials and equipment. Be sure the materials are current. Clients may be turned off by visual images of out-of-date clothing, hairstyles, and equipment, and may consider the information irrelevant to their situation (Falvo, 2004). If what you need is not available, we encourage you to adapt and be creative. Is there some way to improvise or create illustrations? Healthcare institutions are cost conscious, and your employer may appreciate your creativity. In this section, we discuss printed materials, multimedia, and the Internet and World Wide Web.

PRINTED MATERIALS

Printed material is the most widely used source of information given to clients. Examples of common printed materials include pamphlets, brochures, instructional handouts, and booklets. It is common for clients participating in health education classes to expect handouts and to leave with reading material that supplements and enhances their learning. Falvo (2004) recommends having a good supply of written materials on hand for the common health problems seen in clients who are served by your employer or healthcare institution.

There are multiple sources of printed material. Every voluntary health organization such as the American Cancer Society is more than happy to supply you with printed materials. This is also true for local, state, and federal governments, depending on the type of information that you request. Pharmaceutical firms and commercial sources also have printed materials to distribute to clients. When you cannot find exactly what you want from these sources, consider preparing your own materials.

All printed materials are not equal. They need to be evaluated carefully to determine which ones best meet your purposes. You may want to have a committee help you evaluate the printed materials distributed to clients. Things to consider include the philosophy of your department, healthcare institution, or physicians, clients and their needs, availability of appropriate materials, and cost.

If you decide to prepare your own materials, consider the amount of time and cost it requires. You need to conceptualize and write the copy, then arrange for artistic design, layout, printing, and duplicating the material. This process can be lengthy and costly and the effort needs to be worthwhile (Falvo, 2004). It may be not as cost effective to prepare your own materials as it may have at first appeared.

Selecting Printed Materials

As the educator, you are responsible for providing clients with understandable health information (Wood, Kettinger, & Lessick, 2007). Clients vary greatly in their ability to read and translate symbols on a piece of paper into information that is meaningful to them. You may be tempted to depend on printed materials to convey information to clients. This is especially true when you feel pressed for time and depend on the reading materials to enhance the client's knowledge regarding the topic at hand. Brochures, written instructions, and consent forms are often sources of information, many of which are written above the reading level of the average adult client, who cannot read above the eighth grade level (Winslow, 2001).

The essential issues in evaluating written materials are readability and appropriateness (Hasselkus, 2009). It is your responsibility to review all written materials before sharing them with clients. Select those materials that are at a suitable reading level for clients and also appropriate to the learning objectives.

Readability

Readability of written materials refers to the language level (expressed in terms of grade level), layout, and design (Hasselkus, 2009). Readability involves examining the number of syllables in each word and the number of words in each sentence. Words with many syllables require a higher level of reading skill than words of few syllables. Short sentences are easier to read than long sentences.

In selecting written materials, take into consideration the client's background as well as the purpose of the materials. The client's background and educational level provide clues to reading ability; however, most clients read at three to five grade levels below their educational attainment (Doak, Doak, & Root, 1996). Observe the reading materials in the client's room. If none is available, ask the client what his or her favorite reading materials are. Listen to the vocabulary clients use. How simple or complex are the individual words? If the client is employed, try to determine how much reading is required on the job. Answering these questions provides a quick overview of reading ability.

Next consider the purpose of the written materials. What information does the client need that the material is expected provide? What must the material communicate? Is the purpose to supplement your teaching, fill in "gaps" that you did not have time to explain, or is it to expand on a topic of interest? Is the material a set of instructions on how to do a procedure? Is the material designed to encourage or inspire?

Software programs are now available online that can quickly calculate readability. Word processing software evaluates a selected passage according to the formula chosen by the manufacturer. SMOG Analysis and WordsCount Analytics are two such services. The SMOG Calculator estimates the years of education needed to understand a piece of writing (McLaughlin, 1969). WordsCount Analytics provides similar information plus additional readability services. The readability level of any written material can be determined by submitting a representative passage on either Web site and having it evaluated. The following are Web sites that will help you to evaluate the readability of written materials. The SAM site assesses not only readability, but also usability and suitability elements.

- Iowa Department of Public Health's Fry Readability Graph:
  http://www.idph.state.ia.us/health_literacy/common/pdf/tools/fry.pdf
- Harry McLaughlin SMOG Calculator:
  http://www.harrymclaughlin.com/SMOG.htm
- WordsCount (Web site content copyright 2009):
  http://www.wordscount.info/

- SAM (Suitability Assessment of Materials):
  http://www.beginningsguides.net/pdfs/SAM-for-Beginnings.pdf

When the written material is beyond the reading ability of the client, comprehension is decreased and recall is sketchy and inaccurate. The client also may interpret the information differently than what was intended. As a result, the client's motivation to seek further instruction from written sources may be reduced. One way to assess a client's ability to make use of a pamphlet is to have him or her look it over and ask questions about the content.

Example: "I want to give you a pamphlet that explains things clearly. Will you look at this and tell me if it appeals to you?"

Another way is to ask the client to read a pamphlet and report its comprehensibility.

Example: "Tell me what this pamphlet says to you. Is it boring? Confusing?"

Look carefully at the client while he or she is reading. Does the client show signs of tension? Watch the client's eyes. Do his or her eyes move across and down the page in a systematic manner? These answers provide clues to both readability and appropriateness.

Appropriateness

Appropriateness of written materials focuses on the information itself. Is it suitable given the client's health problem and circumstances? Does the physician want the client to have this information? Is the information appropriate to the client's ethnic and cultural values and beliefs (Hasselkus, 2009)? Written materials should be age, gender, and culturally appropriate and respectful (Zarcadoolas, Pleasant, & Greer, 2006). Whatever written materials are given, it is important to assess the client's ability to understand and use the information to improve health and well-being.

Generational differences may influence the type of printed material you give to clients. Something that a young person finds captivating may be insulting to an older client. Whatever the case, you do not want to offend clients by distributing materials that they consider beneath their intelligence.

In the acute care setting, many clients who need instruction are affected by medications they are receiving. It is not unusual for certain drug-induced states and other postsurgical or disease conditions to blur vision and slow intellectual processing.

Visual acuity may be a problem and may be affected by mundane problems, such as the need to put on the client's glasses. Fear and anxiety can lesson reading ability or even make it impossible for the client to grasp the meaning of any printed words. Selecting an appropriate time to discuss and share written materials is as important as selecting appropriate materials. Meal times and visiting hours are times to avoid.

Pamphlets and Brochures

Pamphlets and brochures are attractive, readily available, and often free. You can use them before, during, or after a presentation. Clients can hold them and use them to study and learn at their own pace, thus exercising more control over the learning experience. Voluntary health organizations are a rich source of printed materials, and many are provided in both English and Spanish. Examples include the American Cancer Society, the American Heart Association, and the American Lung Association. Virtually every disease that affects a specific population is served by an organization that provides public education and written materials.

Some Web sites offer print-on-demand health information that is current and cost effective. For example, health information is available from the Joint Commission through the Speak Up initiative (Joint Commission, 2009). These brochures can be downloaded and used as needed. Their brochures are not copyrighted; however, the Joint Commission requires that it be credited as the source of the material. Topics are varied; examples include medication safety, preventing infection, pain management, and preventing medical mistakes.

It is important to give careful consideration to the timing of pamphlet distribution if you are using them in a class. If the pamphlets contain the actual information you wish to discuss, use them as advance organizers and a substitute for note taking. If you decide they are distracting, keep them out of sight until the presentation is completed.

Instructional Handouts and Patient Education Pathways

Instructional handouts refer to information specifically prepared for a client or group of clients served by a specific physician(s) or healthcare institution/agency. They typically cover preparation for diagnostic procedures, following treatment regimens, and follow-up care after a treatment or a procedure. If you are preparing these handouts, you need to have a final draft approved by the physician(s) or your employer. Follow the guidelines for writing instructional materials. Place this information on video or audio media for clients with low health literacy (Roberts, 2008).

Patient education pathways are instructional tools that facilitate client education. They inform clients about what to expect in their course of treatment and their role in recovery and restoration of health, both major goals of the pathways. When shared with clients, pathways are personal educational tools that encourage participation in self-care routines and symptom management. Pathways assume that clients who are well informed and knowledgeable about their treatment are more likely to adhere to the treatment plan. The information provided in the pathways is comprehensive, consistent, and specific to the treatment a client is undergoing. It covers every aspect in the course of treatment; for example, diet, tests, treatments, medications, activities, education, and discharge planning. Patient education pathways are similar to the multidisciplinary critical pathway tools used to manage a client's hospital stay (Clarke, 2002).

Bulletin Boards

Bulletin boards supplement health education. Depending on clients' needs and health topics of interest, bulletin boards can display a variety of information. For example, they can highlight accident prevention, national health awareness months, and announce health fairs. Specific health-related topics are often of interest, such as the nature of heart disease, cancer, and diabetes. Information can be related to the season of the year, such as preventing the common cold/flu during the fall months and healthful eating during holidays. Not only do bulletin boards supplement health education, but they also reinforce information you have taught. The display reminds clients of the important points of your presentation.

Bulletin boards are a type of informal learning that allows clients to learn at their own pace. Place them in conspicuous spots that are suitable for browsing. Keep in mind that pausing and glancing are the usual activities of browsers. Information that is deep or wordy will languish unread or may disappear if someone wishes to really delve into it. High traffic areas are good places for bulletin boards, such as waiting rooms (hospital, clinic, and office), hallways, and cafeterias. If the bulletin board is to be read by children or clients in wheel chairs, lower the height of the board from the normal erect adult's eye-level position.

Bulletin boards display pictures, photographs, tables, graphs, and cartoons as well as text information. Content, text, and graphics should be simple, clear, and at a reading level appropriate for the target population. Determine the central message for the bulletin board and then organize the content to support that message. Organizers, such as headings, should be clearly marked and easy to differentiate from the body of the text.

The font used for headings should be larger than that used for text. The lines of the text should be short enough to scan with sufficient space to separate distinct messages. Paragraphs and sentence length should be short and easy to read. Block style fonts such as Times New Roman, Gothic, and Verdana are easier to read than are script fonts or italics, which resemble handwriting. Use both upper and lower case lettering. Avoid ALL CAP LETTERING AS IT IS DIFFICULT TO READ (Thomas, 2007). It is also perceived as shouting.

Avoid cluttering the board with too much text or graphs and tables. Too much and too complex information are difficult for clients to quickly grasp. Display just the essential information and avoid extraneous information that detracts from your message. The display and text should be current and updated as necessary.

Although bright, primary colors attract children, these colors are difficult for older adults to read. Recall that age-related changes in the eyes make it difficult for older adults to discriminate among the blue, green, and violet colors. The warm colors of red, orange, and yellow are easier for older adults to see (Linton, 2007). Make the background of the bulletin board a light color to avoid the glare that occurs with white backgrounds. Dark color text on a light color back ground is easier for older adults and others to read (Thomas, 2007).

If you have handouts or pamphlets to distribute that reinforce the message on the bulletin board, place them in a folder attached to a lower corner of the board. If the handouts or pamphlets are too bulky or heavy, consider placing a small table next to the bulletin board.

Posters

Many of the suggestions pertaining to bulletin boards also apply to the preparation of posters. Posters are another effective way to communicate health information. They can accompany a presentation or be located in conspicuous places for viewing. Posters are easy to make and also commercially available. They are especially useful for limited periods of time to communicate a specific message such as a health month, workshop announcement, or safety precautions. If posters remain in place too long or they are overused, they lose their ability to attract attention and lead to boredom (Pittman, 2009). Posters are low cost, portable, and allow for self-paced learning.

Posters should use only key words to communicate a message rather than complete sentences. Use bullets or list the essential information by numbers for brevity. If you use a picture, figure, or cartoon it should be clear and large enough to be understood immediately. Illustrations should be appealing to the age, gender, socioeconomic, and cultural characteristics of clients. Sensitivity and delicacy are important, especially if you inject humor.

As with bulletin boards, use appropriate colors and block style fonts rather than script fonts for ease of reading. If your clients are older, use larger and bold fonts. If you are using a poster with a presentation, remember the 6 W formula. It means that the last row of the audience should be no farther from the poster than six times the width of the poster. For example, if the poster is two feet wide, the last row of viewers should be no farther than 12 feet from the poster. For a larger audience, transform the poster into a transparency, slide, or PowerPoint slide.

Flip Charts

The flip chart is versatile because it is portable and is used like a whiteboard/chalkboard. Creative uses of flip charts include composing instantaneous posters, gathering and preserving audience contributions, and having clients write out their thoughts. The flip chart combines the advantages of posters and whiteboards/chalkboards. You can plan ahead and prepare your charts or you can have the blank pages available while teaching for spontaneous use.

If you prepare the flip chart ahead of time, take the time you need to prepare exactly what you want: written information, pictures, cartoons, or a combination thereof. A flip chart also is used as an advance organizer because it allows you to write your outline and have the clients follow along as you move through the presentation.

If you plan to use the flip chart spontaneously as you teach, have a good supply of colorful pens on hand. Spontaneous use is appropriate when you want to elicit responses from the audience or when you want your clients to work in small groups and write their contributions down to be shared later with the larger group. If you use this method, hang the finished charts around the room. When you do this, clients feel like valued contributors to the teaching and learning process. Your flip charts also can be saved for future use. The material you have collected can be transcribed and sent to all the participants. The major disadvantage to using a flip chart is that you must have at least some artistic talent to be effective. Also your audience must be small enough so that everyone can see the flip chart.

Whiteboards/Chalkboards

A whiteboard/chalkboard is available in most classroom settings. It is valuable for making a spontaneous drawing, diagram, or illustration. You can add to or take away from the drawing while using it to explain the meaning or purpose of the topic under discussion. The whiteboard/chalkboard is an excellent device for involving clients. To promote contributions, ask a question and then write down the responses from the clients. Most individuals find it reinforcing to see their words written on the board. The best questions to ask first are those to which everyone can respond, such as questions about personal experience.

> Example: "How can you tell when you are stressed out? What do you do or what have you seen others do when they are stressed out?"

The whiteboard/chalkboard also helps with organizing information. You can link ideas in a circle, or list problems on one side and solutions on the other. The board also allows you to compare and contrast various points of view or to organize contributions from the audience into whatever schema you choose. Whenever possible, transfer complicated ideas to a handout to which clients can refer during your presentation.

When using the whiteboard/chalkboard, determine whether or not your cursive writing is more legible than your printing; use the more readable style. Write a brief notation on the board and then step aside and face the audience. This allows you to maintain contact with your clients and receive their feedback on the clarity of your point. By stepping aside, you also allow clients to copy the message, which means they are able to integrate both visual and auditory stimuli. Stepping aside also keeps you from becoming so involved with your creation on the board that you start talking to the board instead of the clients.

Preparing Your Own Written Materials

Consider preparing your own written materials if nothing suitable is available. When preparing your own, it is important to write at the sixth grade reading level or lower to benefit clients (Winslow, 2001). Do this by shortening words with multiple syllables, eliminating extraneous words, and simplifying sentence structure. Use everyday, plain language consistent with the client's vocabulary; avoid using medical jargon that clouds the health message.

Plain Language is a U.S. government initiative given emphasis by President Clinton in 1998 when he issued an executive memo requiring federal agencies to write in plain language. Plain language requires that written materials be understandable the first time a person reads or hears it so that clients: (1) can find what they need, (2) understand what they find, and (3) can use what they find to meet their needs. Plain language is grammatically correct with accurate word usage and complete sentence structure. It is clear writing that tells clients exactly what they need to know without using unnecessary words. Plain language makes information more informative and easier for clients to understand.

Begin preparing your own teaching materials by assessing the clients carefully. Know who you are writing for and what their needs are. Consider involving selected members of your target audience as a focus group. Also involve selected healthcare providers who plan to use the material. There may be a difference between what the healthcare providers think is most important for clients to know and what the clients actually want to know.

After you identify the content to communicate, focus on the two to three most important points. Begin developing the most important point first and then develop the others one at a time. Do not overload clients with too much information; decide what is essential and focus on that. If you must use technical terms such as the names of diagnostic procedures, be sure to define exactly what you mean. Keep the message and examples concrete, as they are easier for clients to understand. Abstract messages may be difficult to grasp for those with low health literacy (Seligman et al., 2007; Zarcadoolas, Pleasant, & Greer, 2006). It is important that your information is accurate and updated as necessary. As your focus groups (clients and providers) review your material, make changes based on their feedback.

The layout and presentation of your material are important (Pittman, 2009). Consider the general appearance of the text and margins. Text should be limited so that the material does not appear crowded and margins should be ample. The material should have a clear title that indicates its purpose. Use headings, subheadings, and bullets to present the information in a logical and organized format. Using different fonts, bold fonts, highlighting, bullets, and numbers make the text more readable. Add pictures, illustrations, and diagrams to illustrate important points. They often communicate health messages more effectively than does text (Bryan, 2008). Be sure the material is age, gender, and culturally appropriate for your target audience. Color always livens up a message if it is cost effective to add it. The goal in preparing your own written material is to simplify the message while communicating the essential health information. Box 11-1 lists guidelines for writing your own instructional materials.

Evaluating Printed Materials

Printed information must be accurate and from a reliable source. This is important for all printed materials, whether in the form of pamphlets, brochures, or instructional handouts.

BOX 11-1   Guidelines for Writing Instructional Materials

Planning:

- Identify the purpose of the materials.

- Identify the most important points to communicate (two to three).

- Assess the characteristics and needs of the target audience.

- Involve selected members of your target audience as a focus group.

- Involve selected healthcare providers who will use the materials.

Organizing:

- Group like information together.

- Develop each point/group, one at a time.

- Keep paragraphs brief.

Writing:

- Use short, simple sentences that express one idea only.

- Use plain language and familiar words with only one or two syllables.

- Be consistent in how you define and use words.

- Avoid medical jargon, technical terms, abbreviations, and acronyms.

- Write at the fourth to sixth grade reading level.

- Use conversational style with an active voice.

- Use concrete, not abstract, examples.

- Avoid extraneous words.

- Update the material as necessary to maintain currency and relevance.

Appearance and Layout:

- Add pictures, illustrations, and colors that support the message.

- Use pictures and illustrations that are age, gender, and culturally appropriate.

- Use attractive spacing and layout with generous white space.

- Use 12-point type for text.

- Use larger point type, bold or underline to separate headings and subheadings.

- Use bold typeface fonts; avoid script fonts and italics.

- Use highlighting, bullets, and numbers as appropriate.

- Use upper and lower case lettering; avoid all caps.

Always consider the source of the printed materials. Many health and disease-related brochures that healthcare institutions/agencies use are prepared by voluntary health organizations. Examples of reputable voluntary health organizations are the March of Dimes and the American Heart Association. These are accurate and reliable sources of information.

Instructional handouts are usually prepared by a committee in the healthcare institution or by a physician who has approved the content. These are also accurate and reliable sources. In contrast, newspaper and magazine advertisements are less reliable, although not necessarily inaccurate sources of information. Each source must be evaluated on its own merits.

MULTIMEDIA

Video Media

Videotapes and DVDs are excellent instructional tools. Both show action images with sound; however, DVDs are replacing videotapes in popularity and usage. Regardless of format, video is the closest substitute to the actual experience because it stimulates both hearing and sight. Videos evoke imagery and intense emotion as they invite clients to experience the scenes being enacted with the actors. Visual images are more likely to be remembered than information clients read or hear (Doak, Doak, & Root, 1996).

Videos allow clients to observe the action without being direct participants, which is consistent with Bandura's social cognitive theory of how people learn. The actor models the desirable behavior; for example, child-rearing practices or performing a procedure. Videos are also excellent for generating an affective response in the audience and for promoting discussion. Videos can be stopped to discuss a particular action or generate problem-solving options from the audience. They help clients anticipate experiences for which they must prepare; for example, preparation for childbirth. Visual images are also effective with non-English speaking clients.

Videos are easy to store and transport. If you are making a presentation at another location, most facilities have a videocassette recorder (VCR) or DVD player and television monitor. You need to confirm this in case you need to bring your own equipment. Many health departments and community health organizations will lend videotapes and DVDs for presentations. Contact the appropriate agency to determine what is available and reserve your request.

Consider making your own video recording, as they are relatively easy to make if you have access to the requisite equipment. If you are dissatisfied with the results, you can easily remake it. Using a video camera to record a client's performance, such as a team member performing a procedure, is an excellent teaching tool. Clients can then watch their performance and receive immediate and accurate feedback as they attempt to learn a particular procedure. If you make a video recording, keep it to 8 minutes or less, as clients tend to lose interest if it is longer. If the video needs to be longer, stop it periodically and discuss it to keep clients' attention. Videos that tell captivating stories or have multiple scene changes hold clients' interest for longer periods (Doak Doak, & Root, 1996).

As with any learning experience, videos are most valuable if prefaced by advance organizers. An introduction includes its title, its length, a synopsis of the message or story, and what you expect clients to gain from the viewing. It is helpful to tell clients specifically what they should notice and what they are expected to do with the experience afterward: Discuss the plot or perform the procedures. If unfamiliar words are used, introduce them beforehand. Put the words on a transparency, handout, or on the whiteboard/chalkboard before the video is shown.

Audio Media

Audio cassettes, DVDs, and CDs are formats for recording sound. These formats are widely available, as are their respective players. Audio messages are also supported by other portable media players such as the iPod, and the MP3 player. Audio media is especially useful when clients must learn an auditory skill. For example, teaching the parents of an asthmatic child to recognize various breath sounds. By listening to different types of breathing, parents can learn which types of breathing by their child requires an emergency response and which types can be improved with routine treatment.

Audio media are useful for hearing directions when the client cannot look at the speaker. Consider the client who is lying prone while following directions for exercise or relaxation. Many people find it easier to concentrate when their eyes are closed or when they listen to soothing music or directions for creating healing images. Clients can make an audiocassette tape of their favorite therapeutic music or download therapeutic music onto the iPod/MP3 player (Pittman, 2009).

In these days of early discharge, clients often leave the hospital before they or their families are confident of the procedures they must perform at home. Audio recording of health instructions for use after discharge reminds clients of the information that they were taught. For example, by recording your voice during the client's final teaching session, you can talk the client through a procedure with a minimum of extra time and effort. First review with the client the necessary equipment and record this information at the beginning of the tape. Then, as the client performs the procedure, record each step, pausing when the client needs more time with some steps than with others. You should offer words of reinforcement and encouragement during this session. When the client and family go home, they will hear your reassuring words, which are comforting to those who must now handle the procedure on their own. In addition to being a reassuring experience that lowers tension, the familiarity of your voice recreates a mind-set that more closely approximates the last teaching session. This promotes more accurate recall. You need the proper audio equipment for recording a tape or DVD. Most healthcare institutions have the equipment and most families have playback equipment at home.

When you are in community health settings and clients live far away, such as in rural settings, consider depending on the telephone between home visits. Or an audio tape, DVD, or CD could be left with the family containing reminders, complicated instructions, etc.

Audio media have many advantages. They are used with individuals or groups. They are inexpensive, readily available, and can be tailor-made, erased, or remade in the clients language. Also, they help clients develop listening skills. Audio media captures nuances of speech that are impossible to convey in written communication. However, audio media have some drawbacks as well. Listeners find it difficult to listen for more than 15 minutes without other stimuli because they get bored. Remember that tapes, DVDs, and CDs are somewhat fragile and need protection from moisture and temperature extremes.

Computer-Assisted Instruction

Many health maintenance organizations and healthcare institutions/agencies have special areas where clients can access interactive software to supplement health education. Computer-assisted instruction (CAI) is an excellent resource for self-paced learning. It does not become impatient; its pace can be controlled by the client; and it gives immediate, objective, and consistent feedback. The software allows clients to repeat all or part of a lesson and progress at their own rate. Clients acquire information in private, and no one else has to know what they think or how long they take to obtain the expected knowledge. CAI is useful for clients of any age, especially if they can control the pace at which they progress. For younger clients, CAI may evoke the fun and excitement of an arcade game. Self-paced learning takes initiative on the part of clients. The CAI may lead you to expect too much independent learning from clients. If CAI is provided in a healthcare setting, be available to answer questions from clients and assist them with the software as the need arises.

Many interactive Web sites are available on the Internet. For example, the Web site MedlinePlus is a service of the National Library of Medicine (NLM) and National Institutes of Health (NIH). The site offers "Easy to Read" instructional materials that are available in more than 40 languages and interactive health tutorials on topics covered under these categories: Diseases and Conditions, Tests and Diagnostic Procedures, Surgery and Treatment Procedures, and Prevention and Wellness (U.S. National Library and National Institutes of Health, 2006). These sites can be accessed from a client's home.

Interactive bulletin boards serve as a continuing education resource for updating team members (Flournoy, Turner, & Combs, 2000). Short, succinct lessons, messages, and updates can be created for team members. It is self-paced learning that team members use when they have the time and interest.

Digital Camera and Photographs

The digital camera has largely replaced its older counterpart, the 35-mm camera. A digital camera takes video or still photographs by recording images on an electronic image sensor. Images are displayed immediately after they are recorded and can be stored or deleted as desired. Images are printed via inexpensive electronic photo print equipment or taken to any commercial print service.

Digital photos are displayed using a LCD projector, which is suitable for large groups. Everyone in your audience sees the same photo at the same time. Single photographs are best used on an individual basis or in a small group. When they are passed around, however, they may be distracting to the audience.

Slides

Slides, 35 mm, may still be available for health education purposes in some healthcare institutions/agencies. The slides are placed in a carousel and require a slide projector to use. They can also be inserted into a PowerPoint presentation. A slide presentation is excellent for the visual learner and helps to clarify your comments. The order of slides can be replaced or rearranged in the carousel if you change the nature of your presentation. You need to prepare a script to accompany the slide presentation. Slides are easy to store and to transport. Because 35-mm film is no longer being produced, it is wise to learn to use the digital camera.

Objects and Models

Actual objects should be used for demonstration when possible. For example, use a real syringe when you teach self-injections and use a real dressing when you teach how to change a dressing. Models are used when the real object, such as a heart, is not available or not feasible to use. Three types of models are replica, analogy, and symbol.

Replica

A replica is a model that resembles the real object. It is a scaled construction that magnifies the features of the original object. The increased size of the features makes demonstration easier. This type of model can be picked up and manipulated and helps convey the concept of dimensions. Replicas are useful for kinesthetic clients who learn better with hands-on opportunities. For example, clients can take a model of a kidney apart and put it back together again, thus getting a better idea of how the kidney works. By handling the replica, clients are able to control the pace of learning.

A replica can be used to help clients develop a skill. Learning to clean a central line or to examine breasts for lumps are challenging procedures that are best learned on something other than a human being. Replicas exist for practicing these skills, but they are expensive, fragile, and require storage space.

Replicas best serve only a few clients at a time. Compensate for this by using team teaching and placing different replicas at different "stations." Such an arrangement divides the larger group into several smaller ones and allows each station to become an area of concentrated focus with fewer competing stimuli.

Analogy

An analogy is something that has features similar to something else (Merriam-Webster, 2007); it compares the familiar with the unfamiliar for explanatory purposes (Ruhl, 2009). Analogies build on clients' existing knowledge to communicate complex medical concepts. They emphasize a shared quality that helps make something unfamiliar become more understandable. A good analogy is familiar, short, clear, and visual.

When creating an analogy, the unfamiliar concept is the "target," whereas the familiar concept that you want to use for comparison is the "analog." The target and the analog are connected with the words "like" or "as." For example, explaining that the action of the heart is like a pump that moves water. Ruhl (2009) identifies five things to remember when using analogies:

1. Determine the need for the analogy. Use an analogy when you are trying to explain something hard to understand.
2. Confirm that the client understands the analogy. Ask "tell me how you understand what I said . . ." and then have the client explain in his or her own words what you explained.
3. Follow-up with a full explanation and use other instructional materials to augment your explanation.

4. Point out the limitations of the analogy. For instance, it is true that the brain is like a computer, but there are differences of which the client should be aware.

5. Make the client aware that the analogy is just a starting point. Once he or she understands the concepts, use that understanding to move forward.

Ruhl encourages health educators to be creative and spontaneous, adapt analogies to the client's style of language, and build on the common references that clients use.

Analogies demand conceptual sophistication and an ability to understand how things are alike and different. Because not everyone perceives the same way, practice using the analogy on others to find out if they understand the point and if it fits the message you intend to convey.

Symbol

A symbol stands for something else that it represents by association or resemblance. Often a printed or written sign is used to represent an operation, element, quantity, quality, relation, or something invisible (Merriam-Webster, 2007). The treble clef sign and notes on lines are examples of musical symbols. Words are examples of symbols. They are combinations of circles and lines arranged in special patterns to convey a certain meaning. The meaning varies according to the language familiar to the speaker, writer, listener, and reader.

Words are symbolic models that you use to convey a concept or idea to clients. Words are such familiar symbols that you no longer perceive the circles and lines with which words are drawn unless you are dyslexic. If fact, unless you have a photographic mind, you could not even report the exact words on this page. You would probably report the ideas, general concepts, and meanings you attached to what you read.

You may draw diagrams, signs, or cartoons, all of which are attempts to convey meaning through the use of symbols. International traffic signs are examples of such symbols. The picture conveys the meaning. Circles have many meanings. Arranged on top of each other and colored red, yellow, and green, they would be perceived in this country as parts of a traffic light. "Smiley" faces are recognized by most people in this culture as conveying happiness or approval.

The practice of representing something by symbols is so widespread in this culture that it is difficult to describe by example. The symbol + means plus, and the symbol = means equal to. Stick figures can be used by a teacher to symbolize people regardless of artistic talent. The figure can help you focus a client's attention on the desired point. Distinct symbols are used in health care to distinguish between male and female people.

Symbols are gaining widespread application in areas that cater to multilingual groups and international travel. Examples include airports, roadway traffic signs, lodging and food, and handicapped parking symbols. You should avoid using abbreviations that are common among healthcare personnel but are not common to clients. These abbreviations include NPO, PO, and PRN. Although these abbreviations convey meaning to certain groups, they might add confusion to other groups. Figure 11-1 illustrates some common symbols.

Transparencies

Transparencies remain a popular choice for illustrating a presentation and are used as backup to other media, such as PowerPoint presentations. They can be seen with the room lights on. They are useful to highlight important points in a verbal presentation. The highlights can be in the form of brief, well-spaced outlines, pictures, simple drawings, or cartoons. You can prepare transparencies in advance or on the spot in response to interaction with the clients.

You can prepare permanent or nonpermanent transparencies in several ways. To create permanent transparencies, construct a drawing or write text on paper, copy the material in a copy machine, and then run the copy together with a blank transparency through a thermo fax machine. The thermo fax and carbon on the copy interact to

FIGURE 11-1 Common Symbols.
Sources: © AbleStock, © WilleeCole/ShutterStock, Inc.

make the transparency in the presence of heat. The same process is used to create picture transparencies. To create nonpermanent transparencies, use nonpermanent, washable color marking pens. This works well for illustrating as you are presenting. The transparency is reusable as the ink will wash off. Transparencies are relatively inexpensive to purchase and can be stored flat in pocket envelopes that fit a standard note binder.

Transparencies are projected onto a screen via an overhead projector and useful for any size audience. The projector is bulky with a long arm attached that has a mirror and lens that focus and redirect the light forward onto a screen. When a transparency is placed on the projector, the image is directed onto the screen. The projector has a very bright halogen lamp, a fan to cool the machine, and a storage place for additional lamps.

The overhead projector needs to be adjusted before the presentation to ensure a good projected image on the screen. This means adjusting the size of the screen and the distance from the projector to the screen. We recommend that you stand to one side of the projector and look at the audience when giving a presentation. Place the projector so that you can face the audience. The audience looks at the screen while you look at the transparency on the projector to see what the audience sees.

Microsoft PowerPoint Slides

Microsoft PowerPoint is a presentation software program widely used by educators. It is useful for large audiences and requires an LCD projector to display the images onto a screen for viewing. The presentation can be accessed from the computer, a disc, or a flash drive. The room may need to be darkened for best viewing.

To use, identify what you want to illustrate through PowerPoint slides. You can input text, graphics, movies, or other objects on the slides and arrange and rearrange them as you wish. The software provides a template with a variety of formats and backgrounds to create the slides. You can navigate through the slides as you make your presentation. The slides can be printed or you can display the presentation live on a computer. The software is easy to use but requires the proper equipment. See Box 11-2 for help in preparing your presentation.

Story Boards

A story board is an educational tool that is a visual presentation of text or graphic information. Story boards tell a story or explain sequential information (Pittman, 2009). Microsoft PowerPoint software is commonly used for creating story boards. The software provides many options for layout, text, and graphics.

BOX 11-2   Guidelines for Creating and Using PowerPoint Slides

- Choose a format that best illustrates your points with headings and subheadings.
- Choose a plain background to limit the distractions on the slides.
- Choose a soft background color that contrasts with the lettering.
- Use bullets or numbers to separate the information.
- Use upper and lower case lettering; avoid all capitalized lettering.
- List as few words as possible to communicate the message.
- Limit the amount of information on each slide; avoid overcrowding.
- Limit the number of slides so the audience focuses on your comments.
- Advance the slides to match your comments.
- Be sure the hardware and software are operating properly ahead of your presentation.
- Give a copy of the slides to the audience to reinforce learning.

Story boards are easy to develop, edit, and distribute for client education purposes. They are low cost and provide consistent, current information to clients. The development of story boards begins by selecting a health-related topic followed by identifying the essential information to include. A committee can help determine the topic, content, and accuracy. When developed, story boards can be distributed via e-mail, printed, or made into posters with the proper printer (Kisak & Conrad, 2004).

Cartoons

Cartoons can be transferred to a transparency or PowerPoint slide and projected for large groups; or cartoons may be circulated among members of a small group or shared with an individual. Humorous cartoons provide comic relief and make a point much more clearly than many words. Before you decide to use humor, test it out on people similar to your intended audience. Drawings that are intended to be humorous also can evoke unexpected reactions among clients, who may perceive the material differently than you do. Cartoons are not necessarily cross-cultural, so you should show prospective cartoons to someone from the target culture and have them critique it for you. As with photographs, cartoons can be placed in clear plastic covers for protection.

Cell Phones

Cell phones are increasingly popular and often replace land line telephones. Both are used to supplement and reinforce health education. Many healthcare institutions/agencies provide telephone numbers for clients who have concerns. Health advice lines are also available. Telephones are used to follow up with clients to offer encouragement and help with any problems they are having adhering to a treatment regimen.

Cell phones were used creatively in a study of adolescents with Type 1 diabetes. One group kept a food diary, whereas another used the cell phone camera to record their dietary intake. The photographs were downloaded and, along with the food diaries, analyzed. Although there was no significant difference between the two groups, it does demonstrate a novel use of the cell phone to monitor clients (Donald, Franklin, & Green, 2009). In another study, text messaging was shown to be effective in improving self-efficacy and adherence in adolescents with Type 1 diabetes (Franklin, Waller, Pagliari, & Greene, 2006).

INTERNET AND WORLD WIDE WEB

The Internet is a huge global network that connects computers for the purpose of transferring information from one computer to another. It connects millions of private, public, academic, business, and government computers. The Internet is the infrastructure that supports the Web. The Web is a network of hypertext documents called Web pages that are accessed via the Internet. Web pages may contain text, images, videos, audio, and other multimedia. Users are able to easily navigate among these pages with the click of the mouse. The Web was created to display information, whereas the Internet was created to exchange information. The Internet and the Web are not synonymous terms, although they are often used as if they were (Sopczyk, 2008; Wikipedia, 2009).

To access the Web, clients must have a computer, or have access to one, with a telecommunication link and special software to connect to an Internet service provider (ISP). Clients navigate the Web through a browser such as Microsoft Internet Explorer and Netscape Navigator. Once on the Internet, search engines (Google) and directories (Yahoo) are available that allow users to search for specific information and Web sites (Sopczyk, 2008).

The technology and supporting software are developing rapidly and changing daily. By the time that you read this, today's technology will have advanced and the number of health-related Web sites greatly expanded. Nurses who work with this technology need to keep abreast of these changes to assist clients needing health education.

Wikipedia (2009), an online encyclopedia, estimates that by 2009, one fourth of the world's population will use the services of the Internet. The Pew Internet/California HealthCare Foundation survey found that 74% of US adults go online and 61% of these adults look online for health information (Fox & Jones, 2009). The nurse who works as an educator must be computer and information literate to use this medium to assist clients (Sopczyk, 2008).

Because so many clients access the Internet, you should ask them if they are looking at health-related Web sites. If so, ask which ones they find useful and evaluate if they are accessing reliable sources of information. By listening to what the clients have learned about health issues, you have the opportunity to evaluate that knowledge. You can refer clients to reliable Web sites if that is indicated. Clients may have questions about what they are learning or they may be overwhelmed with the amount of information they are finding. Urge clients to use online health information to supplement that given by their healthcare provider and not as a substitute. Many clients misunderstand or misinterpret health information and require clarifying explanations.

eHealth Web Sites

The Web is the newest source for interactive health information, often referred to as eHealth. Electronically available health information includes access to personal health records online, health education libraries, professional health journals, and self-assessment tools. When health information is so widely available and accessible, it has the potential to improve the quality of health if used by clients. It also has the potential to create problems for clients and providers if the health information is inaccurate and influences their decision-making and healthcare practices.

The Internet is advantageous for clients because it is accessed in private in their own homes. Information is read at the clients' speed and convenience. Taking advantage of this technology is more effective for those clients with adequate health literacy skills. Those at the low health literacy level may find accessing and understanding health information on Web sites more challenging.

Clients without a personal computer have free access through public libraries, community centers, or senior centers. Clients who are enrolled in health maintenance organizations, such as Kaiser Permanente, have access to onsite interactive health education software. Electronic sources of health information are available from the Joint Commission through the Speak Up initiative (Joint Commission, 2009) and Medline Plus, both described earlier in this chapter.

The Web has become a source of information and an educational tool for clients with a variety of health issues (Hawn, 2009; Jacobi et al., 2007; Scharer, 2005; Schultz, Stava, Beck, & Vassilopoulou-Sellin, 2003). It puts information and power into the hands of consumers, especially clients with chronic diseases. Half of clients with a chronic disease or disability go online. Of this number, fully 86% have searched for information about health topics (Fox, 2007). Millard and Fintak (2002) found that clients with chronic illnesses frequently access Web sites to get information about their illness and engaged in self-care and self-diagnosis. In a large study, they found that users were skeptical about health care in general. Some users were not satisfied or had experienced problems with access to the healthcare system. Others lacked insurance coverage or found it difficult to obtain health care. Favored health Web sites were those designed specifically for health topics, medical journals, advocacy groups, and academic Web sites. Other ways that clients can access health-related information is through YouTube, Podcasts, and streaming video. A difficulty with Web sites is that clients do not know if the information is reliable.

Evaluating Web Site Information

Almost anything can be found on the Web, so it is important to evaluate each site for accuracy and reliability. Although Web sites can be a source of excellent information, they also can be misleading and provide misinformation. It is your responsibility to thoroughly evaluate each Web site that you recommended to clients. Monsivais and Reynolds (2003) and MedlinePlus offer guidelines for evaluating Web sites.

- What is the source of the information? Is it from an individual or an organization? Examples of reliable sources of information include local, state, and federal government sites, US colleges and universities, professional organizations, and voluntary health organizations. Look at the "about us" Web page for this information. Is there a way to contact the Webmaster?
- What is the quality of the information? The writers of the information should be identified and may be found in "about us" Web page or mission statement. Who are they? Are they recognized experts in the field about which they are writing? Be skeptical; quackery thrives on the Internet. Look for claims that sound too good to be true such as promises about new cures and "secret ingredients."
- What evidence is offered to support the claims? Is it based on medical research conducted by properly credentialed researchers at known healthcare institutions, scientific laboratories, or universities? Is the evidence based on personal

testimony and opinion? If so, are the persons and their credentials identified? Is there a way to contact them? Be skeptical of anonymous testimonials that claim cures and promote treatments.

- How current is the information? Note the date the information was posted and the last time the site was updated. Credible sites provide dates. Does the site provide references and maintain hyperlinks to other credible sites?
- Is the information biased? What is the purpose of the site and who is sponsoring and funding it? Is it by public funds, donations, or supported by commercial advertising? The distinction between the health information and the advertisement should be clear. Web sites can appear to be credible, but may not be to a careful observer. The purpose of many Web sites is to sell a product or recommend a particular treatment (Butler & Foster, 2003). Such a site would not be considered an objective source of information.

When clients search for information on the Web, many options appear and choosing among them is confusing. Talk with clients about how to find credible Web sites. Also urge clients to talk with their healthcare providers about the accuracy of health information they are finding on the Web.

Social Networking Web Sites

Boyd and Ellison (2007) define social network sites as "web-based services that allow individuals to (1) construct a public or semi-public profile within a bounded system, (2) articulate a list of other users with whom they share a connection, and (3) view and traverse their list of connections and those made by others within the system. The nature and nomenclature of these connections may vary from site to site" (p. 2). Although social network Web sites are popular, it is not known how many adults use them to gather or share health information. Most users who access these sites, do so to share updates about themselves or their friends (Fox & Jones, 2009). Facebook, Twitter, and MySpace are examples of social networking sites that are used by clients to share information.

E-mail, short for electronic mail, is used by both healthcare providers and clients, especially in rural areas. It increases the speed of communication and the ability to keep in contact with other clients and providers. Electronic communication also has disadvantages (Sopczyk, 2008). It lacks context, such as facial expression and tone of voice. Communications via e-mail may take more time than expected; e.g., hours or even days to send and receive messages. Although instant messaging does not have this time lag, more information can be communicated via e-mail than is the case with instant messaging. With e-mail there is a written record of the information shared or the advice given. It important that this be accurate and appropriate and a copy of it be placed in the client's record. Although healthcare institutions and agencies take steps to ensure privacy in electronic communications and have guidelines for use, you can never assume that the communications are private.

Hawn (2009) anticipates that social networking sites will become increasingly used by clients and healthcare providers. Hawn reports that through e-mail, instant messaging (IM), or video chat, some clients are now able to contact their physicians directly. It is a way for clients to stay in touch with their physicians. E-mail access to personal physicians and nurse practitioners is now available through some health maintenance organizations, such as Kaiser Permanente and Palo Alto (California) Medical Group. Clients can also make appointments, refill prescriptions, and see

---

BOX 11-3   Choosing a Medium

Questions to ask yourself when choosing a medium:

1. What medium is most appropriate given the learning objectives, teaching content, and teaching strategies?

2. Is sound necessary, or can a silent medium be used?

3. Is motion important, or can still pictures convey the ideas?

4. Is color important, or is black and white more advantageous?

5. Is individual study encouraged?

6. Is the focus on learning as a group?

7. How often is the material likely to need updating?

8. Do you have the technical competence to use this medium?

9. Can you handle common problems with this medium?

10. Do you know where to get help with it?

11. What is realistic for you to accomplish given your budget and time constraints?

12. What resources are necessary in the learning environment to use this equipment, such as a screen, podium, and electrical outlets?

their personal test results online. Some physicians are establishing their own Facebook-like profiles and communicating with clients via secure e-mail message networks. Some are writing blogs about common health topics (Hawn, 2009).

Electronic discussion boards have been useful for clients who are experiencing similar health issues and share common concerns. Clients post their experiences and thoughts on the site and gain the support of other clients experiencing similar problems. Clients exchange helpful messages with each other. It is an effective, relatively inexpensive way to provide social support to clients. Discussion boards are also a promising health resource (Scharer, 2005; Schultz et al., 2003). HealthBoards.com is an example of a social support site (http://www.healthboards.com/). Clients have access to more than 150 message boards that cover a wide range of health topics. This resource may be especially helpful for clients with disabilities or chronic illnesses.

SELECTING INSTRUCTIONAL MATERIALS

When selecting instructional materials, review the learning objectives, teaching content, and teaching strategies and ask how you can best supplement these. Consider the characteristics of your clients and which media would best help them learn. In Box 11-3 we have summarized some questions to ask in this process.

Table 11-1 summarizes the advantages, disadvantages, and helpful hints in using the various types of instructional materials. We hope this is helpful to you in making a selection for your purposes.

TABLE 11-1   Features of Instructional Materials

Type	Advantages	Disadvantages	Helpful Hints
Video media	Good substitute for actual experience. Easily obtainable. Easy to remake and update. Can be stopped and rerun. Familiar to many.	Size of monitor limits audience distance. Technical skill needed. Expensive initial investment.	Need compatible equipment. Can take longer than expected to make a tape/DVD. Store properly.

(continues)

TABLE 11-1 Features of Instructional Materials *(continued)*

Type	Advantages	Disadvantages	Helpful Hints
Audio media	Can be used with individuals or groups. Good for developing listening skills. Accessible. Inexpensive. Can be tailor-made, erased, or remade.	Can be dull if used by itself or for too long a period. Audiocassettes can be damaged easily. Need proper playback equipment.	Store properly. Should be of high audio quality to maintain interest.
Computer-assisted instruction	Client controls the pace. Correct responses reinforced immediately. Incorrect responses retaught immediately. Good for sequential thought processes. Allows client to repeat the lesson if necessary.	Depends on client initiative. Time consuming for client. Time consuming for nurse to monitor. Limited value if nurse is not available for questions. Clients must be visual learners and computer literate. Can be boring.	Select the most user-friendly software available. Spend time with client to ensure comfort with the program.
Digital camera and photographs	Images can be displayed and printed immediately. Images easily stored and deleted. Can be used with taped narration or music.	Expensive initial investment. Single photographs distracting if passed around during presentation. Shows no movement.	Synchronize with a presentation.
Objects and models	Depict the real thing as closely as possible. Can be handled and studied at client's pace. Replicas are static. Analogies are dynamic. Appeal to kinesthetic learners.	Can be bulky and heavy. Inconvenient to transport. Requires storage space. Time consuming. Expensive and fragile. Analogies require conceptual sophistication.	Require advance planning if borrowed. Works well with several stations around a teaching area. Requires a teacher at each station.

(continues)

TABLE 11-1   Features of Instructional Materials (continued)

Type	Advantages	Disadvantages	Helpful Hints
Transparencies	Versatile, inexpensive, and reusable. Teacher can face learners. Eliminates verbal repetition. Can be used with the lights on. Can be used with overlays. Good backup for PowerPoint.	Overhead projector is bulky and needs to be adjusted to the screen. Uses bulbs that often burn out. Transparencies are time consuming to prepare.	Protect transparencies from hand oils and fingerprints. Use multicolor, washable pens.
PowerPoint slides	Easy to format, create, use and stored on disk or flash drive.	Requires expensive equipment and screen. Slides are time consuming to prepare. Must have operational LCD projector and screen.	Be sure equipment is available and working properly. Important to sequence slides and story board.
Story board	Shows still, motion, and sound. Stimulating to audience. Allows audience to follow the presentation.		
Instructional handouts and education pathways	Developed for specific clients and/or healthcare institution. Easily changed and updated. Clients can review at their pace.	Take time to prepare and update. Duplicating takes time.	Require storage space. Keep materials organized and handy for use.
Pamphlets and brochures	Portable and attractive. Can be used before, during, and after a presentation. Can be studied at client's pace. Readily available. Often free.	May overwhelm clients if too many. May contain outdated or irrelevant information. May be culturally inappropriate.	Distribute at the most propitious time. Check for currency of information.

(continues)

TABLE 11-1   Features of Instructional Materials *(continued)*

Type	Advantages	Disadvantages	Helpful Hints
Bulletin boards	Clients can process at own pace. Attracts browsers.	Can get cluttered and outdated. Unsuitable for long or complex information.	Change often. Keep attractive, lively. Contain a minimal number of messages.
Posters	Portable and attractive. Attracts browsers. Can be used before, during, and after a presentation. Can be studied at client's pace. Readily available. Often free.	Time consuming to make. Provide limited viewing. Need a prop. Bulky to carry and store. Useful only to readers.	Change often. Keep attractive, lively. Contain a minimal number of messages.
Flip charts	Versatile, portable. Use like a whiteboard/ chalkboard. May be prepared before or created spontaneously during presentation.	Require artistic talent and good handwriting. Clients may have a limited view.	Have a good supply of black and colored pens. Use masking tape or adhesive to affix flip charts to wall.
Whiteboards/ Chalkboards	Widely available. Useful for spontaneous illustration at the time of client's concern. Offer reinforcement to respondents. Erasable. Allow teacher to add to and take away from illustration. Good back-up aid.	Two dimensional. Messy. Require pen/chalk and an eraser. Require good lighting. Can be time consuming to use. Requires legible writing skills.	May need to supply pens/chalk and eraser. Chalk is messy, especially on dark clothing. Write high on board to avoid writing below clients' line of vision. Divide in half for lengthy lists.

CLIENTS WITH SPECIAL NEEDS

Clients with hearing and visual impairments present special challenges when it comes to the selection of instructional materials and media. Insofar as possible, materials and media should be adapted to the particular needs of each client. It helps to involve the client's family, significant other, or caretaker if that is appropriate and the client is agreeable. They may have suggestions that will facilitate your health teaching.

In Chapter 4 we discussed ways to assess a client's degree of hearing and visual impairment. Depending on that analysis, you need to identify the best way to communicate with hearing impaired and visually impaired clients. We offer some practical suggestions here.

Many clients who are hearing impaired are able to benefit from print media and video recordings. If a client is receptive to print media, choose materials that are appropriate in terms of readability and informative, such as pamphlets and brochures. If the client knows how to write and has the strength to do it, providing paper and pencil may be an effective way to communicate. If the client is computer literate and a laptop computer is available, this may be helpful. Many health-related videos are commercially available and also available online. You can also custom make videos to suit the special needs of your client.

Visual impairment for clients can be mild, moderate, or severe or the client may be blind. You need to know each client's specific capabilities to make an appropriate selection of instructional materials and media. Many clients who are visually impaired are able to benefit from auditory media. If the client is not a reader or has poor literacy, Pittman (2009) recommends using audio media. Audio cassettes, DVDs, and CDs are commercially available and can be custom made to suit the needs of clients. Clients with visual impairments need special equipment to use these media; however, many clients already have recorders and players in their homes.

Clients with limited visual impairment may benefit from print media if the font size is sufficiently enlarged. Background and font colors can be altered to increase readability. Magnifying lamps and hand-held lighted magnifiers are also available to assist these clients.

EVALUATING EFFECTIVENESS OF INSTRUCTIONAL MATERIALS

Evaluate the effectiveness of all instructional materials. Evaluation tools should be specific to the type of materials that you are using to supplement health education. Box 11-4 provides some criteria for evaluating the effectiveness of instructional materials.

BOX 11-4   Evaluating Effectiveness of Instructional Materials

Were the instructional materials:

Teaching Plan:

- Appropriate to the learning objectives?

- Appropriate to the teaching content?

- Complementary to the teaching strategies?

Learners:

- Appealing to visual, auditory, and/or kinesthetic learners?

- Appropriate to the client's level of comprehension?

- Age, gender, and culturally appropriate and sensitive?

- Engaging to the client(s)?

Selection:

- Visually pleasing?

- Suitable to the time constraints of the learning activity?

- Visible in terms of contrast, size, and location?

- Easy to use?

- Accurate and up to date?

- Cost effective and within budget constraints?

COPYRIGHT ISSUES IN USING INSTRUCTIONAL MATERIALS

Copyright laws in the United States protect intellectual property and original works of authorship when they are fixed in a tangible form. This protection exists for both published and unpublished works (US Copyright Office, 2009). Knowing about copyright restrictions is important if you are using certain instructional materials, such as text and images. Instructional materials may be copyrighted or they may be in the public domain. Depending on their source, it is important to know the difference and respond accordingly. If you have any questions about copyright issues, it is best to consult with your employer's legal counsel.

Instructional materials taken from professional journals, magazines, and other published sources always carry a copyright. To make multiple copies, you must seek written permission from the publisher or the owner of the materials. When making the request, allow plenty of time and ask how the copyright owner wants the materials cited. It is important to comply with the copyright owner's citation (Kisak & Conrad, 2004). Copyright law permits an individual to make one copy of a copyrighted document for their own personal use without requesting permission.

Instructional materials in the public domain are not protected by copyright and therefore do not require permission. Examples of materials in the public domain include those first published in a US government document. It also includes commonly used materials in which the ownership is unknown or questionable. Some images are also in the public domain and available for use. Even though no permission is required, credit should always be given to the source of the information.

If you are downloading information from Web sites, be sure to check the copyright information provided on that Web site. Clear guidelines are provided that identify what is and is not copyrighted and any restrictions on the use of the information (Kisak & Conrad, 2004). For example, on the Joint Commission Web site, there is no copyright or reprinting permissions required for the Speak Up materials. However, the Web site asks that the Joint Commission be credited as the source of the materials.

CASE EXAMPLE: MRS. ROSA LOPEZ

We now expand the teaching plan for Mrs. Rosa Lopez by adding suitable instructional materials. See Table 11-2 for these additions; they are in italics. To assist Mrs. Lopez's understanding of hypertension and the importance of limiting sodium intake, we would provide her with culturally appropriate pamphlets such as "Living with Hypertension." We would also have a chart available that explains the mechanism of hypertension and its relationship to excess sodium intake. To help her learn about sodium in foods, we would give her two handouts: "Planning a Low Sodium Diet" and "Foods High in Sodium" that acknowledge her cultural food preferences and traditions. We might also assist her with how to read food labels the next time she is at the grocery store to identify the amount of sodium in the food she chooses. If she accesses the Internet, we would show her how to search the Web for information about low-sodium diets to include meal planning, sample menus, recipes, and snacks. If she is a member of a health maintenance organization, it may offer instructional materials and interactive tutorials over the Internet or at an educational site. To learn how to take her blood pressure, Mrs. Lopez would need to purchase a digital blood pressure monitor for home use that is available from the pharmacy. You will need to instruct

TABLE 11-2   Sample Teaching Plan for Mrs. Rosa Lopez

Learning Objectives	Content Outline	Strategies and Materials	Evaluation
By the end of this lesson, the client will be able to:	Greeting and introductions		Examples are provided in Chapters 12 and 13
1. Explain the relationship between excessive sodium intake and hypertension. (cognitive)	Hypertension Definition Fluid retention Excess sodium intake Role in fluid retention Sodium and salt relationship Sodium is 40% of table salt (sodium chloride) Fluid retention and C-V system	Talking/discussion Answer questions Discussion question: "What is the relationship between sodium intake and hypertension?" Video: *Understanding Hypertension.* Chart: *Hypertension.* Pamphlet: *Living with Hypertension.*	Verbal questions Paper and pencil test
2. Choose to limit the intake of sodium to 2000 mg/day by working with the nurse to prepare a dietary plan. (affective)	Four components of dietary plan: 1. Remove salt shaker from table. 2. Use no salt in cooking. 3. Avoid canned or processed foods that are high in sodium. 4. Use low-sodium seasonings, such as herbs and spices.	Talking/discussion Answer questions Read sample labels for sodium content Discussion question: "How can you incorporate these changes into your meal planning and usual diet?"	Short term: attitude scale Long term: implementation of dietary changes

Handout: Planning a Low Sodium Diet.
Handout: Foods High in Sodium. Assignment: Read food labels when grocery shopping.
Internet search: HMO site or Internet search engines (e.g., Google) for low sodium diets

3. Demonstrate accurately obtaining self-blood pressure reading using home digital equipment without any verbal guidance. (psychomotor)	Techniques for obtaining blood pressure: 1. Read equipment directions 2. Locate brachial artery 3. Place arm in cuff 4. Inflate cuff 5. Release air in cuff 6. Record findings	*Talking/discussion* Demonstrate procedure *Handout: Have client read the printed directions for using the equipment.* *Handout: Steps to Taking Your Blood Pressure.* Have client demonstrate the procedure. Answer questions. Develop recordkeeping system and record the findings for home use.	Blood pressure Checklist to Obtain blood Pressure Record of blood pressure readings

BOX 11-5   **Evidence-Based Nursing Practice**

Kennedy, C., & Chen, J. (2009). Changes in childhood risk taking and safety behavior after a peer group media intervention. *Nursing Research, 58*(4), 264–273.

Purpose: This study examined the effectiveness of a 4-week program for school age children in reducing risk-taking behaviors and increasing safety behaviors.

Method: A two-group, experimental, repeated-measures longitudinal design was used to compare 122 White and Latino children randomly assigned to a media intervention group or a wait-list control group 1, 3, and 6 months after the media intervention.

Results: Children who received the media intervention increased their safety behaviors, but risk-taking behaviors remained unchanged. Findings suggest that interventions that influence children's media experiences help enhance safety behaviors, and that strategies to aid parents in finding media alternatives are relevant to explore.

her ahead of time to purchase this, and perhaps identify sources of funding for the equipment. She will also need paper and a pencil to record the findings.

SUMMARY

In this chapter we introduced health literacy and the importance of considering readability and appropriateness when selecting written materials. We discussed instructional materials under three broad headings: printed materials, multimedia, and Internet and World Wide Web. Instructional materials are designed to help you achieve the learning objectives and supplement your teaching strategies. The materials that you select should be appropriate to you as the teacher and to clients as learners. Each type of instructional material has advantages and disadvantages that must be considered when making a selection.

Clients with special needs include those with auditory and visual impairments who need special consideration. Instructional materials and Web sites need to be evaluated in terms of being reliable and accurate sources of information. Criteria were provided to help in the evaluation process. It is important to remember that some instructional materials are protected by copyright. These implications were discussed.

EXERCISES

Exercise I—Assessing Health Literacy

Purpose: Assess the impact of health literacy on client care.

Directions:

1. Select a client for whom you have cared who was confronted with a major health decision. Identify that decision.
2. List the literacy and decision-making skills the client needed to make a good, informed decision.
3. Share your thoughts with the class.

Exercise II—Writing Health Information

Purpose: Prepare health information for distribution to clients.

Directions: Work in pairs and prepare a handout that includes the purpose, description, rationale, benefits, and instructions for clients for one of the following:

1. Mammography
2. Immunizations
3. Colonoscopy
4. Chest x-ray
5. Blood test

Exercise III—Writing Health Information

Purpose: Increase awareness of client perceptions of medical jargon.

Directions:

1. Look at the words in the left-hand column.
2. In the middle column, write what a client might think the words mean. If you cannot think of a possible client meaning for the word, ask friends who do not have medical backgrounds, or clients who could use some entertainment.
3. In the third column write the medical meaning.
4. In the last column write an alternative word or phrase that would convey the desired meaning.

Medical Terms and Client Understanding

Word	Client Meaning	Medical Meaning	Easier Synonym
Ambulate			
Cancer			
Concussion			
Culture			
Decubitus			
Discharge			
Force fluids			
Fracture			
Heart attack			
Hematocrit			
Hemorrhage			
A negative test			
NPO			
BID			
Reflux			
Stool			
Void			

Exercise IV—Rewriting Health Information

Purpose: Evaluate health information.

Directions:

1. Bring in a health-related written advertisement for a product or medication.
2. Identify the central message of the advertisement. What is explicit? Implicit?
3. What assumptions does the advertisement make about the client's health literacy?

4. At what reading level is the advertisement?
5. Share with others in your class.

SUPPLEMENTAL ONLINE RESOURCES

ProLiteracy:
http://www.proliteracy.org/NetCommunity/Page.aspx?pid=371&srcid=345
and http://www.proliteracy.org/NetCommunity/Page.aspx?pid=370&srcid=191
Institute of Medicine report:
http://www.iom.edu/CMS/3775/3827/19723.aspx
National Center for Education Statistics (NCES):
http://nces.ed.gov/naal/health_results.asp#top
Plain Language: Improving Communications:
http://www.plainlanguage.gov/
Joint Commission:
http://www.jointcommission.org/PatientSafety/SpeakUp/
National Library of Medicine:
http://medlineplus.gov/
SMOG Calculator:
http://www.harrymclaughlin.com/SMOG.htm
WordsCount:
http://www.wordscount.info/

REFERENCES

Boyd, D. M., & Ellison, N. B. (2007). Social network sites: Definition, history, and scholarship. *Journal of Computer-Mediated Communication, 13*(1), article 11. Retrieved 7-10-09 from http://jcmc.indiana.edu/vol13/issue1/boyd.ellison.html.

Bryan, C. (2008). Provider and policy response to reverse the consequences of low health literacy. *Journal of Healthcare Management, 53*(4), 230–241.

Butler, L., & Foster, N. E. (2003). Back pain online: A cross-sectional survey of the quality of web-based information on low back pain. *Spine, 28*(4), 395–401.

Clancy, C. M. (2008). Navigating the health care system. What's your health literacy score? *Agency for Healthcare Research and Quality (AHRQ).* Retrieved 6-22-09 from http://www.ahrq.gov/CONSUMER/cc/cc052008.htm.

Clarke, L. K. (2002). Pathways for head and neck surgery: A patient-education tool. *Clinical Journal of Oncology Nursing, 6*(2), 78–82.

Doak, C. C., Doak, L. G., & Root, J. H. (1996). *Teaching patients with low literacy skills* (2nd ed.). Philadelphia: Lippincott.

Donald, H., Franklin, V., & Greene, S. (2009). The use of mobile phones in dietary assessment in young people with Type 1 diabetes. *Journal of Human Nutrition and Dietetics, 22*(3), 256–257.

Falvo, D. R. (2004). *Effective patient education a guide to increased compliance* (3rd ed.). Sudbury, MA: Jones and Bartlett.

Flournoy, E., Turner, G., & Combs, D. (2000). Critical care nurses read the writing on the wall: Use interactive bulletin boards to teach your nurses. *Nursing Management, 31*(2), 46–47.

Fox, S. (2007). E-patients with a disability or chronic disease. Retrieved 7-2-09 from http://www.pewinternet.org/Reports/2007/Epatients-With-a-Disability-or-Chronic-Disease.aspx.

Fox, S., & Jones, S. (2009). The social life of health information. Retrieved 7-2-09 from http://www.pewinternet.org/~/media//Files/Reports/2009/PIP_Health_2009.pdf.

Franklin, V. L., Waller, A., Pagliari, C., & Greene, S. A. (2006). A randomized controlled trial of sweet talk, a text-messaging system to support young people with diabetes. *Diabetic Medicine, 23*(12), 1332–1338.

Hawn, C. (2009). Report from the field. Take two aspirin and tweet me in the morning: How twitter, facebook, and other social media are reshaping health care. *Health Affairs, 28*(2), 361–368.

Hasselkus, A. (2009). Health literacy. *The ASHA Leader,* January 20, 28–29.

Jacobi, C., Morris, L., Beckers, C., Bronisch-Holtze, J., Winter, J., Winzelberg, A. J., et al. (2007). Maintenance of Internet-based prevention: A randomized controlled trial. *International Journal of Eating Disorders, 40*(2), 114–119.

Joint Commission. (2009). Retrieved 6-16-09 from http://www.jointcommission.org/PatientSafety/SpeakUp/

Kisak, A. Z., & Conrad, K. J. (2004). Using technology to develop and distribute patient education storyboards across a health system. *Oncology Nursing Forum, 31*(1), 131–135.

Levy, M., & Royne, M. B. (2009). The impact of consumers' health literacy on public health. *The Journal of Consumer Affairs, 43*(2), 367–372.

Linton, A. D. (2007). Age-related changes in the special senses. In Linton, A. D., & Lach, H. W. (1997). *Matteson and McConnell's gerontological nursing concepts and practice* (3rd ed., pp. 600–627). St. Louis: Saunders Elsevier.

McLaughlin, G. H. (1969). SMOG grading: A new readability formula. *Journal of Reading, 12*(8), 639–646.

Merriam-Webster's Dictionary and Thesaurus (2007). Springfield, MA: Merriam-Webster Inc.

Millard, R. W., & Fintak, P. A. (2002). Use of the Internet by patients with chronic illness. *Dis Manage Health Outcomes, 10*(3), 187–194.

Monsivais, D., & Reynolds, A. (2003). Developing and evaluating patient education materials. *The Journal of Continuing Education in Nursing, 34*(4), 172–176.

National Center for Education Statistics (NCES). (2003). National Assessment of Adult Literacy (NAAL). Retrieved 6-15-09 at http://nces.ed.gov/naal/health_results.asp.

Pohl, M. L. (1981). *The teaching function of the nurse practitioner.* Dubuque, IA: Wm. C. Brown.

Pittman, T. J. (2009). Teaching tools. In Lowenstein, A. J., Foord-May, L., & Romano, J. C. (eds.). *Teaching strategies for health education and health promotion.* Sudbury, MA: Jones and Bartlett.

Roberts, D. (2008). Nursing antidotes for poor health literacy. *MEDSURG Nursing, 17*(2), 75.

Ruhl, T. S. (2009). How to use analogies. Altoona Family Physicians Residency. Retrieved on 7-17-09 from http://www.altoonafp.org/how_to_use_analogies.htm.

Scharer, K. (2005). An Internet discussion board for parents of mentally ill young children. *Journal of Child and Adolescent Psychiatric Nursing, 18*(1), 17–25.

Schultz, P. N., Stava, C., Beck, M. L., & Vassilopoulou-Sellin, R. (2003). Internet message board use by patients with cancer and their families. *Clinical Journal of Oncology Nursing, 7*(6), 663–667.

Seligman, H. K., Wallace, A. S., DeWalt, D. A., Schillinger, D., Arnold, C. L., Shilliday, B. B., et al. (2007). Facilitating behavior change with low-literacy patient education materials. *American journal of Health Behavior, 31*(suppl 1), S69–S78.

Sopczyk, D. (2008). Technology in education. In Bastable, S. B. *Nurse as educator: Principles of teaching and learning for nursing practice* (pp. 515–552). Sudbury, MA: Jones and Bartlett.

Thomas, C. M. (2007). Bulletin boards a teaching strategy for older audiences. *Journal of Gerontological Nursing, 33*(3), 45–52.

US Copyright Office, 2009. Retrieved 7-6-09 from http://www.copyright.gov/.

US National Library and National Institutes of Health. (2006). *MedlinePlus guide to healthy Web surfing*. Retrieved 6-16-09 from http://www.nlm.nih.gov/medlineplus/tutorial.html.

Wikipedia. (2009). History of the Internet. Retrieved 7-2-09 from http://en.wikipedia.org/wiki/Internet and http://en.wikipedia.org/wiki/History_of_the_Internet

Winslow, E. H. (2001). Patient education materials: Can patients read them, or are they ending up in the trash? *American Journal of Nursing, 101*(10), 33–38.

Wood, M. R., Kettinger, C. A., & Lessick, M. (2007). Knowledge is power: How nurses can promote health literacy. *Nursing for Women's Health, 11*(2), 180–188.

Zarcadoolas, C., Pleasant, A. F., & Greer, D. S. (2006). *Advancing health literacy: A framework for understanding and action*. San Francisco: Jossey-Bass.

PART V

Client Education Outcomes

CHAPTER 12

Formative Evaluation

Quality is never an accident.
It is always the result of intelligent effort.
—John Ruskin (1819 to 1900)

OBJECTIVES

Upon completion of this chapter you will be able to:
- Identify at least three purposes for evaluation.
- Distinguish between the purview of formative and summative evaluation.
- Identify the three components of formative evaluation.
- Describe the evaluation of the teaching and learning process to include learning objectives, content, teaching strategies, and instructional materials.
- Discuss the significance of client adherence in health education.
- Describe the barriers and facilitators that affect client adherence.
- Describe the evaluation of the learning environment to include the facility, temperature, seating, and equipment.
- Evaluate the nurse/client interaction in terms of attitudes, communication, and satisfaction.

KEY TERMS

adherence	formative
attitudes	instructional materials
communication	interaction
compliance	learning objectives
content	strategies
effectiveness	summative
evaluation	

INTRODUCTION

The final step of the teaching and learning process is evaluation. Evaluation means to determine the value, significance, worth, or condition of something by careful appraisal and study (Merriam-Webster, 2007). Applied to health education, evaluation is the process of judging the effectiveness of your teaching efforts. Everything you have studied to this point has a bearing on evaluation. Chapter 1 introduced the Client Education Model that is the conceptual framework for this text, and now we are ready to address the final component of the model, Client Education Outcomes. The model shows two distinct aspects of client education outcomes: formative and summative evaluation. This chapter discusses formative evaluation and the next chapter, Chapter 13, discusses summative evaluation, both equally important aspects of evaluation.

Formative evaluation is ongoing during teaching and learning activities. It involves evaluation of the teaching and learning process, evaluation of the learning environment, and evaluation of the nurse/client interaction as it is occurring. Summative evaluation occurs at the conclusion of the teaching and learning process and involves evaluation of client learning, evaluation of program effectiveness, and evaluation of integration of learning into daily living (Slavin, 2009). Formative evaluation seeks to know, "How are we doing?" whereas summative evaluation seeks to know, "How did we do?"

PURPOSES OF EVALUATION

Evaluation serves many purposes. It is important for both nurses as educators and clients as learners as it informs them about the progress in learning as well as the effectiveness of the teaching and learning process. Evaluation is feedback that tells clients and nurses if their time and effort together has been well spent (Slavin, 2009).

Evaluation is about judging and providing a basis for making those judgments (Morrison, Ross, Kemp, & Kalman, 2007). Evaluation tells us the degree to which the learning goals and objectives have been met, not met, or if they were appropriate (Falvo, 2004). Evaluation tells us whether or not the content was suitable and the teaching strategies and instructional materials effective. Evaluation in health education provides evidence about:

1. Client learning
2. Effectiveness of the teaching and learning process
3. Teacher effectiveness
4. Cost/benefit of health education programs

Redman (2007) identifies additional purposes of evaluation, noting that it can motivate clients and reinforce their correct behavior as well as reinforce educators for effective teaching. Evaluation is also useful in working with team members. It helps to determine if team members are safe and competent to deliver nursing care and perform nursing procedures.

Evaluation provides credibility and accountability to individual client education efforts and to health education programs taught to groups of clients. It is vital to the institution's education department to document the importance and effectiveness of teaching and learning. This includes documenting client learning, the time teaching takes, and the positive, cost-effective results of the time investment. In addition to the preceding political and financial factors, nurses as educators need to be aware of the legal responsibilities of documentation. The absence or presence of nursing notes is important and documents the clients' responses to teaching and learning. Documentation also provides for continuity of teaching efforts as it serves as a communication tool among health team members (Rankin, Stallings, & London, 2005).

OVERVIEW OF FORMATIVE EVALUATION

Formative evaluation is ongoing during the teaching and learning process. It involves making adjustments to an educational activity as it is occurring if that is indicated. It is about making refinements and adjustments mid-way through teaching to better meet the learning objectives and needs of clients (Falvo, 2004). As you are teaching, it is important to know if clients are responding and learning. This means being sensitive to the suitability and level of the teaching content as well as the teaching strategies and instructional materials.

Formative evaluation is about how clients are progressing in learning. As you are teaching clients, attend to feedback about how you can improve as a teacher. Feedback for the teacher is information that occurs during the process of teaching and learning that increases the effectiveness of that process (Slavin, 2009). Feedback given to clients during the process of learning is more helpful than feedback that is delayed until the conclusion of the lesson.

Review the Client Education Model in Chapter 1, specifically the Client Education Outcomes portion of the Client Education Model. In Box 12-1 you will find the Client Education Outcomes: Formative Evaluation portion of the Client Education Model. It is the framework for the next section of this chapter.

BOX 12-1   Client Education Outcomes: Formative Evaluation

- **Evaluation of the teaching plan**
  - Learning objectives
  - Content-strategies-materials
  - Client adherence
- **Evaluation of the learning environment**
  - Facilities
  - Temperature
  - Seating
  - Equipment
- **Evaluation of the nurse/client interaction**
  - Attitudes
  - Communication
  - Satisfaction

EVALUATION OF THE TEACHING PLAN

Formative evaluation of the teaching plan includes an ongoing assessment of the clients' progress in achieving the learning objectives. It also includes assessing the effectiveness of the teaching content, teaching strategies, and instructional materials. This section focuses on these components of evaluation.

Learning Objectives

In Chapter 9 you learned how to write learning objectives in the cognitive, affective, and psychomotor domains. Now you need to evaluate how clients are doing in achieving the learning objectives. Were the learning needs of clients accurately assessed and established in the first place? Because formative evaluation is ongoing during the teaching and learning process, your role is to assess how clients are progressing in meeting the learning objectives.

Observation of Behavior

Assessment of clients' progress in learning is done in one of several ways. The first is direct observation of behavior for verbal and nonverbal cues to learning (O'Brien, 2007). For example, listen to the clients' reaction to the learning objectives and questions that they ask about them. Is something not clear? Is there a word or phrase that is misunderstood? What is their nonverbal behavior telling you? Do their facial expressions show anxiety, curiosity, or interest? Do the clients appear overwhelmed? Roll their eyes in puzzlement?

If you are teaching a client how to perform a psychomotor skill, a good way to assess the client's progress is to observe the client performing it. For example, if you are teaching a client to change a dressing, demonstrate the procedure and then ask the client to do the same. Demonstration/return demonstration, taught in Chapter 10, is an effective way to observe the client's progress in mastering psychomotor skills. It provides immediate feedback about how well the client is learning. It is an opportunity for you to reinforce what the client is doing right and correct any mistakes that the client is making. Practice with feedback is how much of human learning occurs.

Direct Questioning

Direct questioning is another way to assess client progress in learning. Ask direct questions related to the content you are teaching. By asking a question, you pick up any gaps or misunderstandings immediately and clarify the information. For example, if you are teaching a hospitalized client about medications to be taken after discharge, you could ask, "How often should you take this medication at home?" to see if the message is understood. A related question is, "What side-effects of the medication should you report to the physician?" If you are teaching a client about nutrition, you could ask, "What foods are best to include on a daily basis?" and "What foods are best to avoid or take in limited quantities?"

Direct questioning provides clues about each client's learning style and general ability level. The language a client uses to answer the questions offers important clues to the senses through which the client learns more easily.

Examples: "I get it."
"I see your point."
"I hear you."

If a client makes one of these statements, consider the possibility that the client learns most easily in the kinesthetic or visual or auditory modes respectively.

Questions also help clients to anticipate the future. Listening to their answers helps you to evaluate their ability to transfer the learning to their living situation.

> Examples: "How will you be able to do this when you get home?"
> "What will you do if . . . ?"

There are disadvantages to asking questions. Questioning takes time and energy, and it is less suitable for a large group because you cannot quiz each client. Questions in a discussion group may bring up tangential topics that digress from the subject matter. Formulate your questions ahead of time if you are teaching a group of clients. When the clients are not responding as you anticipate, consider rephrasing the question. Perhaps the question was not clear or meant something different to clients than you intended. Questioning is an art that requires preparatory thought on the part of the teacher.

When using questioning, avoid expecting clients to read your mind. Remember that people are trained to give teachers and other authority figures exactly what they want to hear. Question should contain all of the information necessary for clients to understand the context and to decipher what is needed or missing.

Questions that require only a "yes" or "no" are of limited value in evaluation. Usually you learn very little useful information from such questions.

> Examples: "Do you understand these directions?"
> "Do you know the circumstances under which you should call your physician right away?"

These questions allow clients to say "yes" because the nurse may look harried and clients do not want to be bothersome. Clients may also say "yes" to avoid giving the impression that they are stupid.

Open-ended questions require clients to think through an answer and are much better than questions that result in a simple "yes" or "no" answer.

> Examples: "Would you explain to me in your own words what these directions say?"
> "Tell me how you plan to manage your [wound care, medication schedule, diet, etc.] at home."

It is also important to avoid putting clients at risk for giving a socially unacceptable answer. For instance, most young parents would answer "yes" if the visiting nursed asked the following question:

Example:	"Are you doing everything they told you to do in the hospital for your baby?"

A more informative and tactful approach would be the following:

Examples:	"When you come home with a new baby, it is impossible to recall everything they told you to do. Tell me what you remember and I can help fill in the gaps."
	"All babies are different; is your baby anything like the ones they described in your parenting classes?"

Teaching Content

Observe clients in the process of learning and consider the content as an area needing modification. Is the content consistent with the learning objectives? Is the content appropriate to this client? Is the content too complex for the client to understand or is it too simplistic and insulting? Only by observing for verbal and nonverbal cues to their behavior, asking questions, and listening to their responses will you be able to determine this.

When working with young clients or those who have trouble understanding how the human body works, it may be helpful to draw an analogy to something with which they are familiar. For example, when teaching about basic nutrition, describe how the body is like a finely tuned car engine in which each part needs to function properly for it to work. Car engines need a fuel source, functioning components, and an exhaust system, just like the human body. Another frequent analogy is comparing clogged arteries in arteriosclerosis and atherosclerosis with pipes that are clogged with drainage. Fluids (blood) do not flow efficiently and smoothly when obstructed.

Teaching Strategies

While teaching, consider your approach to teaching the content. How is your approach being received by clients? Is it helping them learn or is it frustrating to them? For example, in teaching about diet, you could show pictures of the food pyramid and identify healthful and unhealthful foods and food portions. Or, you could have cutouts of foods and have clients place the foods in the recommended hierarchy of the pyramid. The second strategy results in more effective and lasting learning.

Clients' level of participation is important to evaluate (Rankin, Stallings, & London, 2005). Do the clients ask questions? Do clients participate by contributing their thoughts and experiences? Did you build on their previous knowledge and experiences that bear on the teaching content? Were their social roles and developmental tasks respected? Were they given practice time if you taught a psychomotor skill?

The strategies you select depend, to some degree, on the resources, materials, and equipment that you have available for teaching. Consider what is available and use your creativity and select the strategies that promote the best learning.

Instructional Materials

Instructional materials supplement the teaching and learning process and enhance client learning. As with teaching strategies, you are constrained by the instructional materials that are available. Many healthcare institutions today have an abundance of health education pamphlets and handouts to distribute to clients. In formative evaluation, your role is to assess the suitability of the written materials given to clients. Ask yourself, "is this the most helpful material for the clients at this time?" "Is this material written at the clients' reading ability level?" "Are the clients benefitting from this written material?"

Tutorial programs are available at some healthcare institutions to promote client education. Be available as clients interact with these programs to answer questions and monitor their learning progress. Again, listening to their responses and answering their questions provides the ongoing feedback you need to evaluate learning.

Client Adherence

Of great importance to any health education program is whether or not clients have benefitted from what they are learning. This area of concern is known as client adherence, formerly known as compliance. Adherence refers to the degree to which clients are following the agreed-upon recommendations of the healthcare provider (Chisholm-Burns & Spivey, 2008). Adherence is not an either/or situation. For example, nonadherence to medication may include not taking a medication as prescribed or missing doses, or discontinuing or lowering the dose of the medication because of undesirable side-effects. Nonadherence to a diet includes failure to consistently follow the dietary guidelines.

The word *adherence* suggests a collaborative relationship between nurses and clients, whereas the word *compliance* suggests an obedient relationship. When clients are called noncompliant, it implies that nurses and healthcare providers know what is best for clients and expect them to follow orders. When clients do not comply, they are at fault. Adherence implies a cooperative relationship that is based on shared responsibility. A cooperative relationship respects the clients as independent, intelligent, and autonomous individuals who are active participants in promoting, retaining, and restoring their health (Lutfey & Wishner, 1999).

Scope of Nonadherence

Nonadherence takes many forms, such as not keeping appointments, not taking medications as prescribed, not following dietary recommendations, and not engaging in healthy life style practices, e.g., exercise and diet. It also includes the failure to follow recommended treatment regimens such as hot/cold applications, changing bandages, and returning for follow-up visits. Adherence is important if clients are to receive the maximum benefits from treatment and health education. Medical treatments and medications are ineffective if not taken as prescribed. This can result in worsening of the client's health problem and its impact on the family, increase healthcare costs, and even result in preventable death (Dubiel, Cwynar, Januszewica, & Grodzicki, 2005; Osterberg & Blaschke, 2005).

Statistics on nonadherence vary widely and differ in reference to specific health problems. For example, DiMatteo (2004) conducted a meta-analysis of adherence to medical treatment and found the average nonadherence rate was 24.8%. Adherence was highest in clients with HIV, arthritis, gastrointestinal disorders, and cancer. Adherence was lowest in clients with pulmonary disease, diabetes, and sleep disorders. Other researchers reported a meta-analysis that showed an average nonadherence rate of 25% overall for breast cancer screening and treatment (Magai, Consedine, Neugut, & Hershman, 2007). Another group reported on studies that estimate 30% to 60% of clients showed some degree of nonadherence in taking oral medications as prescribed, including failure to fill prescriptions (Miaskowski, Shockney, & Chlebowski, 2008). Adherence to medication is higher in clients with acute diseases and less so in clients with chronic diseases, such as hypertension, diabetes, and hyperlipidemia, in which the goal is to control rather than cure the disease.

Nonadherence is a major public health problem in this country that places a financial burden on the healthcare system in terms of hospital and nursing home readmissions and overuse of health services (Vermeire, Hearnshaw, Van Royen, & Denekens, 2001). Unhealthy life styles, such as smoking, excessive intake of alcohol, sedentary life style, and poor diet have consequences for the individual, family, society, and the healthcare system. Healthy life styles have a positive impact on health and decrease the risk of developing cancer, heart disease, stroke, and other serious illnesses.

Barriers to Adherence

Clients who are nonadherent are so for a variety of reasons. Clients choose the health behaviors in which they will engage. Generally the choice is a trade-off among a variety of influences in their lives. For example, dietary modifications may be difficult to follow if there is insufficient money to buy food. Or, it may be impractical to prepare the food as instructed. Perhaps the rationale for behavior change does not make sense to the client. It is also possible that a client's social network does not offer enough reinforcement to sustain a behavioral change, such as quitting smoking. It may be that the client does not like the side-effects of a medication and does not understand the reason to continue taking it. This is especially true when the disease does not cause symptoms such as hypertension and hyperlipidemia. It also may be that the healthcare provider failed to adequately understand and address the client's needs.

Nonadherence was studied from the perspective of demographic factors, psychological factors, social factors, and client/providers interaction factors, and no clear patterns have emerged (Lutfey & Wishner, 1999). *Demographic factors* such as age, sex, race, income, marital status, and educational level do not consistently correlate with adherence (Magai et al., 2007; Vermeire et al., 2001). This may seem confusing because education does appear to be correlated with health-promoting behaviors. However, we know that knowledge of health and illness is not enough to motivate lasting change and relinquish addictions. For example, some healthcare providers smoke, abuse substances, suffer from eating disorders, and avoid getting flu vaccines, even though they know the risks of such behavior. *Psychological factors* related to nonadherence include forgetting, not wanting to use medications, unpleasant side-effects of medications, lack of motivation, inability to understand instructions, being uncooperative, or psychiatric illness such as depression. Individual perceptions about how clients see their susceptibility to disease or severity of disease are important, as illustrated in the Health Belief Model. *Social factors* related to nonadherence include the lack of family member/peer support, poor family cohesiveness, stigma of the disease, different approaches to treatment, difficulty navigating the healthcare system, living conditions, and financial limitations. Finally, consider *client/provider interaction factors* may be related to nonadherence. For example, the nurse or provider may be rushed, does not clearly explain the rationale for the treatment, or directs rather than collaborates with clients. Why clients do not adhere is an individual matter.

Predictors of Nonadherence

Nurses as educators can anticipate nonadherence from clients under certain circumstances. Knowing who is likely to nonadhere to a treatment regimen alert nurses to assess clients more carefully and provide additional education if indicated. Predictors of nonadherence guide nurses and include clients with chronic diseases that require long-term treatment, clients who are not responding as expected to therapy, and clients who have a history of not adhering. Other predictors include clients who do not believe the treatment will be helpful, lack the support of family and friends, unpleasant side-effects from the treatment, and complex medication regimens. Also less likely to adhere are clients who have psychological problems such as depression or those who have poor communication with the provider (Miaskowski et al., 2008). See Figure 12-1 for a summary of factors that deter adherence.

Facilitators of Adherence

The literature offers rich resources for strategies to foster adherence. This section looks at adherence through a discussion of health education, the nurse/client interaction, stages of behavioral change, and locus of control.

Health Education

Our basic assumption is that if we as educators provide relevant health information, clients will adhere to the recommendations. We know that is not true in all cases; however, nurses are obligated to provide accurate, relevant, and timely health information. Information is the basis for making behavioral and life style changes. This is what the role of nurses as educators is all about.

If clients are motivated to learn and you have their attention, teach them about the nature of their health problem and the purpose of the treatment regimen. Teach them about the importance of following the treatment regimen and its rationale. Point out the positive signs of progress and the side-effects of treatment. Reinforce the physician's directions. Often clients ask nurses questions they do not want to bother the

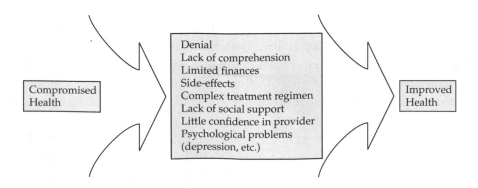

FIGURE 12-1   Factors That Deter Adherence.

physician with. Rains, Penzien, and Lipchik (2006) recommend limiting the major points to three to four, while teaching and using simple, everyday language. Use pictures or models to facilitate learning along with written instructions. Ask clients to restate your major points and reinforce the clients when they have done so successfully. Repetition of the message aids learning and emphasizes the points you make.

Always listen to the client's perspective. It is in listening that nurses determine how clients understand the message and perceive their health status and how the message fits into activities of daily living. There may be good reasons why clients do not adhere, and nurses need to know what these are (DiGiacomo, 2008). By listening to clients you see the barriers to adherence from the client's perspective. Sometimes clients are overwhelmed with the complexity of their medication schedule. Consider, for example, the challenges clients with HIV face who must adhere to antiretroviral therapy to suppress viral replication and avoid developing resistance. The treatment involves expensive medications with complex dosing schedules that may cause food interactions and side-effects (Osterberg & Blaschke, 2005).

If appropriate, involve and educate family members about clients' needs. This fosters adherence. For example, teaching a male client about a low sodium diet does little good if his wife, who does all of the cooking, does not participate in learning. Be sensitive to roles and responsibilities in families and use clinical judgment in working with them. Conflicting roles and responsibilities may mean family members are not available to help (Miaskowski et al., 2008). Review, for example, the challenges of the "sandwich generation" discussed in Chapter 6, in which parents are attempting to meet the needs of their children as well as the needs of their aging parents. Many factors influence family involvement in the care of a family member.

Nurse/Client Interaction

The nurse/client interaction is important in fostering adherence. The nurse collaborates with clients who need to make behavioral changes to retain, promote, or restore health. It is a relationship of equals who mutually respect each other and work together to achieve the common goal of adherence. This shared decision making and open communication are effective strategies in fostering adherence (Robinson, Callister, Berry, & Dearing, 2008).

Listening to clients, nurses gain insight into how they view the necessary changes and adjustments that must be made. Based on these insights, nurses offer suggestions for clients to consider. Be persuasive in helping clients see the importance of making a behavioral change. As educators, nurses are better informed about the consequences of not changing (Falvo, 2004). If you determine that clients are having trouble with the treatment regimen and unwilling or unlikely to adhere to it, notify the physician (Miaskowski et al., 2008).

Stages of Behavioral Change

When clients are confronted with the need to change behavior or adhere to a treatment regimen, they have decisions to make. Behavioral and life style changes usually do not happen instantly; rather, change is a process that occurs over time. Prochaska Redding, and Evers (2001) proposed a model of behavioral change that is useful in health education. They posit that behavior change occurs in a series of stages: precontemplation, contemplation, preparation, action, maintenance, and termination, as illustrated in Table 12-1 (Prochaska & Norcross, 2001; Prochaska et al., 2008). Actions to support behavioral changes are included in the table.

Locus of Control

As you work with clients, assess how they see their role in promoting, retaining, or restoring their health. The concepts of locus of control and self-efficacy are interrelated and important to adherence. Recall the concept of self-efficacy discussed in Chapter 3, which is a person's belief that he or she is capable of performing successfully to attain specific goals (Bandura, 1986). Before clients can adhere to any treatment regimen, they must have confidence that they are capable of doing what is required of them. Locus of control refers to beliefs about the source of control over one's life, whether it is within or external to the individual (Slavin, 2009). Locus of control is perceived differently in cultural groups. Clients who have an internal locus of control believe that success or failure results from their own efforts and abilities. They believe they have some control over their health and are more likely to adhere to the treatment regimen and health recommendations. Clients who have an external locus of control believe that success or failure is beyond their control; that is, it is caused by fate, luck, or other people's actions. These clients are less likely to have confidence in their ability to control their state of health. Clients with an internal locus of control and a high sense of self-efficacy are more likely to be receptive to health education and adhere to health recommendations.

In summary, as you teach clients, stress the importance of their role in promoting, retaining, and restoring health. Remember that adherence requires collaboration among nurses, providers, and clients. Clients make the final decision about whether or not to implement health recommendations. Do your best to empower clients and support their role in assuming responsibility for their health. Nurses should respect the decisions clients make.

TABLE 12-1	Prochaska and Colleagues' Stages of Behavioral Change	
Stage	**Characteristics**	**Nurse as Educator Role**
Precontemplation	Client is unaware of the problem, but others are aware of it	Supportive, nurturing role
Contemplation	Client is aware of the problem; thinks about changing within next 6 months. Contemplates pros and cons.	Encouraging client to examine/gain insight into problem
Preparation	Client intends to change soon, within the next month. Has a plan of action but has not yet made that decision.	Coaching role as client makes plans to change. Suggest programs: weight loss, smoking cessation, etc.
Action	Client takes the time and makes effort to modify behavior. Lasts up to 6 mos.	Consultant role, providing advice and guidance
Maintenance	Client maintains change and prevents relapse. Lasts beyond 6 mos.	Consultant role, providing advice and guidance
Termination	Client fully committed to behavioral change—100% confident of ability to maintain the change.	Reinforcing success.

EVALUATION OF THE LEARNING ENVIRONMENT

Formative evaluation of the learning environment includes assessing the facility for lighting, temperature, seating, noise, available equipment, and any other environmental factors that have a bearing on teaching effectiveness.

Facility

Much health education occurs on an informal basis and captures that "teachable moment" described in earlier chapters. Enhance the moment by creating a quiet environment for teaching and giving clients full attention and eye contact. These are important considerations wherever you are teaching, whether in the hospital, long-term care facility, private home, school, or worksite. Do your best to evaluate the environment and make necessary changes.

When health education is formal, that is, held in a classroom or special area for teaching, you need to assess the impact of the facility and its resources on teaching and learning (Rankin, Stallings, & London, 2005). As with informal teaching, formal teaching occurs in the hospital, long-term care facility, school, worksite, and community settings. Client comfort and the absence of distractions are your primary concerns.

Client comfort is ensured by having good lighting, a room temperature suitable for learning, and sufficient and comfortable seating. It is also important to ensure that the facility is quiet, without distracting environmental noise. Formative evaluation involves paying attention to these factors as you are teaching. For example, is lighting needed for taking notes if you darken the room for a video? Is the room getting too warm and causing clients to doze? Too cold and clients are shivering? Can you open a window or adjust the thermostat? Are clients fidgeting in their chairs because the chairs are uncomfortable? Can you pause for a moment and have everyone stand up and move? Are clients distracted by noises in the environment or private conversations going on in the class? These are all factors that you can do something about while teaching to maximize client learning.

Equipment

There is always the possibility that the equipment you need is not available or operational in the facility. For this reason, we advise you to carry an extension cord and any other back-up portable equipment that you may need such as an overhead projector. If you are using special equipment, be sure that you know how to operate it ahead of your presentation. It is disconcerting to clients when nurses have to take time away from teaching to fuss with equipment that is not working properly. It is important to plan ahead and check out what equipment is needed and what equipment the facility offers. This includes making sure that the microphone is working. The working condition of the equipment should be assessed and, if possible, projectors, microphones, etc. should be set up ahead of time.

EVALUATION OF THE NURSE/CLIENT INTERACTION

Attitudes

Attitudes are contagious, especially when nurses are encouraging clients to learn new information and adopt new ways of living. Attitudes are established during the introduction to learning and continue to be influential during the process of learning. Positive attitudes build curiosity, interest in, and enthusiasm for what you are teaching. Negative attitudes present new learning as matter-of-fact, a kind of take-it or leave-it approach that is uninteresting, and perhaps boring to clients. The bottom line is that attitudes matter and how you feel about your role and conduct yourself as an educator sends a message to clients. Nurses should model positive attitudes toward learning and constantly self-assess while teaching.

Communication

In addition to attitudes, how nurses communicate is important. Encouragement is an essential trait of educators, especially when clients are learning new information. Making new connections, drawing analogies, showing how new learning fits into what clients already know are important forms of communication. Help clients think through their situations. Asking clients questions fosters dialog, especially questions that require critical thinking such as, "What would you do if . . . ?" "Why should this be done first . . . ?"

The process of communication includes prompting clients when appropriate, coaching them as they learn new information, and guiding them in learning essential information versus nonessential information. During the process of formative evaluation, nurses need to be adaptable. If communication is ineffective, consider what would be a better approach and change what you are doing as you are doing it. This is what effective educators do—adapt in midstream when it is indicated.

Satisfaction

It is important that clients and family are satisfied with the health education process. Satisfaction is important when educating clients and families about health (Falvo, 2004; Rankin, Stallings, & London, 2005). Dansky and Miles (1997) suggested that satisfied clients are more likely to maintain relationships with providers. Other important outcomes are that satisfied clients are more likely to keep appointments, comply with treatment, and refer other patients to their providers (Chung, Hamill, Kim, Walters, & Wilkins, 1999).

CASE EXAMPLE: MRS. ROSA LOPEZ

Formative evaluation of the interaction with Mrs. Rose Lopez begins with reviewing the learning objectives and critiquing the teaching and learning process as it is ongoing. For example, by the end of the lesson, the cognitive objective is to have Mrs. Lopez able to explain the relationship between excessive sodium intake and hypertension. An example of midcourse correction might be to notice that Mrs. Lopez preferred the videotape instruction to viewing charts and pamphlets. Consequently we would focus on the videotape and reinforce its message.

In evaluating the affective objective, choose to limit the intake of sodium to 2000 mg/day by working with the nurse to prepare a dietary plan, we would ask, "How do you plan to incorporate these changes into your meal planning and usual diet?" Note the strength of Mrs. Lopez's desire and willingness to limit excessive sodium intake. Depending on her response, we would follow up with suggestions for how she could accomplish this. We would also ask how these dietary changes would help control her high blood pressure. We would reinforce Mrs. Lopez's correct responses and reteach if her responses demonstrate a lack of understanding. It also might be helpful for Mrs. Lopez to talk with clients with a similar diagnosis to gain practical meal planning suggestions.

The psychomotor objective is to demonstrate accurately obtaining self-blood pressure reading using home digital equipment without any verbal guidance. We would have Mrs. Lopez read the equipment directions as we demonstrate how to take the blood pressure using her own digital equipment. Mrs. Lopez would then perform a return demonstration and record the findings following the procedure checklist. She would be given a checklist handout of the steps to follow at home in obtaining her blood pressure, after which she would be given an opportunity to evaluate her own performance. During this time Mrs. Lopez would be given an opportunity to ask questions and be given feedback to guide her learning.

In the formative evaluation process, we would encourage Mrs. Lopez, listen to her concerns, correct misunderstandings, and assure accurate skill performance. When necessary, misinformation would be corrected by reviewing and reteaching any missed or misunderstood content.

BOX 12-2   Evidence-Based Nursing Practice

Greenberg, M. E. (2000). Telephone nursing: Evidence of client and organizational benefits. *Nursing Economics, 18*(3), 117–123.

Purpose: This study described the outcomes of an established Telephone Nurse Service. Outcomes were assessed from the perspective of the client and the organization.

Method: This descriptive study examined 120 phone calls to the Telephone Nurse Service in a Southwestern clinic over 1 month. Calls were handled by trained and experienced RNs using approved written clinic-specific protocols. Follow-up phone questions were asked of clients.

Results: 80% of callers surveyed reported that if they had not been able to speak to the nurse they would have sought medical care elsewhere.

SUMMARY

This chapter begins the discussion of the final phase of the teaching and learning process: evaluation. Evaluation of client education has two aspects, formative and summative; this chapter discussed formative evaluation. Formative evaluation is ongoing during the process of teaching and learning. As the educator, you are continuously monitoring the effectiveness of the teaching plan with attention to the learning objectives, content, teaching strategies, and instructional materials. You are also attending to the learning environment as well as the quality of the interaction with clients. The desired outcome of all health education is client learning. Formative evaluation asks "how are we doing and are the clients learning?" Answering that question and facilitating client learning by making necessary changes during the process of teaching and learning are your responsibilities as educator.

EXERCISES

Exercise I—Evaluation of the Teaching and Learning Process

Purpose: Apply formative evaluation to the teaching plan.

Directions: Divide into small groups. Discuss the following situations and describe how you would handle each one as the educator.

1. You are teaching a hospitalized client ready for discharge about the importance of taking an antibiotic as prescribed. The client speaks little English. The client learning objective is to explain the purpose of the antibiotic. You have progressed with your teaching, feel very positive about it, and are about to conclude when the client asks you what the word "antibiotic" means.

2. You are in the middle of teaching a group of older clients about improving their memory. At the beginning of the class you distributed several handouts and now notice that some of them are reading the materials and not listening to you. You think about asking the class to refrain from looking at the materials until later or stopping where you are in your presentation and discussing the materials, or some other alternative.

3. You are teaching a class on benefits of exercise to a group of older clients. You enlisted an assistant to demonstrate the exercises while you point out the benefits of each one. Your assistant does not show up and you are expected to go ahead with the class.

Exercise II—Evaluation of the Learning Environment

Purpose: Apply formative evaluation to the learning environment.

Directions: Divide into small groups. Discuss the following situations and describe how you would handle each one as the educator.

1. You are having a conversation with a mother whose 2-year-old child is going home from the hospital. The child is still sick and crying. You are trying to teach the mother the discharge instructions but the child's crying is disrupting your communication.
2. You plan to lead a bereavement discussion group and have arranged the chairs in the room in a circle so everyone can see each other. Several individuals come late to the session and slip into the back of the room and sit in the chairs lining the wall. Several group members have turned around to look at them, disrupting the discussion at a sensitive point.

Exercise III—Evaluation of the Nurse/Client Interaction

Purpose: Apply formative evaluation to the nurse/client interaction.

Directions: Divide into small groups. Discuss the following situations and describe how you would handle each one as the educator.

1. Have each person share a personal experience about learning new information or a skill. Then identify the teacher behaviors during the experience that facilitated learning and teacher behaviors that interfered with learning.
2. Discuss how you would change the behaviors that interfered with learning into behaviors that facilitate learning. In other words, how would you have handled the situation to achieve a better outcome?

SUPPLEMENTAL ONLINE RESOURCES

American Academy of Family Physicians:
http://www.aafp.org/fpm/20050600/44five.html
Science Daily:
http://www.sciencedaily.com/releases/2007/07/070721194716.htm
e-pill Medication Reminders:
http://www.epill.com/statistics.html

GigaNano, LLC, BioMedical Consultants:
http://www.patientcompliance.net/
HSM Group:
http://www.hsmgroup.com/info/compli/compli.html

REFERENCES

Bandura, A. (1986). *Social foundations of thought and action: A social cognitive theory.* Englewood Cliffs, NJ: Prentice Hall.

Chisholm-Burns, M. A., & Spivey, C. A. (2008). Pharmacoadherence: A new term for a significant problem. *American Journal Health-Systems Pharmacists, 65*(April 1), 661–667.

Chung, K. C., Hamill, J. B., Kim, H. M., Walters, M. R., & Wilkins, E. G. (1999). Predictors of patient satisfaction in an outpatient plastic surgery clinic. *Annals of Plastic Surgery, 42*(1), 56–60.

Dansky, K. H., & Miles, J. (1997). Patient satisfaction with ambulatory healthcare services: Waiting time and filling time. *Hospital and Health Services Administration, 42,* 165–176.

DiGiacomo, M. (2008). Patient adherence: Sharing the responsibility. *PT Magazine, 16*(7), 28–30.

DiMatteo, M. R. (2004). Variations in patients' adherence to medical recommendations: A quantitative review of 50 years of research. *Medical Care, 42*(3), 200–209.

Dubiel, M., Cwynar, M., Januszewica, & Grodzicki, T. (2005). Patient's education in arterial hypertension. *Blood Pressure, 14*(Suppl 2), 53–56.

Falvo, D. R. (2004). *Effective patient education a guide to increased compliance* (3rd ed.). Sudbury, MA: Jones and Bartlett.

Lutfey, K. E., & Wishner, W. J. (1999). Beyond "compliance" is "adherence." *Diabetes Care, 22*(4), 635–639.

Magai, C., Consedine, N., Neugut, A. I., & Hershman, D. L. (2007). Common psychosocial factors underlying breast cancer screening and breast cancer treatment adherence: A conceptual review and synthesis. *Journal of Women's Health, 16*(1), 11–23.

Merriam-Webster's Dictionary and Thesaurus (2007). Springfield, MA: Merriam-Webster, Inc.

Miaskowski, C., Shockney, L., & Chlebowski, R. T. (2008). Adherence to oral endocrine therapy for breast cancer: A nursing perspective. *Clinical Journal of Oncology Nursing, 12*(2), 213–221.

Morrison, G. R., Ross, S. M., Kemp, J. E., & Kalman, H. K. (2007). *Designing effective instruction* (5th ed.). Hoboken, NJ: John Wiley and Sons.

O'Brien, P. G. (2007). Patient and family teaching. In Lewis, S. L., Heitkemper, M. M., Dirksen, S. R., O'Brien, P. G., & Bucher, L. *Medical-surgical nursing* (7th ed., pp. 53–65). St. Louis: Mosby.

Osterberg, L. & Blaschke, T. (2005). Adherence to medication. *New England Journal of Medicine, 353,* 487–497.

Prochaska, J. O., & Norcross, J. C. (2001). Stages of change. *Psychotherapy, 38*(4), 443–448.

Prochaska, J. O., Redding, C. A., & Evers, K. E. (2008). The transtheoretical model and stages of change. In Glanz, K., Rimer, B. K., & Viswanath, K. (eds.). *Health Behavior and health education: Theory, research, and practice* (4th ed.). San Francisco: Jossey-Bass.

Rains, J. C., Penzien, D. B., & Lipchik, G. L. (2006). Behavioral facilitation of medical treatment for headache—Part II: Theoretical models and behavioral strategies for improving adherence. *Headache The Journal of Head and Face Pain, 46,* 1395–1403.

Rankin, S. H., Stallings, K. D., & London, F. (2005). *Patient education in health and illness* (5th ed.). Philadelphia: Lippincott Williams & Wilkins.

Redman, B. K. (2007). *The practice of patient education a case study approach* (10th ed.). St. Louis: Mosby Year Book.

Robinson, J. H., Callister, L. C., Berry, J. A., & Dearing, K. A. (2008). Patient-centered care and adherence: Definitions and applications to improve outcomes. *Journal of the American Academy of Nurse Practitioners, 20,* 600–607.

Ruskin, J. (1918 to 1900), In Knowledgeable Quotes: Knowledge quotes reference (2009) retrieved July 9, 2009 at http://www.ceolibrary.org/quotes/qualityquotes.htm.

Slavin, R. E. (2009). *Educational psychology theory and practice* (9th ed.). Upper Saddle River, NJ: Pearson Education.

Vermeire, E, Hearnshaw, H., Van Royen, P., & Denekens, J. (2001). Patient adherence to treatment: Three decades of research. A comprehensive review. *Journal of Clinical Pharmacy and Therapeutics, 26,* 331–342.

CHAPTER 13

Summative Evaluation

What gets measured gets done.
If you don't measure results, you can't tell success from failure.
If you can't see success, you can't reward it.
If you can't reward success, you're probably rewarding failure.
If you can't recognize failure, you can't correct it.
If you can demonstrate results, you can win public support.
—Osborne, D. & Gaebler, T., 1992, pp. 146–155.

OBJECTIVES

Upon completion of this chapter you will be able to:
- Identify the three components of summative evaluation.
- Distinguish between measurement and evaluation.
- Describe how the evaluation of client learning is accomplished.
- Distinguish between direct and indirect measurement methods.
- Describe four sources of error in measurement.
- Select measurement techniques best suited for cognitive, affective, and psychomotor objectives.
- Describe how the evaluation of program effectiveness is accomplished.
- Discuss the importance of cost and evidence-based practice in evaluation.
- Describe how to evaluate the integration of learning into daily living.
- Summarize the impact health education can have on a community.

KEY TERMS

adherence	measurement
choice	reinforcement
collaboration	sources of error
evaluation	summative
formative	

INTRODUCTION

This chapter is about summative evaluation. Summative evaluation occurs at the conclusion of teaching and learning and involves evaluation of client learning, evaluation of program effectiveness, and evaluation of integration of learning into daily living (Morrison, Ross, Kemp, & Kalman, 2007; Slavin, 2009). With summative evaluation, we want to determine, "How did we do?" This chapter explores each of these components of summative evaluation.

OVERVIEW OF SUMMATIVE EVALUATION

After any teaching effort, it is important for nurses as educators to pause, look back, and reflect on what has been accomplished and what they can learn from their efforts. Nurses need to ask, What worked well and what did not? Which practices should be continued and which should be abandoned? Was it really worth the effort in terms of time, energy, and cost? Did clients really benefit? Did life style changes become a part of clients' activities of daily living? Summative evaluation seeks to answer these questions. The components of summative evaluation are listed in Box 13-1. They are the evaluation of client learning, evaluation of program effectiveness, and evaluation of integration of learning into daily living. The chapter addresses each component in depth.

Summative evaluation involves making comparisons between what is effective and what is not. It focuses on evaluating the effectiveness of teaching to include learning objectives, teaching strategies, and instructional materials (Falvo, 2004). For example, summative evaluation helps to determine whether learning objectives stated one way are easier for clients to grasp than when they are stated another way. It also helps to compare the effectiveness of different strategies such as videos versus discussion to teach a particular topic. Summative evaluation helps to compare the effectiveness of different instructional materials; for example, is having models and equipment to manipulate more effective than having pictures of the same?

After each teaching session or at the conclusion of a series of health education sessions, compare the evaluation results of the present session with those of the past. This informs you of what is effective and ineffective about each component of the teaching plan. This information provides an overall picture of the effectiveness of a single teaching session or multiple sessions. Summative evaluation also provides information about accountability that is useful in evaluating the entire health education program and justifies the program's continuation.

BOX 13-1   Client Education Outcomes: Summative Evaluation

- **Evaluation of client learning**

  - Measurement

  - Direct measurement methods

  - Indirect measurement methods

- **Evaluation of program effectiveness**

  - Course/program evaluation

  - Evidence-based nursing practice

  - Cost

- **Evaluation of integration of learning into daily living**

  - Client adherence

  - Impact on the community

  - Justification for health dollars

EVALUATION OF CLIENT LEARNING

At the conclusion of a teaching and learning session, educators want to know if clients learned the content. Did clients achieve the knowledge, attitudes, and skills specified in the learning objectives? Did clients learn what was intended? How well did they learn and did the learning improve their health in any demonstrable way? In this section we discuss how to answer these questions.

Measurement

To evaluate something, set up criteria against which to compare the results of evaluation. Measurement means gauging the dimensions, quantity, or capacity of something by comparing it with some kind of standard (Merriam-Webster, 2007). Measurement ranges from the concrete, such as clients learning to take their own pulse, to the abstract, such as learning better ways to handle stress. Both phenomena are important; however, the former is much easier to measure than the latter. Methods of measurement

FIGURE 13-1   Direct and Indirect Measurement Continuum.

are ordered along a continuum from direct to indirect at opposite ends, as illustrated in Figure 13-1.

Measurement involves both observation and recording of behavior, regardless of whether the measurement is direct or indirect. *Direct measurement* is the most accurate when it takes place in the actual situation and, ideally, occurs over time. It is direct observation of the behavior being measured. For example, nurses make observations at the hospital bedside, in the home, or at the worksite. Direct observations are also obtained from equipment and monitors that measure things such as vital signs, oxygen levels, blood glucose, etc.

Indirect measurement is not as accurate as direct measurement. It occurs when the educator creates substitute situations or takes incomplete samples of behavior. For example, if you role play with clients, you create substitute situations that imitate, or substitute for, the real one. When you give clients paper-and-pencil tests, you attempt to measure cognitive processes indirectly. No one knows what thinking is or what it looks like. Therefore, you must infer from what clients write whether or not they have thought about, retained, and gained the knowledge and understanding you hoped they would grasp.

Measurement methods are also categorized as being objective or subjective (Lorig & Associates, 2001). Examples of *objective measures* include observables such as vital signs, weight, blood glucose, cholesterol levels, wound healing, hospital readmissions, and class attendance. *Subjective measures* are data from human observers (clients, providers, educators) and are therefore considered biased measures. These measures are less reliable, as there are multiple explanations for client behavior. There may be extenuating circumstances that effect whether the client is able to successfully meet the objectives, and these circumstances may be unknown to the observer. For example, a provider reports that an overweight client has little interest in weight reduction when in fact the client does not understand how to diet. The provider assumes the client is not motivated to learn about weight reduction because the client discarded reading material that she was given, when in fact the client has low health literacy skills. Another example is of the client as observer. The client, who chain smokes, reports that he stopped smoking, when in fact he cut down to one to two cigarettes a day.

Sources of Error in Measurement

Error is always possible in measurement, and the more indirect the measurement, the more likely it will be that errors will occur. Redman (2007) notes the following common sources of error: indirect measurement, the complexity of behavior, observer bias, and sampling error. A brief description of each source of error follows.

Indirect Measurement

Indirect measurement provides a false picture of how a client would react unless the nurse observes that person in the actual situation. The saying, "He talks a good game" indicates that many people know the difference between talking about a situation and actually handling it. Because your time with clients is limited, your only choice may be to measure the learning objectives by indirect means, such as oral quizzes and paper-and-pencil tests. Keep in mind that these methods are indirect, from which you infer the degree of client learning.

Complex Behavior

Behavior, by nature, is complex. The causes of behavior, especially thought patterns, feelings, and attitudes, are difficult to identify for both the observer and the client exhibiting the behavior. As an educator, you may not be able to discover what, if any, impact the learning had on clients. A client may act agreeable just to please you, or he or she may choose not tell you all of the variables involved in a failure to learn. Indeed, clients themselves may not be fully aware of all of the factors that help or hinder their learning.

Observer Bias

Humans are limited in the amount of stimuli they can notice. Observers draw conclusions based on their own perceptions, culture, and past experiences. This can lead to making erroneous inferences and conclusions about client learning. One advantage of working with colleagues is that it can help balance the perceptions of individual clients. How others see a particular client influences your perceptions. When you team teach, you and your colleagues give balanced views of the clients. If a colleague tells you a client, a family, or team member is difficult to deal with, you are likely to approach that individual in a different manner. This can lead to bias, but it can also lead to a collaborative effort to help the client learn. Approach each individual with openness.

Sampling

Sampling is obtaining a small picture of the client's behavior that is representative of all of the learning you provided. From this sample, you infer that the client has or has not mastered the learning objectives. Sampling error occurs when the sample you choose to measure is not representative of client learning. Clients may have learned A, B, and C; but if you measure D, E, and F, you get a false picture of the client's learning and achievements.

The period of time during which you choose to measure the behavior can also be misleading. For example, you form a different perception of your client's willingness and ability to do range-of-motion exercises if you test him early in the morning rather than waiting until later in the day. It is not possible to observe all the required behaviors. Therefore, your task is to select behavioral samples that are as representative as possible and relevant to the variables that are most critical. In general, you can compensate for measurement errors by using a variety of measurement methods.

Direct Measurement Methods

Remember that measurement methods must be consistent with the learning objectives. You cannot test everything you have taught or that clients have learned, so you must select a representative sample to test (Slavin, 2009). Direct measurement of behavior is achieved through video recordings, rating scales, check lists, evaluation rubrics, and anecdotal notes.

Observation of Behavior

Direct observation occurs when the nurse observes clients demonstrating mastery of psychomotor skills. For example, you observe a client properly using crutches with no axillary pressure and no loss of balance. Another example is observing how skillfully a client removes a dressing, cleans the wound, and applies a fresh dressing without contamination. Both examples are direct observations of client behavior.

Direct observation also involves nurses using the senses. For example, the nurse listens to breath sounds through a stethoscope after a guided session of turning and deep breathing. Or the nurse counts the client's pulse and respiration rate to observe the impact of a relaxation exercise. Direct observations of client responses are documented by using a checklist designed for specific procedures, which is discussed later in this chapter.

Video Recordings

Direct observation of behavior is also achieved through video recordings. Video recordings offer the advantage of accuracy. The video camera observes and records what happened, rather than depending on the nurse's interpretation of what happened. The recording is useful in that both the nurse and clients get accurate feedback by watching it. This is especially useful when teaching health team members new psychomotor skills. The recording can be studied at length for feedback to improve performance.

Video recordings are helpful when clients role play new affective behaviors, such as improving interpersonal communications. Families who are puzzled by their communication difficulties can sometimes gain insight into their patterns when viewed from a different perspective. Video recording helps decrease defensiveness and increases objectiveness as they watch themselves.

Video recordings are effective for teaching health team members how to interact with clients who are depressed, anxious, or hostile. They are also effective for nurses who are new in the role of educator and for experienced nurses who want to improve teaching performance. It is much easier to accept feedback from observing a video recording of one's performance rather than an instructor's critique.

Rating Scales

Rating scales on surveys and questionnaires use a Likert scale to rate client responses. For example, a rating scale asks if clients strongly agree, agree, disagree, or strongly disagree with a number of specific items. Another rating scale asks how clients would evaluate items on a scale that ranges from 1 to 5, in which #1 means no confidence and #5 means total confidence. There are variations of this scale depending on what you want to know. For example, #1 could mean "did not help me" at the low end and #5 "helped me a great deal" at the high end of the scale.

Rating scales are given to clients to fill out at the conclusion of a teaching session, course, or program to evaluate their satisfaction with the teaching experience. They provide insight into the clients' perceptions of learning effectiveness. They also provide helpful feedback to improve the teacher's performance. Rating scales are used for statistical purposes. Collating the results and determining the mean and standard deviation for each item on the rating scale provides instructive information. These data collected over time provide useful feedback to evaluate clients' perceptions of teaching and learning effectiveness. Figures 13-4 and 13-5 are sample rating scales to evaluate learning objectives and teacher evaluation that are shown later in this chapter.

Checklists

Checklists are more precise tools than rating scales because they identify each of the desired behaviors and provide space for recording the presence or absence of each behavior. In creating a checklist, identify the critical elements of the desired behaviors and exclude nonessential ones. For example, when measuring a mother's bonding behavior include observations such as whether she looks at, touches, and talks to the infant rather than whether she has the most updated equipment. Another example is teaching a client to give a self-injection. It is not critical how the client arranges the placement of equipment on a tray. It is critical, however, that the sterility of the equipment is maintained. Figure 13-2 is a sample checklist of critical requirements for giving an injection. The learning domain is psychomotor and the learning objective is: "The client will perform an injection accurately according to the steps of the procedure."

Assistance from colleagues is valuable in developing a checklist. They can try out the checklist to refine the items and wording. Because clients do not "pass" until they can do every step correctly, it is important to establish the number of times clients must exhibit the correct behaviors to ensure that they have mastered the task.

Evaluation Rubrics

An evaluation rubric is a measurement tool that combines features of the rating scale and checklist that are useful for evaluating team members' performance when a team member is your client (see Figure 13-3). The example uses Benner's (1984) five levels of proficiency (novice, advanced beginner, competent, proficient, and expert) to evaluate nurses in their role as educators. The evaluator notes the level of proficiency at which the team member is performing each criterion. The evaluator then writes an anecdotal note in the space provided. An alternative rating scale that could be used instead of Benner's levels is: beginning, developing, proficient, and independent. Whichever rating scale is used, a committee of nurses in the healthcare institution should define the rating levels. There should be broad agreement of the definition of the scope of skills and responsibilities for each level. The criteria in the example are samples of what could be included in the rubric.

Anecdotal Notes

An anecdotal note is a brief vignette of a client's behavior at a particular moment in time. This type of note is used in psychiatric facilities because it helps observers de-

Name of Client: _____						
Behavior			**Dates**			**Comments**
1. Selects appropriate equipment.						
2. Identifies action, use, side effects, and dosage range of medication.						

3. Maintains sterility:
  a. of equipment.
  b. in administration.						

4. Prepares accurate dosage:
  a. verifies dosage prescribed.
  b. draws up correct dose.
5. Selects acceptable injection site.						

6. Injects at appropriate angle:
  a. 30- to 60-degree angle for SQ
  b. 90-degree angle for IM
7. Aspirates plunger before injecting.						

8. Injects medication.						
9. Disposes of needle safely.						

FIGURE 13-2   Checklist for Giving an Injection.

tect changes in clients' behaviors over time and the circumstances under which changes occurred. For example, an adolescent client hospitalized for severe behavior problems was cooperative with her therapist away from the hospital, but was obstinate and defiant with caregivers on the psych unit. The nurse must determine:

1. What is the client's behavior with her family and friends?
2. What is the gender of the therapist and other caregivers? Does the gender of the caregiver make a difference?
3. How are the therapist's interactions with the client different from that of the staff?

It is crucial for various caregivers on the unit to use the observations as important data for evaluation. They should not automatically jump to the conclusion, "The client always acts just fine for me." (The hidden implication is, What are the rest of you doing wrong?)

Criterion	Novice	Advanced beginner	Competent	Proficient	Expert	Notes
Communicates learning objectives				Yes		Clearly stated at outset
Presents accurate information		Yes				Much improved over previous session
Uses appropriate teaching strategies		Yes				Tried another strategy when the first was ineffective
Uses appropriate handouts			Yes			Distributed two handouts written in client's native language
Answers questions	No					Needs to take the time to answer questions
Seeks feedback periodically	No					Needs to pause and seek feedback
Maintains eye contact		Yes				Fairly consistent eye contact
Definitions of these terms should be created by a committee of professional nurses in the healthcare institution/agency using the tool: Novice, Advanced beginner, Competent, Proficient, and Expert.						

FIGURE 13-3   Evaluation Rubric.

Anecdotal notes must be recorded consistently over time for the caregivers to pick up client behavior patterns and changes. They should be pertinent to the learning objectives with related comments. They should also clearly and specifically describe client behavior and be free of bias or derogatory terms. The first example illustrates an inappropriate comment.

Example: "The client is obnoxious and uncooperative."

It would be better to restate such an observation as:

Examples: "The client refuses to get out of bed until . . .
"When client is reminded about the importance of exercise to his recovery, he avoids eye contact and does not respond."

This latter example may create a climate of investigation rather than disapproval.
If nurses are curious rather than judgmental, they will more likely discover clues that
help create a learning environment conducive to success. If they maintain an attitude
of curiosity, they are more likely to discover if there are disparities between clients'
goals and nurses' goals.

Indirect Measurement Methods

Indirect measurement methods must be consistent with the learning objectives. Develop questions that provide evidence of how well clients achieved the learning objectives. Indirect measurement of behavior includes direct questioning and written
measurement.

Direct Questioning

Direct questioning is an effective way to determine a client's level of understanding of
what you taught. It is useful in both formative and summative evaluation; however, it
is more often used in formative evaluation when teaching is ongoing. Its use in summative evaluation is limited to oral quizzes, which have little application in health education. Direct questioning is also used to obtain oral feedback from clients at the
conclusion of a teaching session or program to learn what was most and least helpful.

Written Measurement

So far we have considered measurement involving direct transactions with clients in
which you have observed the learning directly or asked clients for their perceptions of
the learning that took place. A more indirect technique to gather evidence of learning
is written measurement; however, there are prerequisites to using this method for
evaluation. For example, to use a written measurement tool, clients must be able to
read and have the ability to see. A well-educated client taking medications that cause
double vision cannot participate in written measurement, nor can clients whose reading glasses are unavailable. Clients who are bilingual but read only in another language, or clients who are so weak that they cannot write, are inappropriate subjects
for written evaluation.

One of the main advantages of written measurement is its efficiency in terms of time and energy. One person (not necessarily the nurse educator) can distribute a written measurement tool to many people at once. The data can be analyzed at the evaluator's convenience and can be easily stored along with the conclusions. In this computer age, written measurement tools for evaluation are part of software educational programs.

Test Construction

To construct an effective test, you need to keep many variables in mind. A good test covers all of the relevant material and relates directly to the learning objectives. Because you cannot ask everything on a test, the test should include a representative sample of what was taught (Gronlund & Brookhart, 2009). Testing is sampling what clients have learned.

Any test should be relevant to the clients in terms of their life experience and health literacy level. If the clients' reading skills are limited, use very simple words and supplement them with pictures. If they are unable to understand written directions, give the directions orally. Reviewing a couple of sample items with clients helps them to understand your expectations. Many clients are more confident if you show them what you want them to do. Be aware that clients may read directions only as a last resort.

A good test uses different types of items, such as true-or-false, multiple choice, matching, fill-in-the-blank, and short answer essay to test learning in a variety of ways. True-or-false and fill-in-the-blank questions are good for testing knowledge of facts. Matching questions are good for testing recall of related concepts. Multiple choice questions are good for distinguishing myths from reality, as well as measuring some levels of problem solving, inference, and making generalizations. Short answer essay questions reveal the clients' thinking processes. They also provide clues to the clients' use of the information you taught. In Box 13-2 you will find guidelines for writing test questions.

When preparing test questions, avoid using the exact words you used while teaching so as to measure understanding rather than memory. The use of "giveaway" words should also be avoided, although they can be used as distracters in the questions. "Never," "always," and "all" are usually false; "generally," "mostly," and "usually" are usually true. If words such as these are used, the test may measure the test-wise skills of clients rather than their attainment of the learning objectives. Be clear about what you want to measure.

True-or-false questions are good for testing common misperceptions about health and illness. These questions test recognition of information rather than recall.

BOX 13-2   Guidelines for Writing Test Questions

1. Group questions according to type: true-or-false, matching, multiple choice, fill-in-the-blank, and short answer essay.

2. State general directions at the beginning of the test: "This test is designed to measure what you know about how to take care of yourself. It will help us plan further teaching." (For clients with low literacy say, "Please take this test. The results will tell us what else we need to teach you.")

3. State specific directions before each group of questions.

4. Indicate where to record the answer and provide a place for the clients' answers.

5. Use vocabulary that fits the reading level of the clients.

6. Make the directions as clear and as short as possible.

7. Underline or bold the directions and special words.

8. Make all multiple choice options similar in length.

9. Put the multiple choice question and answer options on the same page.

10. Make all multiple choice options grammatically parallel.

The advantage is that they are easy to write. The disadvantage is that clients have a 50% chance of selecting the correct answer regardless of their knowledge. If used, write out T or true and F or false in front of the question and instruct clients to circle the correct answer. When clients have to write either T for true or F for false, sometimes it is difficult to decipher their handwriting.

Each multiple choice question has three parts: the stem, the correct answer, and the distracters. The stem is the lead-in sentence or question to which the client must then fit the correct answer. The distracters are other possible but incorrect answers (Slavin, 2009). Myths and plausible answers are good distracters. A good test question is grammatically consistent with all of the possible answers. All answer options should be about the same length. Inconsistencies in length can give clues to the correct answer. Clients guess the right answer by looking for the best grammatical fit in matching or multiple choice questions. If all of the options begin with the same word or phrase, then that word or phrase should be stated only once at the end of the stem. See the example in Box 13-3. Try to avoid negatively stated items. If you use negative items, be sure to underline the negative. An example of this is test question 2 in Box 13-3.

BOX 13-3   Example of Multiple Choice Questions

1. Which of the following statements is true about parenthood? It is a/an:

    a. Impossible role for most couples.

    b. Demanding but growth enhancing experience.

    c. Essential element of a healthy marriage.

    d. Necessary for a well-rounded, fulfilled life.

2. Effective crutch walking includes all of the following _except:_

    a. Avoiding slippery surfaces so that you remain stable.

    b. Keeping the crutch snug in your armpits by learning on them.

    c. Practicing until you have developed a smooth rhythm.

    d. Placing your most important items in a fanny pack.

A table of random numbers helps to list answers in a random manner because it is easy to slip into a predictable pattern for listing correct responses. Another way to randomize the sequence of choices in multiple choice questions is to arrange answers alphabetically.

In a matching question the number of answers should be longer than the column of items presented for identification or description (Slavin, 2009). If the number of answers is exactly the same as the number of test items, then the question is testing the client's ability to use logic and the process of elimination, rather than testing the client's knowledge.

Fill-in-the-blank questions should contain blanks that are all the same size. If the blanks vary in size, mind reading is encouraged. Clients will try to guess what word you had in mind when constructing the test. If you choose to provide a list of the correct words, then it too should contain distracters.

Short answer essay questions are good because clients can answer them in their own words. Reading their answers, you learn about the clients' perceptions about the health issue and gain insight into their thinking. For health education purposes, the answer to the question should take only a few sentences.

Questions should be grouped according to the type of question. If they are not, clients must switch mental processes to answer each type. For example, all true-or-false questions should be grouped together and all multiple choice questions should be together. If the test is likely to produce some anxiety, it may help to start it with some easy items. This helps to measure clients' learning rather than how they think when stressed.

Making test directions clear is a challenging task. A good way to clarify the directions is to have them critiqued by someone who knows the subject. Sometimes clients need "helps" and "hints." This is especially true when a written tool is used to test children. Include a grading scale if clients are to grade themselves; a key can be included at the bottom upside down or on the back page.

Pretests and Posttests

The pretest is useful for assessing the clients' current knowledge about a subject and their learning needs. The results of the pretest allow nurses to construct the knowledge base for teaching and avoid repeating what clients already know. Pretests are also good for piquing the curiosity of clients. One possible disadvantage of pretests is that they are often perceived as threatening. This threat may be outweighed by the fact that pretests are helpful as self-diagnostic tools.

At the conclusion of the teaching session, administer a posttest. The posttest should be the same as the pretest to determine the gains made as a result in the teaching session. The results of both pre- and posttests are compared to measure client learning. Some test services design equivalent pretests and posttests. This means that although the tests are not exactly alike, they test the same knowledge or skills. The process for developing equivalent tests is lengthy, expensive, and must be done with populations of significant size. This involves sophisticated statistical analysis that is beyond the scope of this text.

Choosing Appropriate Measurement Tools and Techniques

Cognitive, affective, and psychomotor learning objectives require different measurement tools and techniques. To determine which are best, ask which are most appropriate for the learning objective you are measuring. For example, which are most appropriate to measure cognitive learning? The most appropriate tools to use here are oral questions and written measurement. These methods are indirect because you cannot measure cognition (thinking) directly.

How do you measure changes in clients' attitudes or feelings? You may be able to question them directly if they trust you. Their willingness to share is affected by the quality of the nurse/client relationship. Direct observation is also an excellent technique because you can infer much from clients' behavior. Clients are not always fully aware of or willing to admit their attitudes and feelings. However, a client's behavior may give clues if you are an astute observer. Video recordings done with client's permission, and anecdotal notes are two good ways to capture the needed data. Written measurement in the form of an attitude scale or opinion survey also may be useful. The use of open-ended questions is yet another way to measure attitudes and feelings. Many factors influence a person's willingness to admit attitudinal change or lack of change.

How do you decide whether or not clients can perform a psychomotor skill at a satisfactory level? Direct observation is the main method for evaluating the attainment of psychomotor skills. If performance is being evaluated, the video recording is an excellent tool. Checklists and rating scales are also useful because they enable you to remain objective with a previously constructed and well-thought-out list. Checklists also reduce the likelihood that crucial elements of the desired performance will be neglected.

EVALUATION OF PROGRAM EFFECTIVENESS

Course/Program Evaluation

Developing a plan to evaluate course/program effectiveness begins when program planning is done (Falvo, 2004). Program planning begins with the assessment of client needs, which is the basis for creating health education programs to address those needs. Program evaluation is usually broad in scope, covering an entire department or a specific program; however, it can also refer to a single course (Worral, 2008).

The purpose, scope, and context of evaluating a program must be clearly defined. In contemplating program evaluation, consider the questions that you want answered (Lorig & Associates, 2001). Do you want to know a program's overall effectiveness? Or the clients' perceptions of the degree to which the learning objectives were taught? Do you want to know the clients' level of satisfaction with the program? Or whether the cost of the program was worth the outcomes? Is the purpose of the evaluation to justify the expenditures of time and money by the health education department? Or is it to identify the program's strengths and weaknesses?

Also consider the intended audience for the evaluation and how the evaluation report will be used. The report may be intended for the healthcare institution/agency management accreditation bodies, or for internal use by the health education staff. The intended use of program evaluation may be to improve services or justify additional funding.

The data that you gather must be consistent with the questions that the program evaluation is designed to answer (Lorig & Associates, 2001). For example, if a health education course was designed for staff to reduce hospital-acquired infections, then you would collect data about the infection rate before and after the teaching intervention to determine its impact. If a program was designed to reduce hypertension in clients, you would collect blood pressure readings and medication usage before and after the teaching session to determine its impact.

To conduct program evaluation, you need the services of someone who is knowledgeable about program evaluation, research design, types of quantitative and qualitative data to collect, and statistical analysis. A discussion of that level of program evaluation is beyond the scope of this text. For our purposes, we will focus only on the evaluation of learning objectives and teacher evaluation.

Evaluating learning objectives is done in one of several ways. Figure 13-4 illustrates a typical rating scale for evaluating learning objectives. The form is customized by listing each learning objective to be evaluated. Each learning objective is then rated on a 3- or 5-point scale. When using a form like this, include open-ended questions, leaving ample space for clients to provide written responses. Open-ended questions require clients to provide a more thoughtful response than does a checklist. For example, to gain additional information from the clients, ask questions like these:

1. What content was the most helpful for you? (variations: What was the most important thing you learned? Name the two most important things you learned.).
2. What content was the least helpful for you? (variations: What was the least important thing you learned? Name the two least important things that were taught.).
3. What content was not covered that you think should have been? (variation: What content would you like to see covered in this course in the future?)
4. What would be helpful for us to know that would make the course better?

At the time the form to evaluate learning objectives is administered, also administer a teacher evaluation form such as that shown in Figure 13-5. We have used this form on numerous occasions and found it very helpful for nurses as educators. Administer both evaluation forms on the last day of the class while everyone is still present. The forms should be administered by the department secretary or someone other than the nurse who taught the course. The nurse should leave the room when the forms are distributed. Responses are confidential and clients should not be asked to sign their names to the forms. Once clients have completed the forms, the responses can be tabulated and then shared with the nurse who taught the course and the head of the health education department.

List each learning objective here	0	1	2	3	4	5
1.						
2.						
3.						
4.						

Descriptors for the key can vary.
For example, the stem can read
"To what degree did this course help
you achieve the learning objective?"
and the key could be a 3-point rating
scale: not at all, somewhat, and a lot.

Key:
0 = not applicable
1 = did not help me achieve this objective
2 = helped me less than I expected
3 = helped me about what I expected
4 = helped me more than I expected
5 = definitely helped me achieve this objective

FIGURE 13-4   Sample Form to Evaluate Learning Objectives

Evidence-Based Nursing Practice

Increasingly, nurses are expected to implement teaching strategies and practices that have been shown through research to be effective. It is important to use the strongest evidence when making health education decisions (Worral, 2008). Evidence-based nursing practice was introduced in Chapter 1, and we have included examples of current research relevant to health education throughout this text. Applying research findings informs the decisions and choices you make about health education and helps clients achieve the best possible healthcare outcomes.

Cost

Cost is an important component of program evaluation. Cost of health education can be measured by one of two methods: cost-benefit analysis and cost-effectiveness analysis (Nelson, 2008). Cost-benefit analysis looks at the relationship between the cost of a health education program and its outcomes. Cost can be direct (e.g., salaries, materials, and equipment) or indirect (e.g., heating, lighting, space, and housekeeping). Outcomes include cost reduction, net savings, and measurable impacts on client care (Falvo, 2004). Cost-benefit analysis asks: Did the health education program

Teacher Evaluation Form

Speaker: _____

Evaluator: _____

Key:
0 = not applicable
1 = definitely below average
2 = slightly below average
3 = average
4 = slightly above average
5 = definitely above average

0 1 2 3 4 5

Objectives — Were the objectives:
Clearly presented to the clients?
Evident throughout the presentation?

Content — Was the content:
Clearly explained?
Accurate?
At the right vocabulary level?
Appropriate to the audience's background?

Strategies — Were the strategies:
Appropriate for the content?
Appropriate for the audience?

Teaching aids — Were the materials:
Appropriate to the context?
Appropriate to the objectives?
At the client's level of comprehension?
Pleasing to the eye?
Visible (contrast, size, and location)?
Used in a practiced manner?

Performance — Did the teacher:
Dress appropriately to the clients and topic?
Maintain eye contact with the audience?
Speak in a clear audible voice?
Use a pace appropriate to the audience?
Stay attuned to the audience?
Give recognition for contributions?
Allow time for questions?
Seek feedback periodically?
Show preparation by smooth performance?

Comments:

FIGURE 13-5   Teacher Evaluation Form
Babcock and Miller, (1994). Client education: Theory & practice. St. Louis: Mosby.

lower the cost of providing care to a specific group of clients? For example, was the number of bed sores reduced? Did fewer clients develop postoperative pneumonia? Were there fewer readmissions for diabetic clients? If the cost is less than the savings, the program is a cost benefit to the institution.

Cost-effectiveness analysis looks at the financial impact of an educational program on clients' health behavior. Behavioral changes are more difficult to measure because they are less observable and quantifiable. Cost effectiveness is determined by comparing the results of different health education programs on changes in clients' health behaviors. The educational intervention that has the greatest impact on improving health behavior is considered to be the most effective. For example, which weight management program was most effective for clients needing to lose weight? Documenting this information contributes to the overall evaluation of health education programs.

That health education is effective in reducing cost and encouraging client adherence is no longer in dispute. For example, cardiovascular disease is the major cause of morbidity and mortality among the elderly and a major contributor to the cost of care (Plan targets seniors with high cholesterol, 2008). Health education can play a major role in reducing this cost and promoting, maintaining, and restoring health among the elderly. For example, Koelling, Johnson, Cody, and Aaronson (2005) conducted a randomized, controlled trial of 223 clients with systolic heart failure. The treatment group received a 1-hour, one-on-one education session with a nurse educator at the time of discharge, while the control group received the standard discharge process. The education intervention group received detailed information about heart failure (etiology, rationale for and actions of medications, dietary restrictions, self-care behaviors, and what to do if symptoms worsened). The control group received the standard discharge teaching. The education intervention group reduced rehospitalization for heart failure by 51%. Overall, rehospitalization or death for the education intervention group was reduced by 35% at the 6-month follow-up when compared with a control group. The total cost for patients in the education intervention group was $2823 per patient lower that the cost for patients in the control group, a significant savings.

EVALUATION OF INTEGRATION OF LEARNING INTO DAILY LIVING

All of our health education activities are for naught if the client and community does not benefit in some substantial, measurable way. Summative evaluation seeks to know the long-term outcomes of health education activities. In this section we look at long-term client adherence, the impact on the community, and justification for health education dollars.

Client Adherence

The topic of client adherence was introduced in Chapter 12 on formative evaluation. We now address long-term adherence; that is, to what degree clients have integrated what they learned into their daily living activities. This is the true test of adherence. We are interested in the behavior and life style changes that persist long after the completion of the health education intervention. In other words, do clients maintain these changes when they return to their homes and usual routines? The best way to determine adherence is to observe clients in their home when they are unaware of your presence. This is unrealistic, so we have to employ other methods to gain this information.

If you are working in a clinic or doctor's office, reinforce health teaching at each visit with the client. Rather than asking, "Are you exercising as you were advised?" ask, "Tell me how you are working your exercise program into your daily routine." The client will usually answer yes to the first question and will likely give a more thoughtful and accurate response to the second. Provide written information and brochures to supplement your teaching and encourage adherence. Other strategies include postcards or letters reminding clients about appointments and screening tests. Sometimes support staff will telephone clients to remind them about appointments or follow up.

Follow-up questionnaires can be sent to clients at different time intervals after discharge. This can be done at 6-month, 1-year, or 2-year intervals depending on the level of follow-up information desired. Questions can be constructed that indicate the level of adherence to the treatment regimen. This same process and data gathering can be done by telephone interviewing. Another option is completing a questionnaire via e-mail if clients are Internet connected.

Instruct clients to keep a log of their progress in adhering to a treatment regimen. For example, have clients record their medications, exercise activities, or weight management (DiGiacomo, 2008). This gives clients an active role in the treatment plan and motivates them to assume responsibility for adherence. Contracts between clients and providers based on mutually agreed-upon goals may be used to ensure client commitment to the desired change.

Sometimes clients are referred to support groups who are grappling with the same health issues. Support groups are powerful motivators and a source of encouragement provided by others who are dealing with the same health issue. Voluntary health organizations can be a source of information as well as support if the client needs more information (Miaskowski, Shockney, & Chlebowski, 2008).

If clients are not following the recommended changes, you need to find out why (Rankin, Stallings, & London, 2005). Nonadherence could be for good reasons rather than simply being unwilling. It may be caused by financial factors such as a medication regimen that is too expensive or inflexible. It may be that clients do not know how to substitute recommended foods for foods that they can afford and are available locally. It may be that clients simply misread or misunderstood the discharge directions. The only way nurses will know is to ask and then listen to what clients say. Once you know the reasons for nonadherence, you can make suggestions that are appropriate and acceptable to clients.

Impact on the Community

A healthy community is everyone's concern. Each area in the United States has a public health agency charged with monitoring the community's health to include such things as communicable diseases and morbidity and mortality rates. Based on these data, community health initiatives are undertaken and health education programs are developed.

Of national importance in the United States today is the increasing rates of obesity among the population. Obesity contributes to the development of cardiovascular disease and diabetes, resulting in increased healthcare costs and early mortality. Other health issues in the community include stop-smoking programs, healthy nutrition (especially in the schools), and promotion of exercise and activities for all ages, including the elderly. Health fairs are another example of effective programs designed to increase healthy behaviors in communities. Health fairs offer early detection of disease and health education on many topics related to healthful living.

The Healthy People 2010 (2009) health indicators identify the major health concerns in the United States at the beginning of the Twenty-first century. These are areas that require client education to address the most significant preventable threats to health and wellness. The health indicators are: physical activity, overweight and obesity, tobacco use, substance abuse, responsible sexual behavior, mental health, injury and violence, environmental quality, immunization, and access to health care. Nurses as educators work with many different stakeholders to provide age-specific, culturally appropriate and linguistically competent health education to address the Healthy People 2010 indicators.

A significant barrier to promoting, retaining, and restoring health is the healthcare system's focus on caring for people after they have become sick or harmed. Solutions to this problem begin with addressing illness or harm before they occur and concentrating on prevention. Prevention is an essential aspect of a community approach and is supported by a report released by the Trust for America's Health in July 2008. This report found that a small investment in disease prevention could result in significant savings in US healthcare costs. The report, entitled *Prevention for a Healthier America: Investments in Disease Prevention Yield Significant Savings, Stronger Communities*, concluded that an investment of $10 per person per year in proven community-based programs to increase physical activity, improve nutrition, and prevent smoking and other tobacco use could save the country more than $16 billion annually within 5 years. This is a return of $5.60 for every $1 invested (Trust for America's Health, 2008). This research supports the need for a continued focus on health education.

Not only is prevention an important alternative approach that uses health education, but there also must be systems designed to identify, review, and disseminate information about health education interventions and programs. Increasingly, federal agencies are recognizing the value to the public and healthcare organizations of classification systems that summarize the best current evidence-based research about the effectiveness and utility of healthcare interventions and programs. Not only is more research needed, but systems of disseminating current research about interventions and programs are also needed. As a nurse, you may have opportunities to participate in research that contributes to advances in client education. We encourage you to take advantage of these opportunities to contribute to the body of nursing knowledge.

Justification for Health Dollars

Health care in the United States is expensive, and funding for it competes with multiple other needs at the national and state levels. Funding needed to support Medicare, Medicaid, and other health-related programs increases each year. It is a concern that challenges the best minds as our leaders search for solutions.

Nonadherence to medical regimens is a significant public health problem having a major financial impact on the United States healthcare system. Nonadherence is estimated to cost $100 billion each year in the United States and is responsible for 10% of hospital admissions and 23% of nursing home admissions (Aliotta, Vlasnik, & Delor, 2004; Dezii, 2000; Vermeire, Hearnshaw, Van Royen, & Denekens, 2001). The largest proportion of this cost (70%) appears to be a result of decreased productivity and premature death, with direct medical costs accounting for the remaining 30% (Dezii, 2000).

Nonadherence to treatment is not confined to the United States. It is a worldwide problem identified by the World Health Organization (WHO). The WHO

(2003) states that "poor adherence to treatment of chronic diseases is a worldwide problem of striking magnitude and the consequences of poor adherence to long-term therapies are poor health outcomes and increased health costs" (p. 11). Solutions are needed that reach a very large audience.

Client adherence to treatment is that crucial aspect of clinical care that links the intentions of healthcare providers with the expectations and capabilities of clients. The most effective prescribed medication is of little value if the prescription is not filled or the recommended dosages, frequency, and duration are not adhered to. Client education is an essential component for addressing issues of adherence. Nurses teach clients about their diagnoses, how to care for themselves, and how to acquire information for making informed decisions that meet their individual needs. Informed clients are more likely to cooperate with treatment regimens and demonstrate better management of health problems than clients who are not informed (Oermann, Masserang, Maxey, & Lange, 2002). Health teaching informs clients of their choices, treatment options, risks and benefits and consequences of nonadherence.

CASE EXAMPLE: MRS. ROSA LOPEZ

We now illustrate how to measure each of the learning objectives for Mrs. Lopez. The cognitive objective, "Explain the relationship between excessive sodium intake and hypertension" can be measured in several ways. We would ask Mrs. Lopez to verbalize the relationship or give her a brief paper-and-pencil test. The test questions can be true-or-false, multiple choice, short answer essay, or fill-in-the-blank. See Table 13-1 for sample questions.

The affective objective, "Choose to limit the intake of sodium to 2000 mg/day by working with the nurse to prepare a dietary plan," would be evaluated in several ways. The short-term measure is to have her fill out an attitude scale, as seen in Box 13-4. Another approach would be to have Mrs. Lopez construct a meal plan from a list of foods to determine her choices. The long-term measure would be whether or not she makes the dietary changes resulting in lower blood pressure. To determine this she records her blood pressure on a chart. Dietary changes should result in lowered blood pressure readings. The ability to take her own blood pressure is a psychomotor skill, so the chart measures her success in the affective domain.

The psychomotor objective, "Demonstrate accurately obtaining self-blood pressure reading using home digital equipment without any verbal guidance" can be evaluated by observing Mrs. Lopez's performance. The steps of the procedure are shown in the checklist in Box 13-5.

Mrs. Lopez would be considered successful when you observe her complete each step of the procedure correctly. We would have her perform the procedure once initially to check her familiarity with the procedure. She would be tested once. If she does not perform correctly, then we would repeat the procedure until she is accurate and is comfortable with the procedure. Mrs. Lopez would use the chart shown in Box 13-6 to record her daily blood pressure readings. Each time she comes in for a weekly

---

TABLE 13-1 Sample Test Questions for Mrs. Rosa Lopez

Sample True-or-False Questions

Directions: Circle T if the statement is true. Circle F if any part of the statement is false.

T F 1. It is OK to add a small amount of salt to my food at the dinner table.

T F 2. Processed and canned foods are low in sodium.

T F 3. Excess sodium intake can cause body fluid retention.

T F 4. Excess fluid retention can result in the elevation of blood pressure.

Sample Multiple Choice Question

Directions: Put an X in front of the one best answer.

1. A sodium restricted diet is important in the treatment of hypertension because it:

_____ a. minimizes excess fluid retention.

_____ b. results in fluid accumulation.

_____ c. expands the blood capillaries.

_____ d. increases urinary output.

Sample Short-Answer Essay and Fill-in-the-Blank Questions

Directions: Fill in the blanks to make the statement correct. The missing words are listed at the bottom.

1. Although _____ sodium in your _____ is important to make a regular part of your _____ routine, it may not _____ the need for medication. Dietary changes will help you to control _____ accumulation and may help you _____ your blood _____.

Possible missing words:

daily   pressure   diet

limiting   style of life   eliminate

rate   fluid   reduce

2. In 25 words or less, describe the relationship among sodium, fluid retention, and hypertension.

BOX 13-4   Sample Attitude Scale for Mrs. Rosa Lopez

Directions: Place an X in the column that most closely describes your feelings toward each of the statements. Be as honest as you can; this information is for you.

Statement	Agree	Neutral	Disagree
1. I am too busy to worry about meal planning.			
2. Altering my diet requires making too many changes.			
3. I can tell when my blood pressure is up.			
4. I am worried about stroke or heart disease.			
5. Everyone must die of something sometime.			
6. Proper diet can have a positive effect on my life.			
7. My children are cooperating with my dietary changes.			
8. I like salty snacks when I watch television.			

BOX 13-5   Sample Checklist for Taking the Blood Pressure

_____ Reads digital blood pressure equipment directions.

_____ Arranges the digital blood pressure equipment on a table by a chair.

_____ Locates the brachial artery.

_____ Places arm in the cuff.

_____ Inflates the cuff according to equipment directions.

_____ Releases air in the cuff according to equipment directions.

_____ Records the systolic and diastolic pressure, the pulse, and the date.

BOX 13-6   Sample Chart for Recording Blood Pressure

Systolic Reading													
Diastolic Reading													
Pulse													
Date													

checkup, her readings would be reviewed and her blood pressure checked to assess her progress. We would expect to find similar readings to our own. If they are similar, we would consider her performance successful. Because some digital blood pressure equipment also calculates the pulse rate, we also have included a row on the chart to record the pulse, too.

Adherence for Mrs. Lopez

If Mrs. Lopez adheres to the teaching plan, she would incorporate the dietary changes into her meal planning and daily diet. She would also be taking her blood pressure and recording it daily. At her clinic visits, we would take her blood pressure and compare our readings with hers.

If Mrs. Lopez tells us she is not adhering, our first response would be to reinforce her honesty and talk about the perceived barriers. After listening to her story, we would help her identify options to surmount the problems. As we identify these options, we might preface them with, "Have you thought about . . . ," or "How would . . . work for you?"

For illustrative purposes, we create a problem interfering with Mrs. Lopez's adherence. She says she is too busy with her employment, her children, and volunteering to implement all of the dietary changes. She removed the salt shaker from the table, adds no salt in cooking, avoids canned or processed foods high in sodium, and uses low-sodium seasonings such as herbs and spices in her cooking, but she enjoys munching on salty snacks in the evening as she watches television. We would then focus on her enjoyment of salty snacks. Some options include finding snacks that are satisfying but devoid of the sodium content. We would do this by giving her a handout listing low-sodium snacks or showing her how to search the Internet for such listings. For example, we would suggest unsalted nuts, crackers, rice cakes, granola bars,

---

BOX 13-7   Evidence-Based Nursing Practice

Oermann, M. H., Webb, S. A., & Ashare, J. A. (2003). Outcomes of videotape instruction in clinic waiting area. *Orthopaedic Nursing, 22*(2), 102–105.

Purpose: This study examined the effectiveness of general health-promotion teaching for patients in the waiting room of a clinic, using focused videotape instruction.

Method: An experimental design was used with 215 subjects in waiting rooms of clinics in a university medical center in the Midwest. Subjects were randomly assigned to two groups: one group received the focused videotape instruction, and the control group did not receive the intervention.

Results: There was a significant gain in knowledge for patients who viewed the videotape in the waiting room, and they were more satisfied with their education compared with the control group. This study supports focused video instruction as an effective and efficient teaching intervention for disseminating health information in the waiting area.

---

and fresh and dried fruits. We might also suggest keeping her mind and hands busy with a craft as she watches television, such as knitting or embroidery, or by taking a daily evening walk.

SUMMARY

Summative evaluation is the final step in the teaching and learning process. Summative evaluation focuses on evaluation of client learning, evaluation of program effectiveness, and evaluation of the integration of learning into daily living. It is important to use the results of evaluation to improve health education and your effectiveness as an educator. This chapter has covered the details of the evaluation of client learning to include measurement, sources of error in measurement, and direct and indirect measurement methods. Selecting specific measurement tools are affected by the domain (cognitive, affective, and psychomotor) of the learning objectives. A variety of tools are available from which to choose.

We believe effective client education will lead to behavioral and life style changes. Clients who want to promote, retain, and restore their health may need to modify what they are doing and adopt healthier ways of living. The challenges you face as an educator are influenced by client assessment data that you have collected and how you use that data to provide meaningful, interesting, and motivating health education.

We urge you to keep in mind the power of warmth and caring as motivating forces to help clients change. Remember that clients are in charge of their own behavior and live with the consequences of their choices. You can provide an interesting, stimulating, and timely health messages, but you cannot enforce adherence. Your role is that of teacher and guide, not health enforcer.

EXERCISES

Exercise I—Evaluate a Test by Finding the Flaws

Purpose:
- Make an inference about the purpose of this test.
- Apply guidelines for proper test construction.

Directions:

1. Find all of the flaws in this test and state your rationale for each.
2. Rewrite the test to improve the form, clarify questions, and to maintain the purpose of the test.
3. Share your perceptions of the test's purpose with your peers.
4. State the rationale for your conclusion.

Critical Care Unit in the Hospital of St. Anywhere

Directions: Circle the statements you feel to be true:

1. The damage in the heart attack is caused by:
   a. Too much fat in the blood.
   b. Too much blood in the heart chambers.
   c. Too little blood to the heart muscles.
   d. No heart damage; only damage is a clot in a blood vessel.
2. The pain involved in a heart attack is from:
   a. Heart irritability.
   b. Too little oxygen to the heart muscle.
   c. Too little blood to the heart chambers.
   d. Damaged heart muscle.
3. The damage to the heart muscle from a heart attack is:
   a. Similar to a deep cut.
   b. Similar to a muscle sprain.
   c. Similar to a bruise.

4. The healing of the heart following an attack is:
   a. Never really complete, there is always a scar that is subsequently weaker than the natural heart muscle.
   b. Totally complete, leaving no trace or damage.
   c. Leaves a scar.

Directions: Mark T for true; F for false.

_____   5. After a heart attack a client will not return to his or her previous level of physical activity.
_____   6. After a heart attack one's sex life always has to be reduced (in future years).
_____   7. It was my last meal that led to my heart attack.
_____   8. Even an occasional cocktail is bad for your heart.
_____   9. High blood cholesterol signals a proneness to heart attack.
_____ 10. About medication:
   a. You should not become dependent on them as a "crutch."
   b. It may help to carry nitroglycerin tablets in your pocket.
   c. Once you leave the hospital, medications you are given in the hospital are not to be changed in the future by your doctor.

Exercise II–Program Evaluation

Purpose: Investigate program evaluation in a healthcare institution/agency.

Directions:

1. Working in pairs, interview the head of the education department in a local healthcare institution/agency.
2. Prepare interview questions that are consistent with the content discussed in this chapter. Sample questions you can ask:
   a. How do they conduct program evaluation?
   b. Do they have a program evaluation model that they frequently use?
   c. What common indicators do they track?
   d. Describe the health education program being evaluated. What is the purpose of this particular evaluation? What do they hope to learn by the report? Who will read the evaluation report? What types of decisions will be based on the report?
3. Report your findings in class.

Exercise III—Client Adherence

Purpose: Gain insight into client adherence issues.

Directions:

1. Working with your instructor, identify a client for whom you have provided nursing care and health education.
2. Obtain permission to do a follow-up interview with the client either by telephone or by visiting the client at home.
3. Prepare interview questions that are directly related to the health education that you provided.
4. Interview the client.
5. Report in class your findings about the client's adherence to the health education recommendations that you had provided. Was the client adhering to the recommendations? If not, why not? If not, did the reasons surprise you? Were the reasons different from those described in this chapter?

SUPPLEMENTAL ONLINE RESOURCES

American Heart Association:
http://www.americanheart.org/presenter.jhtml?identifier=3043441
The HSM Group:
http://www.hsmgroup.com/info/compli/compli.html
Health Belief Model:
http://www.tcw.utwente.nl/theorieenoverzicht/Theory%20clusters/Health%20
Communication/Health_Belief_Model.doc/
Theory of Planned Behavior:
http://people.umass.edu/aizen/tpb.html
World Health Organization, Adherence to Long-Term Therapies: Evidence for
Action:
http://www.who.int/chp/knowledge/publications/adherence_introduction.pdf
Locus of Control:
http://wilderdom.com/psychology/loc/LocusOfControlWhatIs.html
True/False Questions:
http://teachingacademy.wisc.edu/archive/Assistance/course/true.htm
How to Prepare Multiple Choice Test Items (BYU):
http://testing.byu.edu/info/handbooks/betteritems.pdf

Pretest/Posttest Comparison:
http://www.alnresearch.org/HTML/AssessmentTutorial/Strategies/
    PrePostComparison.html

REFERENCES

Aliotta, S. L., Vlasnik, J. J., & Delor, B. (2004). Enhancing adherence to long-term medical therapy: A new approach to assessing and treating patients. *Advanced Therapy, 21*(4), 214–231.

Babcock, D. E. & Miller, M. A. (1994). Client education: Theory & practice. St. Louis: Mosby.

Benner, P. (1984). *From novice to expert.* Menlo Park, CA: Addison-Wesley.

Dezii, C. M. (2000). Medication noncompliance: What is the problem? *Managed Care, 9*(9 Suppl), 9–12.

DiGiacomo, M. (2008). Patient adherence: Sharing the responsibility. *PT Magazine, 16*(7), 28–30.

Falvo, D. R. (2004). *Effective patient education a guide to increased compliance* (3rd ed.). Sudbury, MA: Jones and Bartlett.

Gronlund, N. E., & Brookhart, S. M. (2009). *Gronlund's writing instructional objectives* (8th ed.). Upper Saddle River, NJ: Pearson Education.

Healthy People 2010. (2009). US Department of Health, Education and Welfare, Public Health Service. Washington DC: US Government Retrieved on May 23, 2009 from http://www.healthypeople.gov/LHI/lhiwhat.htm.

Koelling, T. M., Johnson, M. L., Cody, R. J., & Aaronson, K. D. (2005). Discharge education improves clinical outcomes in patients with chronic heart failure. *Circulation, 111*(2), 179–185.

Lorig, K., & Associates (2001). *Patient education: A practical approach* (3rd ed.). Thousand Oaks, CA: Sage.

Merriam-Webster's Dictionary and Thesaurus (2007). Springfield, MA: Merriam-Webster, Inc.

Miaskowski, C., Shockney, L., & Chlebowski, R. T. (2008). Adherence to oral endocrine therapy for breast cancer: A nursing perspective. *Clinical Journal of Oncology Nursing, 12*(2), 213–221.

Morrison, G. R., Ross, S. M., Kemp, J. E., & Kalman, H. K. (2007). *Designing effective instruction* (5th ed.). Hoboken, NJ: John Wiley and Sons.

Nelson, M. J. (2008). Ethical, legal, and economic foundations of the educational process. In Bastable, S. B. *Nurse as educator: Principles of teaching and learning for nursing practice* (3rd ed., pp. 25–49). Sudbury, MA: Jones and Bartlett.

Osborne, D. & Gaebler, T. (1992). *Reinventing government how the entrepreneurial spirit is transforming the public sector.* Reading Way, MA: Addison-Wesley Publishing Company, Inc.

Oermann, M. H., Masserang, M. Maxey, M., & Lange, M. (2002). Clinic visit and waiting: Patient education and satisfaction. *MedSurg Nursing*, October. Retrieved July 9, 2009 from http://find articles.com/p/articles/mi_m0FSS/is_5_11/ai_n18614291/.

Plan targets seniors with high cholesterol (2008). *Case Management Advisor, 19*(10), 112–113.

Rankin, S. H., Stallings, K. D., & London, F. (2005). *Patient education in health and illness* (5th ed.). Philadelphia: Lippincott Williams & Wilkins.

Redman, B. K. (2007). *The practice of patient education: A case study approach* (10th ed.). St. Louis: Mosby Year Book.

Slavin, R. E. (2009). *Educational psychology: Theory and practice* (9th ed.). Upper Saddle River, NJ: Pearson Education.

Trust for America's Health (2008). *Prevention for a healthier America: Investments in disease prevention yield significant savings, stronger communities.* Retrieved on July 17, 2009 from http://healthy americans.org/reports/prevention08/.

Vermeire, E, Hearnshaw, H., Van Royen, P., & Denekens, J. (2001). Patient adherence to treatment: Three decades of research. A comprehensive review. *Journal of Clinical Pharmacy and Therapeutics, 26,* 331–342.

World Health Organization, (2003). Adherence to long-term therapies: Evidence for action. Report #WHO/MNC/03.01.

Worral, P. S. (2008). Evaluation in healthcare education. In Bestable, S. B. *Nurse as educator: Principles of teaching and learning for nursing practice* (3rd ed., pp. 383–427). Sudbury, MA: Jones and Bartlett.

INDEX

Pages followed by t or f denote tables and figures respectively.